IEEE Recommended Practice for Electric Systems in Health Care Facilities

Published by
The Institute of Electrical and Electronics Engineers, Inc

Dedication

Richard Burgess and John R. Geyer died unexpectedly during the summer of 1984 after completing their chapters. Because of their leadership in developing the White Book, this publication is dedicated to their memory.

IEEE Recommended Practice for Electric Systems in Health Care Facilities

Sponsor

Power Systems Engineering Committee
of the
IEEE Industry Applications Society

Approved March 21, 1985

IEEE Standards Board

Approved July 26, 1985

American National Standards Institute

IEEE Power Engineering Seminars

The IEEE sponsors seminars on the Color Books and other power engineering standards throughout the year.
Our seminars include:
- Protection and Co-Generation Plants Paralleled with Utility Transmission Systems
- Health Care Facilities Power Systems
- Planning, Design, Protection, Maintenance, and Operation of Industrial and Commercial Power Systems
- Electric Power Supply Systems for Nuclear Power Generating Stations
- Large Storage Batteries — Nickel-Cadmium and Lead

IEEE-sponsored seminars and training programs may also be brought to your plant. For details, write to the IEEE Standards Seminar Manager, 445 Hoes Lane, PO Box 1331, Piscataway, NJ 08855-1331 USA. In the US and Canada call us Toll Free at 1-800-678-IEEE and ask for Standards Seminars and Training Programs. Our fax number is 201-562-1571.

Third Printing
December 1990

ISBN 0-471-82747-9

Library of Congress Catalog Number 85-081787

© Copyright 1986 by

The Institute of Electrical and Electronics Engineers, Inc
345 East 47th Street, New York, NY 10017 USA

February 28, 1986   *SH10256*

Foreword

(This Foreword is not part of ANSI/IEEE Std 602-1986, IEEE Recommended Practice for Electric Systems in Health Care Facilities.)

The purpose of the IEEE White Book is to promote the use of sound engineering principles in the design and operation of health care facilities. By alerting electrical engineers, designers, and health care operating personnel to the many problems that are encountered in the design and operation of health care facilities, it is hoped that this book will help in the development of concern for the professional aspects of health care facility engineering. While the IEEE White Book provides extensive discussion on each of the major electrical considerations in the design and operation of health care facilities, the IEEE Recommended Practice for Electric Systems in Health Care Facilities is not planned as a complete handbook. It does, however, direct the engineer to texts, periodicals, and references for health care facilities, and in particular, it acts as a guide through the myriad of codes, standards, and recommended practices published by IEEE and other voluntary and governmental bodies.

Initial planning for a recommended practice on electric systems in health care facilities was begun in 1975; however, those first steps were not very productive, and serious consideration was given to abandoning the project or reducing its scope and treating the matter as a single chapter within the IEEE Gray Book on electric systems in commercial buildings. At the very point when the activity appeared to founder, a new chairman accepted the challenge of the project. On October 1, 1979, a reorganized working group, under Hugh O. Nash, Jr, met in Cleveland, Ohio. Nineteen members attended the 1979 meeting. By the time the revitalized activity was fully under way, a total of 53 contributors had been recruited. Included were consultants, design professionals, enforcement officials, electrical and medical manufacturers, and representatives from both the public and private sectors of the health care industry.

Developed within the Power Systems Engineering Committee of the Industrial and Commercial Power Systems Department of the IEEE Industry Applications Society, this Recommended Practice was produced in accordance with consensus procedures of the Institute of Electrical and Electronics Engineers. Under those procedures, accredited by the American National Standards Institute, all concerned parties are assured of an opportunity to participate in development of the document, and resolution of differing viewpoints is subjected to the scrutiny of all participants. The process is necessarily a slow one, but the resulting product can be relied on to meet the needs of professionals throughout the industry and to reflect sound engineering approaches.

It is the intent of the Power Systems Engineering Committee to maintain this recommended practice so that it continues to remain consistent with the state of the art. Comments and suggestions for future revisions are gratefully solicited. They should be directed to:

Secretary
IEEE Standards Board
345 East 47th Street
New York, NY 10017

When the IEEE Standards Board approved this standard on March 21, 1985, it had the following membership:

Electric Systems in Health Care Facilities

First Edition

Electric Systems in Health Care Facilities

Working Group Members and Contributors

Hugh O. Nash, Jr., *Chairman*

Chapter 1 — Introduction: Hugh O. Nash, Jr., *Chairman*

Chapter 2 — Load Requirements and Energy Management: Lester H. Smith, Jr., *Chairman*; Al B. Marden, Anthony J. Scalone, John G. Talbot

Chapter 3 — Electrical Power Distribution Systems: Mark Martyak, *Co-Chairman*, Paul J. Savoie, *Co-Chairman*; René Castenschiold, Harold S. Cohen, Marvin Fischer, John R. Geyer*, Stephen Maskell, Vinod Wadhwa

Chapter 4 — Planning for Patient Care: John R. Geyer*, *Chairman*; James P. Bosley, Ray Heintel, James Johnson, Corwin Mitten, Richard Nalbert, Robert Pattison

Chapter 5 — Emergency Power Systems: Lawrence F. Hogrebe, *Chairman*; Dick Donnell, James L. Duke, Ed Goodpaster, Ralph Loeb, Jack Ripley, James E. Tyson, Jr.

Chapter 6 — Electrical Safety and Grounding: Jerry Frank, *Chairman*; Richard M. Burgess*, Edward Castwell, Bill Drake, J. Park Goode, Tony LoPinto, Jim Meyers, Allan Morse, Richard Nalbert, Blair A. Rowley, John Swope, Richard Troth, Jim Turner, George Webb

Chapter 7 — Lighting for Health Care Facilities: L.J. Maloney, *Chairman*; Tom Clevenger, William Fisher, H.G. (Casey) Jones, Richard Troth

Chapter 8 — Communication and Signal Systems: James R. Duncan, *Chairman*; Greg S. Batie, Douglas Bors, Robert H. Brown, Bernard Cerier, James L. Duke, John R. Geyer*, Irving Mande, Gaylen G. Marshall, David Moore, Hugh O. Nash, Jr., James L. Pettee

Chapter 9 — Medical Equipment and Instrumentation: Richard M. Burgess*, *Chairman*; Mort Levin, John Lyman

*Deceased

Contents

1. Introduction

1.1 General Discussion. IEEE Std 602-1986, IEEE Recommended Practice for Electric Systems in Health Care Facilities, commonly known as the IEEE White Book, is published by the Institute of Electrical and Electronics Engineers, Inc. (IEEE) to provide a recommended practice for the electrical design for health care facilities. It has been prepared on a voluntary basis by design engineers, health care end users, and electrical and medical manufacturers functioning as the White Book Working Group within the IEEE Commercial Buildings Power Systems Committee.

This recommended practice will probably be of greatest value to the power oriented engineer with limited health care experience. It can also be an aid to all engineers responsible for the electrical design of health care facilities. However, it is not intended as a replacement for the many excellent engineering texts and handbooks commonly in use, nor is it detailed enough to be a design manual. It should be considered a guide and a general reference on electrical design for health care facilities.

1.2 Health Care Facilities. The term "health care facility," as used here, encompasses buildings or parts of buildings that contain hospitals, nursing homes, residential custodial care facilities, clinics, and medical and dental offices. Buildings or parts of buildings within an industrial or commercial complex, used as medical facilities, logically fall within the scope of this book. Thus the specific use of the building in question, rather than the nature of the overall development of which it is a part, determines its electrical design category. Today's health care facilities, because of their increasing size and complexity, have become more and more dependent upon safe, adequate, and reliable electrical systems. Every day new types of sophisticated diagnostic and treatment equipment, utilizing microprocessors or computers, come on the market. Many of these items are sensitive to electrical disturbances and some require a very reliable power source. Invasive medical procedures such as cardiac catheterization have become routine in today's hospital. Such procedures make electrical safety extremely important. Moreover, new medical and surgical procedures are constantly being developed. In addition to the special safety and reliability requirements, health care facilities have unique life safety and communication requirements, because patients are generally unable to care for themselves or evacuate themselves in the event of an emergency. For these reasons, perhaps no area of design or construction is changing as fast as health care facilities.

1.3 IEEE Publications. The IEEE publishes several standards similar to the IEEE White Book, prepared by the Industrial Power Systems Department of the IEEE Industry Applications Society.[1]

[1] ANSI/IEEE Std 142-1982, IEEE Recommended Practice for Grounding of Industrial and Commercial Power Systems.

[2] ANSI/IEEE Std 241-1983, IEEE Recommended Practice for Electric Power Systems in Commercial Buildings.

[3] ANSI/IEEE Std 399-1980, IEEE Recommended Practice for Power System Analysis.

[4] ANSI/IEEE Std 446-1980, IEEE Recommended Practice for Emergency and Standby Power Systems for Industrial and Commercial Applications.

[5] ANSI/IEEE Std 493-1980, IEEE Recommended Practice for the Design of Reliable Industrial and Commercial Power Systems.

[6] IEEE Std 242-1975, IEEE Recommended Practice for Protection and Coordination of Industrial and Commercial Power Systems.

The IEEE Recommended Practice for Electric Power Systems in Commercial Buildings, commonly known as the Gray Book, will be of particular importance as a reference book to the hospital designer because of the many similarities between commercial buildings and health care facilities.

1.3.1 Industry Applications Society. The IEEE is divided into 31 groups and societies which specialize in various technical areas of electrical engineering. Each group or society conducts meetings and publishes papers on developments within its specialized area. The Industry Applications Society (IAS) presently encompasses 23 technical committees covering electrical engineering in specific areas (petroleum and chemical industry, cement industry, glass industry, industrial and commercial power systems, and others). Papers of interest to electrical engineers and designers involved in the field covered by the IEEE White Book are, for the most part, contained in the *Transactions* of the IAS.

ANSI/IEEE Std 241-1983 is published by the IEEE on behalf of the Commercial Buildings Committee of the Industrial Power Systems Department of the Industry Applications Society acting through the Gray Book Working Group. Individuals who desire to participate in the activities of the committees, subcommittees, or working groups in the preparation or revision of texts such as this should write or call IEEE Standards Office, 345 East 47 Street, New York, NY 10017.

---

[1] These documents can be obtained from the Institute of Electrical and Electronics Engineers, Service Center, 445 Hoes Lane, Piscataway, NJ 08854.

1.3.2 Engineering in Medicine and Biology Society. Another IEEE group of interest to the electrical engineer involved in health care facility design is the Engineering in Medicine and Biology Society (EMBS). The EMBS *Transactions* and the EMBS *Magazine* include articles on the physiological effects of electrical shock and other subjects pertinent to electrical safety. Articles dealing with electrical equipment and instrumentation also appear in the EMBS *Transactions.*

1.4 Professional Registration. Most regulatory agencies require that design for public buildings be prepared under the jurisdiction of state-licensed professional architects or engineers. Information on such registration may be obtained from the appropriate state agency or from the local chapter of the National Society of Professional Engineers.

To facilitate obtaining registration in different states under the reciprocity rule, a national professional certificate is issued by the National Bureau of Engineering Registration[2] to engineers who obtained their home-state license by examination. All engineering graduates are encouraged to start on the path to full registration by taking the engineer-in-training examination as soon after graduation as possible. The final written examination in the field of specialization is usually conducted after four years of progressive professional experience.

Clinical Engineering Certification is available through an International Commission. When available, the hospital's clinical engineer should be involved in the electrical design process.

1.5 Codes and Standards

1.5.1 National Electrical Code and Other NFPA Standards. The electrical wiring and design recommendations in the National Electrical Code (NEC), ANSI/NFPA 70-1984, are vitally important guidelines for health care facility engineers. The NEC is revised every three years, and care should be taken to use the edition that is current and adopted by the authority having jurisdiction of enforcement (AHJ) at the time of construction. The NEC is published and available from the National Fire Protection Association (NFPA) and the American National Standards Institute (ANSI).[3] It does not represent a design specification but only identifies minimum requirements for the safe installation and utilization of electricity in the building. It is strongly recommended that the introduction to the NEC, Article 90, covering purpose and scope, be carefully read. The NFPA *Handbook*, of the *National Electrical Code*, sponsored by the NFPA, contains the complete NEC text plus explanations. This book is edited to correspond with each edition of the NEC.

The NFPA publishes the following related documents containing requirements on electrical and medical equipment and systems:

(1) ANSI/NFPA 20-1983, Standard for the Installation of Centrifugal Fire Pumps.

---

[2] PO Drawer 1404, Columbia, SC.

[3] ANSI/NFPA publications can be obtained from the Sales Department, American National Standards Institute, 1430 Broadway, New York, NY 10018, or from Publication Sales, National Fire Protection Association, Batterymarch Park, Quincy, MA 02269.

(2) ANSI/NFPA 53M-1979, Manual on Fire Hazards in Oxygen-Enriched Atmospheres.

(3) ANSI/NFPA 70B-1983, Recommended Practice for Electrical Equipment Maintenance.

(4) ANSI/NFPA 70E-1983, Standard for Electrical Safety Requirements of Employee Workplaces.

(5) ANSI/NFPA 71-1982, Standard for the Installation, Maintenance, and Use of Central Station Signaling Systems.

(6) ANSI/NFPA 72A-1979, Standard for the Installation, Maintenance, and Use of Local Protective Signaling Systems.

(7) ANSI/NFPA 72B-1979, Standard for the Installation, Maintenance, and Use of Auxiliary Protective Signaling Systems.

(8) ANSI/NFPA 72C-1982, Standard for the Installation, Maintenance, and Use of Remote Station Protective Signaling Systems.

(9) ANSI/NFPA 72D-1979, Standard for the Installation, Maintenance, and Use of Proprietary Protective Signaling Systems.

(10) ANSI/NFPA 72E-1984, Standard on Automatic Fire Detectors.

(11) ANSI/NFPA 75-1981, Standard for the Protection of Electronic Computer/ Data Processing Equipment.

(12) ANSI/NFPA 77-1982, Recommended Practice on Static Electricity.

(13) ANSI/NFPA 78-1983, Lightning Protection Code.

(14) ANSI/NFPA 99-1984, Standard for Health Care Facilities.

(15) ANSI/NFPA 101-1985, Code for Safety to Life from Fire in Buildings and Structures.

(16) NFPA 101 HB85, Life Safety Code Handbook.

(17) NFPA FPH1581, Fire Protection Handbook.

ANSI/NFPA 99-1984 replaces NFPA 3M, 56A, 56B, 56C, 56D, 56E, 56G, 56HM, 56K, 76A, 76B, and 76C. NFPA 56A (Inhalation Anesthetics—1978) and 76A (Essential Electrical Systems—1977) are adopted by enforcement authorities for health care facilities and may still be in force in some areas.

The National Electrical Code and other selected NFPA codes are generally adopted by local and state governments for enforcement by electrical and building inspectors and fire marshals.

1.5.2 Health Care Codes and Standards. Additional electrical requirements for health care facilities are included in the Accreditation Manual for Hospitals published by the Joint Commission for the Accreditation of Hospitals (JCAH). Hospitals seeking JCAH accreditation must undergo an inspection semi-annually by JCAH examiners. Accreditation depends on the hospital's conformance with the requirements included in the accreditation manual.

The Department of Health and Human Services publishes a standard entitled, Guidelines for Construction and Equipment of Hospitals and Medical Facilities.[4]

---

[4] This publication can be obtained from the Superintendent of Documents, US Government Printing Office, Washington, DC 20402.

This standard includes electrical requirements which must be satisfied by any facility seeking reimbursement from the Federal Government.

Electrical designers working on projects for the Veterans Administration, armed services, and other government agencies must be aware that these agencies generally publish standards for electrical design. These standards or guidelines can be obtained from the appropriate agency.

1.5.3 Local, State, and Federal Codes and Regulations. While most municipalities, counties, and states use the NEC without change, some have their own codes. In some instances the NEC is adopted by local ordinance as part of the building code, with deviations from the NEC listed as addenda. It is important to note that only the code adopted as of a certain date is official, and that governmental bodies may delay adopting the latest code. Federal rulings may require use of the latest NEC regardless of local rulings, so that reference to the enforcing agencies for interpretation on this point may be necessary.

Some city and state codes are almost as extensive as the NEC. It is generally accepted that in the case of conflict, the more stringent or severe interpretation applies. Generally the entity responsible for enforcing the code has the power to interpret it.

Failure to comply with NEC or local code requirements can affect the owner's ability to obtain a certificate of occupancy and may have a negative effect on insurance.

In most states health care construction comes under the jurisdiction of a state health department. In some instances the state will have its own hospital or health care code with specific electrical requirements.

Both state and local authorities may adopt and enforce one of the model building codes written by a regional building officials group. These include the Standard Building Code, the Uniform Building Code, and the National Building Code.

Legislation by the US Federal Government has had the effect of giving standards, such as those of the American National Standards Institute (ANSI), the impact of law. The Occupational Safety and Health Act, administered by the US Department of Labor, permits federal enforcement of codes and standards. The Occupational Safety and Health Administration (OSHA) has adopted the 1971 (or later) NEC for new electrical installations and equipment within the scope of subpart S—Electrical—of OSHA regulations and also for major replacements, modification, or repair installed after March 5, 1972. A few articles and sections of the NEC have been deemed by OSHA to apply retroactively.

A number of states have enacted legislation embodying various energy conservation standards such as ANSI/ASHRAE/IES 90A-1980, Energy Conservation in New Building Design. Such standards establish energy or power budgets that materially affect architectural, mechanical, and electrical designs.

1.5.4 Standards and Recommended Practices. A number of organizations in addition to the NFPA publish documents which affect electrical design. Adherence to these documents can be written into design specifications.

The American National Standards Institute (ANSI) approves the standards of many other organizations. ANSI coordinates the review of proposed standards among all interested affiliated societies and organizations to assure a consensus approval. It is in effect a clearinghouse for technical standards of all types.

Underwriters Laboratories, Inc[5] (UL) is a non-profit organization, operating laboratories for investigation with respect to hazards affecting life and property, materials and products, especially electrical appliances and equipment. In so doing, they develop test standards. Equipment which has been tested by UL, and found to conform to their standards, is known as listed or labeled equipment.

The National Electrical Manufacturers Association[6] (NEMA) represents equipment manufacturers. Their publications serve to standardize the manufacture of, and provide testing and operating standards for electrical equipment. The design engineer should be aware of any NEMA standard which might affect the application of any equipment specified by him.

1.6 Handbooks. The following handbooks have, over the years, established reputations in the electrical field. This list is not intended to be all-inclusive, and other excellent references in addition to those listed in 1.3 are available, but are not listed here because of space limitations.

(1) *Applied Protective Relaying* (Westinghouse Electric Corporation, 1976). The application of protective relaying to commercial-utility interconnections, protection of high-voltage motors, transformers, cables, are covered in detail.

(2) *ASHRAE Handbook* (American Society of Heating, Refrigerating, and Air Conditioning Engineers[7] [ASHRAE]). This series of reference books in four volumes, which are periodically updated, details the electrical and mechanical aspects of space conditioning and refrigeration.

(3) BEEMAN, D.L., editor. *Industrial Power Systems Handbook.* New York: McGraw-Hill, 1955. A text on electrical design with emphasis on equipment, including that applicable to commercial buildings.

(4) CROFT, T., CARR, C.C., and WATT, J.H. *American Electricians' Handbook.* 9th edition. New York: McGraw-Hill, 1970. The practical aspects of equipment, construction, and installation are covered.

(5) *Electrical Maintenance Hints* (Westinghouse Electric Corporation, 1974). The preventative maintenance procedures for all types of electrical equipment and the rehabilitation of damaged apparatus are discussed.

(6) *Electrical Transmission and Distribution Reference Book* (Westinghouse Electric Corporation, 1964). All aspects of transmission, distribution, performance, and protection are included in detail.

(7) FINK, D.G. and BEATY, H.W. *Standard Handbook for Electrical Engineers.* 11th ed. New York: McGraw-Hill, 1978. Virtually the entire field of electrical engineering is treated, including equipment and systems design.

(8) *IES Lighting Handbook* (Illuminating Engineering Society[8] [IES]: Application Volume, 1981; Reference Volume, 1984). All aspects of lighting, including see-

---

[5] 333 Pfingsten Road, Northbrook, IL 60020.
[6] 2101 L Street, NW, Washington, DC 20037.
[7] Publication Sales, 1791 Tullie Circle, NE, Atlanta, GA 30329.
[8] 345 East 47th Street, New York, NY 10017.

ing, recommended lighting levels, lighting calculations, and design, are included in extensive detail in this comprehensive text.

(9) *Lighting Handbook* (Westinghouse Electric Corporation, 1976). The application of various light sources, fixtures, and ballasts to interior and exterior commercial, industrial, sports, and roadway lighting projects.

(10) McPARTLAND, J. (and the editors of *Electrical Constructions and Maintenance* magazine). *How to Design Electrical Systems.* New York: McGraw-Hill, 1968.

(11) McPARTLAND, J. and NOVAK, W. *Electrical Design Details.* New York: McGraw-Hill, 1960. This reference offers the young engineer insight into the systems approach to electrical design.

(12) SMEATON, R.S., editor. *Motor Applications and Maintenance Handbook.* New York: McGraw-Hill, 1969. Contains extensive, detailed coverage of motor load data and motor characteristics to better coordinate electric motors with machine mechanical characteristics.

(13) SMEATON, R.S., editor. *Switchgear and Control Handbook.* New York: McGraw-Hill, 1977. Concise, reliable guide to important facets of switchgear and control design, safety, application, and maintenance including high- and low-voltage starters, circuit breakers, and fuses.

(14) *Underground Systems Reference Book* (Edison Electric Institute,[9] 1957). The principles of underground construction and the detailed design of vault installations cable systems and related power systems are fully illustrated; cable splicing design parameters are thoroughly covered.

A few of the older texts may not be available for purchase, but are available in most professional offices and libraries.

1.7 Periodicals. *Spectrum*, the basic monthly publication of the IEEE, covers all aspects of electrical and electronic engineering with limited material on health care facilities. This publication, however, does contain references to IEEE books and other publications, technical meetings and conferences, IEEE group, society, and committee activities, abstracts of papers and publications of the IEEE and other organizations and other material essential to the professional advancement of the electrical engineer. The *Transactions* of the Industry Applications Society and the Engineering in Medicine and Biology Society of the IEEE can be useful to health care electrical engineers.

Following are some other well-known periodicals:

(1) *ASHRAE Journal,* American Society of Heating, Refrigerating and Air-Conditioning Engineers.

(2) *Biomedical Electronics,* 455 Mount Arlington, NJ 07856.

(3) *Biomedical Engineering,* 233 Spring Street, New York, NY 10013.

(4) *Consulting Engineer,* Barrington, IL 60010.

(5) *Electrical Construction and Maintenance,* McGraw-Hill, 1221 Avenue of the Americas, New York, NY 10020.

(6) *Electrical Consultant,* One River Road, Cos Cob, CT 06807.

---

[9] 1111 19th Street, NW, Washington, DC 20036.

(7) *Fire Journal*, National Fire Protection Association, Batterymarch Park, Quincy, MA 00269.

(8) *Health Care Systems*, 1515 Broadway, New York, NY 10036.

(9) *Hospitals*, American Hospital Publishing, Inc., 211 E. Chicago Avenue, Chicago, IL 60611.

(10) *IAEI News*, International Association of Electrical Inspectors, 802 Busse Highway, Park Ridge, IL 60068.

(11) *Journal of Clinical Engineering*, 1351 Titan Way, Brea, CA 92621.

(12) *Journal of the Operating Room Research Institute*, 100 Campus Road, Totowa, NJ 07512.

(13) *Lighting Design and Application*, Illuminating Engineering Society, 345 East 47th Street, New York, NY 10017.

(14) *Modern Healthcare*, 740 N. Rush St., Chicago, IL 60611.

(15) *Plant Engineering*, 1301 South Grove Avenue, Barrington, IL 60010.

(16) *Professional Engineer*, National Society of Professional Engineers, 2029 K Street Northwest, Washington, DC 20006.

(17) *Specifying Engineer*, Cahners Publishing Company, 5 South Wabash Avenue, Chicago, IL 60603.

1.8 Manufacturers' Data. The electrical industry through its associations and individual manufacturers of electrical equipment issues many technical bulletins, data books, and magazines. While some of this information is difficult to obtain, copies should be made available to each major design unit. The advertising sections of electrical magazines contain excellent material, usually well illustrated and presented in a clear and readable form, concerning the construction and application of equipment. Such literature may be promotional; it may present the advertiser's equipment or methods in a best light and should be carefully evaluated. Manufacturer's catalogs are a valuable source of equipment information. Some manufacturers' complete catalogs are quite extensive covering several volumes. However, these companies may issue condensed catalogs for general use. A few manufacturers publish regularly scheduled magazines containing news of new products and actual applications. Data sheets referring to specific items are almost always available from the sales offices. Some technical files may be kept in microfilm for use either by projection or by printing at larger design offices. Manufacturers' representatives, both sales and technical, can do much to provide complete information on a product.

Manufacturers of specialized hospital electrical equipment often publish design and installation recommendations and technical updates. This is particularly true of isolation panel, standby system, and transfer switch manufacturers.

1.9 Safety. Safety of life and preservation of property are two of the most important factors in the design of the electrical system. This is especially true in health care facilities because of public occupancy, thoroughfare, high occupancy density and patients—some of them critically ill or injured. In many health care facilities the systems operating staff has limited technical capabilities and may not have any specific electrical training.

Various codes provide rules and regulations as minimum safeguards of life and property. The electrical design engineer often needs to provide greater safeguards than outlined in the codes according to his best judgment, while also giving consideration to utilization and economics.

Personnel safety may be divided into five categories

(1) Safety for maintenance and operating personnel.
(2) Safety for the general public.
(3) Safety for general patients.
(4) Safety for critical patients or patients subject to invasive procedures.
(5) Safety for anesthetized patients.

Safety for maintenance and operating personnel is achieved through proper design and selection of equipment with regard to enclosures, key-interlocking, circuit breaker and fuse interrupting capacity, the use of high-speed fault-detection and circuit-opening devices, clearances from structural members, grounding methods, disconnecting means and identification of equipment.

Safety for the general public requires that all circuitmaking and breaking equipment as well as other electrical apparatus be isolated from casual contact. This is achieved by using locked rooms and enclosures, proper grounding, limiting of fault levels, installation of barriers and other isolation, proper clearances, adequate insulation, and other similar provisions outlined in this standard.

Safety for general patients requires all of the design features used for protecting the general public as well as special provisions to minimize potential difference between any two conducting surfaces likely to come in contact with the patient directly or indirectly. A green ground conductor is required for all patient care areas to keep potential below 500 mV under normal conditions.

Potential differences in critical care areas must be kept below 40 mV under normal conditions. However, the designer must be aware that even with #10 ground conductors connected to form an equipotential grounding system, potential differences higher than 40 mV can be generated during fault conditions. Equipotential grounding or other special protective systems such as isolation transformers are used in critical care areas to protect catheterized patients from electric shock through an exposed catheter.

Patients under anesthesia are treated as critical patients. Where flammable anesthesia is used, isolation transformers and a properly grounded conductive floor shall be provided. All wiring in the hazardous area must be installed as required for Class 1 Division 1 locations.

The National Electrical Safety Code (NESC), ANSI C2, 1984 edition, is available from the IEEE and ANSI. A cloth-bound hardcover edition may be obtained from John Wiley & Sons Inc, New York. It covers outdoor distribution systems, supply and communications systems, overhead lines, high-voltage systems, and other items related to the supply of building power.

Circuit protection is a fundamental safety requirement of all electrical systems. Adequate interrupting capacities are required in services, feeders, and branch circuits. Selective, automatic isolation of faulted circuits represents good engineering. Tripping schemes for the emergency system must be selective, so that faults on adjacent branches or systems or faults on the emergency system itself do not disrupt service to unaffected emergency system circuits—especially if interruption of these circuits can jeopardize the lives or safety of patients. Physical protection of wiring by means of approved raceways under all probable conditions of exposure to electrical, chemical, and mechanical damage is necessary.

Circuits on the emergency system shall be installed in metallic raceway. Circuits to patient care areas shall be installed with a green ground conductor and should be installed in metallic raceway to insure physical protection and to provide redundant grounding. Such raceways should be of sufficient size for future expansion. Additional raceways and spare conductors for future use may be installed within allowable financial constraints. If the raceways are properly constructed and bonded, they can minimize power interruptions. The design engineer should locate equipment where suitable ambient temperatures exist and ventilation is available. The operation of fault-detection and circuit-interruption devices under conditions of abnormal voltage and frequency should be assured.

1.9.1 Appliances and Equipment. Improperly applied or inferior materials can cause electrical failures. The use of appliances and equipment listed by the Underwriters Laboratories, Inc, or other approved laboratories is recommended. The Association of Home Appliance Manufacturers[10] (AHAM) and the Air-Conditioning and Refrigeration Institute[11] (ARI) specify the manufacture, testing, and application of many common appliances and equipment.

High-voltage equipment is manufactured in accordance with NEMA, ANSI, and IEEE standards; and the engineer should make sure that the equipment he specifies conforms to these standards. Properly prepared specifications can prevent the purchase of inferior or unsuitable equipment. The lowest initial purchase price may not result in the lowest cost after taking into consideration operating, maintenance, and owning costs. Value engineering is an organized approach to identification of unnecessary costs utilizing such methods as life cycles, cost analyses, and related techniques.

1.9.2 Operational Considerations. When the design engineer lays out equipment rooms and locates electrical devices, he cannot always avoid having some areas accessible to unqualified persons. Dead-front construction should be utilized whenever practical. Where dead-front construction is not available, all exposed electrical equipment should be placed behind locked doors or gates. This will result in a reduction in electrical failures caused by human error, as well as improved safety.

A serious cause of failure, which is attributable to human error, is unintentional grounding or phase-to-phase short circuiting of equipment which is being worked upon. By careful design such as proper spacing and barriers, and by enforcement of published work-safety rules, the engineer can minimize unintentional grounding and phase-to-phase, and ground faults in the distribution equipment. High-quality workmanship is an important factor in the prevention of

---

[10] 20 North Wacker Drive, Chicago, IL 60606.
[11] 1501 Wilson Boulevard, Arlington, VA 22209.

electrical failures. Therefore, the design should incorporate features that are conducive to good workmanship.

Selective coordination of overcurrent devices is important in health care facilities, especially for critical care areas of hospitals. The system must be studied for both high and low level faults. It is also important to consider the different levels of available short circuit current available from utility and standby sources.

Ground fault protection schemes on large service mains on grounded 480 volt systems will help to minimize damage from arcing ground faults. Arcing ground faults or "burndowns" can cause total destruction of electrical equipment, jeopardizing patient safety by fire and loss of electrical service. By providing one or more additional steps of ground fault protection downstream, designers can insure that otherwise harmless ground faults (such as in the powerhouse or kitchen) will not take out the hospital main or patient care areas of the hospital. Ground fault systems should be tested for selective tripping to insure proper and safe operation.

1.10 Maintenance. Maintenance is essential to proper operation. The installation should be so designed that building personnel can perform most of the maintenance with a minimum need for specialized services. Design details should provide proper space and accessibility so that equipment can be maintained without difficulty and excessive cost.

The engineer should consider the effects of a failure in the system supplying the building. Generally, the external systems are operated and maintained by the electrical utility, though at times they are a part of the health care facility distribution system.

In health care facilities where continuity of service is essential, suitable emergency and standby equipment should be provided. Such equipment is needed to maintain minimum lighting requirements for passageways, stairways, and to supply power to critical patient care areas and essential loads. These systems are usually installed within the building, and they include automatic or manual equipment for transferring loads on loss of normal supply power or for putting battery- or generator-fed equipment into service.

Although applicable codes determine the need for standby or emergency generating systems in health care facilities, they are generally required in any facility that keeps acutely ill patients overnight, performs invasive procedures, administers anesthesia, or otherwise treats patients unable to care for themselves during an emergency. High rise health care facilities regardless of type should have on site emergency or standby generators.

Electrical engineers should consider the installation of bypass/isolation switches in conjunction with automatic transfer switches to permit maintenance on a deenergized transfer switch without jeopardizing patient safety. The isolation/bypass switch permits removal of the transfer switch from the circuit while providing for manual transfer to the normal or emergency source.

Even with isolation/bypass switches, it is possible for a load side circuit breaker to fail killing power to all or part of the critical branch. For this reason it is often wise to provide some normal circuits in critical patient care areas.

1.11 Design Considerations. Electrical equipment usually occupies a relatively small percentage of the total building space, and in design it may be easier to relocate electrical service areas than mechanical areas or structural elements. Allocation of space for electrical areas is often given secondary consideration by architectural and related specialties. In the competing search for space, the electrical engineer is responsible for fulfilling the requirements for a proper electrical installation while at the same time recognizing the flexibility of electrical systems in terms of layout and placement.

Today, architectural considerations and appearances are of paramount importance in the design of a health care facility. Aesthetic considerations may play an important role in the selection of equipment, especially lighting equipment. Provided that the dictates of good practice, code requirements, and environmental considerations are not violated, the electrical engineer may have to compromise in his design to accommodate the desires of other members of the design team.

1.11.1 Coordination of Design. The electrical engineer should work closely with professional associates, such as the architect, the mechanical engineer, the structural engineer, and the civil engineer. He is also concerned with the building owner or operator who, as clients, may take an active interest in the design. More often the electrical engineer will work directly with the coordinator of overall design activities, usually the architect. He should cooperate with the safety engineer, fire protection engineer, the environmental engineer, and a host of other concerned people, such as interior designers, all of whom have a say in the ultimate design.

The electrical designer should become familiar with local rules and know the authorities having jurisdiction over the design and construction. The designer should always contact the authorities having jurisdiction and all applicable utilities before beginning design. Local contractors are usually familiar with local ordinances and union work rules and can be of great help in avoiding pitfalls. Union work practices may, for reasons of safety or other considerations, discourage the use of certain materials and techniques.

In performing electrical design, it is essential, at the outset, to prepare a checklist of all the design stages that have to be considered. Major items include temporary power, access to the site, and review by others. It is important to note that certain electrical work may appear in nonelectrical sections of the specifications. For example, furnishing and connecting of electric motors and controls may be covered in the mechanical section of the specifications. Another notable example would be elevators which are usually specified by the architect. The electrical engineer should make it his business to see that the proper starter, fireman's recall system, and emergency sequencing of elevators are specified.

Electrical engineers working on health care projects should have a working knowledge of medical gas systems because medical gas outlets often share consoles and headwalls he specifies. He should also be familiar with medical gas alarm systems. For administrative control purposes, the electrical work may be divided into a number of contracts, some of which may be under the control of a general contractor and some of which may be awarded to electrical contractors.

Among items with which the designer will be concerned are preliminary cost estimates, final cost estimates, plans or drawings, specifications (which are the written presentation of the work), materials, manuals, factory inspections, laboratory tests, and temporary power. He may well be involved in providing information on how electrical considerations affect financial justification of the project in terms of owning and operating costs, amortization, return on investment, and related items.

1.12 Other Considerations. Those involved in the design of health care facilities should understand the process by which drawings are issued for bidding and construction. The designer should also have some knowledge of shop drawing review, estimating, and contract administration. For more information see the Introduction (Chapter 1) to the IEEE Gray Book.

Design and construction of health care facilities are a team process involving engineers, architects, construction managers, general contractors, subcontractors and equipment vendors. In recent years the contractors and construction managers have become increasingly involved in the design process. In order to successfully complete a health care project, it is important to involve contractors who have a successful track record in health care construction. The larger and more complex the project the more important it is to have contractors who are skilled and experienced in the specialized construction techniques required for medical facilities.

2. Load Requirements and Energy Management

2.1 General Discussion. As with other building types, the determination of loads to be served by the electrical system is fundamental to health care facility design. Equally important is the economic application of materials, labor, and electrical devices to serve identified loads. As a goal, the completed facility should serve the initial loads, provide a margin for incremental growth, and foster the efficient use of energy.

2.1.1 Loads. One of the purposes of this chapter is to aid the designer in estimating loads usually found in health care facilities and to show the range of power typically required by these loads.

2.1.2 Groups of Loads. The cumulative effect of groups of individual loads is one of the determinants of distribution system design. This chapter will provide data from operating health care facilities that will be useful in projecting total load demand. Similarly, a profile for one type of facility will be presented. The reader is cautioned that such data should be viewed within the narrow scope in which it is presented. That is, the data is indicative of a specific building at a specific point in time and cannot be extrapolated necessarily into a typical profile.

2.1.3 Load Growth. Patterns of health care have changed rapidly in recent years, and as the biological sciences continue to advance, altering patterns may be expected in the future. Such changes impose on health care facilities the need to adapt to changing demands of many kinds. The designer of electrical systems should plan for inevitable change and should anticipate incremental growth of loads during the useful life of the facility. In fact, the designer's recognition of the dynamic nature of health care facilities may result in extended useful life. Obviously, the type of health care facility affects the level of change that may be anticipated. Teaching hospitals are more prone to change than community general hospitals, and the latter more so than custodial care facilities.

2.1.4 Energy Utilization. Electrical system design affects the energy required to operate a facility over its useful life. This consideration should be balanced with the loads to be served as the design is created. Another purpose of this chapter is to present data that will help reduce the unknowns faced by the designer, resulting in a more energy efficient facility. Additionally, techniques of energy management will be discussed.

2.2 Loads vs. Facility Type. There are many types of health care facilities, some of which are identified in the introduction. Load density for the total building will vary as the type varies.

Teaching and general hospitals may be expected to offer the broadest spectrum of load types and to yield the highest concentration of load per gross square foot. Conversely, minimal care and custodial care facilities will produce generally low concentrations of load.

Outpatient screening clinics and physicians' offices will be similar to commercial office buildings, except that screening clinics sometimes will include extensive laboratory and radiology facilities.

Psychiatric hospitals, nursing homes, minimal care and custodial care facilities share a common bond since large portions of each will be devoted to patient accommodations. While the similarity will stop there in most cases, the load density (watts per gross square foot) will be influenced significantly by their residential character.

Load density is related to other variables in addition to facility type. As an example, choice of fuel for heating and air conditioning will exert considerable influence on loads.

2.3 Lighting Loads. Lighting for health care facilities is presented in Chapter 7. Loads imposed by the lighting systems will be a function of several variables, among which are:

(1) Tasks to be performed
(2) Quality and quantity of illumination required
(3) Choice of lighting sources.

Lighting design for some areas will be similar to that for other commercial buildings. Other spaces will require the application of specialized lighting techniques. Among the latter are patient rooms, intensive care units, nurseries, and surgical and obstetrical suites.

In all cases, task lighting techniques should be applied, in the interest of energy management and of optimum distribution system capacity.

2.3.1 Loads by Function. For initial calculations, lighting connected loads may be estimated relying on the designer's previous experience or they may be estimated using the IES lighting power budget technique. Readers should refer to the references for this chapter and to the body of Chapter 7 for more on this subject.

2.3.2 Lighting Demand. As with other types of loads, demand factors may be applied to lighting connected load when determining distribution system component capacity. The appropriate factor will depend upon some or all of the following:

(1) Function performed in the area served
(2) Means of lighting control, that is, switching, dimming
(3) Hours of operation for the area served.

As an upper limit, the continuous load supplied by a lighting branch circuit should not exceed 80% of the branch circuit rating. For good design practice, the continuous load supplied should not exceed 70% of the branch circuit rating.

ANSI/NFPA 70-1984 [2][12] permits the use of lighting demand factors in calculating lighting load on feeders. Refer to Table 220-11. However, designers should develop their own factors based on the characteristics of a specific project, consistent with restraints imposed by code authorities.

The factors shown in Table 1 may be used in sizing the distribution system components shown and should result in a conservative design. The factors should be applied to connected lighting load in the first step, and then, to the product resulting from previous steps as the designer proceeds through the system.

2.4 Power Loads. Power loads may be divided into broad categories:

(1) Building equipment
   (a) Heating, ventilating, air conditioning
   (b) Transportation (elevators, escalators, trolleys)
   (c) Auxiliary pumps (fire, sump, clinical air and vacuum, pneumatic tube)
(2) Functional equipment
   (a) Kitchen
   (b) Data processing
   (c) Communication systems
   (d) Office machines and copy equipment
(3) Medical equipment
   (a) X-ray
   (b) Radiation therapy
   (c) Laboratory
   (d) Surgery
   (e) Intensive care, recovery, emergency
   (f) Physical and occupational therapy
   (g) Inhalation therapy
   (h) Pharmacy
   (i) Materials management
   (j) Medical records.

NOTE: Major loads occur in the first two categories, and these loads are similar to those in other types of commercial buildings. The third category is unique to health care.

Table 1
Factors Used in Sizing Distribution System Components

Distribution System Component	Lighting Demand Factor
Lighting panelboard buss and main overcurrent device	1.0
Lighting panelboard feeder and feeder overcurrent device	1.0
Distribution panelboard buss and main overcurrent device	
First 50 000 W or less	0.5
All over 50 000 W	0.4
Remaining components	0.4

---

[12] The numbers in brackets correspond to those in the references at the end of this chapter.

2.4.1 Building Equipment. The types of heating, ventilating, and air conditioning systems chosen for a specific building will have the greatest single effect on electrical load. First, the choice of fuel will be critical. If natural gas, fuel oil, or coal is chosen, electrical loads will be lower than would be the case if electricity were chosen. Second, the choice of refrigeration cycle will have considerable impact. If absorption chillers are chosen, electrical loads will be lower than those imposed by electric centrifugal or reciprocating chillers. Early discussions between mechanical and electrical designers will be advantageous in planning the electrical distribution system.

For initial estimates, before actual loads are known, the factors shown in Table 2 may be used to establish the major elements of the electrical system serving HVAC systems.

Elevators usually are large loads, but since only a few are required in most health care facilities, elevators do not represent a large portion of total load. For preliminary design of the distribution system in buildings of up to twelve stories, assuming vertical speeds up to 450 ft/min, 4500 lb capacity, the following loads may be used:

Electric traction elevators, each	35–50 hp
Hydraulic elevators, each	40–75 hp

Hydraulic elevators ordinarily will not be employed in buildings higher than seven stories and speeds usually will be limited to 150 ft/min. However, capacities

Table 2
Factors Used to Establish Major Elements of the
Electrical System Serving HVAC Systems

Item	Unit
Refrigeration Machines:	kVA/Ton of Chiller Capacity
Absorption	
Centrifugal	1.00
Reciprocating	
Auxiliary Pumps & Fans:	
Chilled Water Pumps	0.08
Condenser Water Pumps	
Absorption	
Centrifugal/Reciprocating	0.07
Cooling Tower Fans	
Absorption	
Centrifugal/Reciprocating	0.07
Boilers:	kVA/Boiler Horsepower
Natural Gas/Fuel Oil	0.07
Coal	
Boiler Auxiliary Pumps:	kVA/Boiler Horsepower
Deaerator	0.10
Auxiliary Equipment:	kVA/Bed
Clinical Vacuum Pumps	0.18
Clinical Air Compressors	0.10

may be higher than 4500 lb. Actual loads should be obtained from the elevator vendor once vertical transportation requirements have been defined sufficiently to permit calculation.

Escalators are not used frequently in health care facilities but may be employed in a few buildings. For initial estimates, escalator load will approximate 25 hp for each landing served above the first.

Horizontal and vertical transportation systems for food, supplies, and materials using automated trolleys or carts are found in a few large health care facilities. Pneumatic tube systems are more common and may be employed as the sole means of transport for small supplies and paper records or as one component in a materials handling system. Automated trolleys or carts impose relatively small loads (less than 10 hp) at numerous locations but will usually be combined with dedicated elevators whose loads will be similar to a service elevator. Pneumatic tube systems are powered by vacuum pumps or exhausters located in a few central locations. Motor drives will vary depending on the extent of the system but are under 10 hp (many, less than 3 hp).

2.4.2 Functional Equipment. Equipment of this type usually consists of numerous small loads except that used in kitchens and except for some office copiers. The effect on the electrical system is to require panelboard space and multiple branch circuits but low load density.

The choice of fuel in the kitchen is the major determinant. If natural gas is the primary fuel, electrical loads will be lower on a watts per square foot basis than where electricity is the primary fuel. Preliminary planning should address this question early. For estimating purposes, the following factors may be used. In calculating kitchen floor area include cooking and preparation, dishwashing, storage, walk-in refrigerator/freezer, food serving lines, tray assembly and offices.

Primary Fuel	Watts/Square Foot
Natural Gas	25
Electricity	125

Computer equipment is employed in several areas of the typical hospital. As a minimum, stand-alone systems for patient and general accounting and for laboratory analyses may be anticipated. However, it is common to find these integrated into hospital-wide management information systems today. Such systems use multiple input stations throughout the hospital, all intended to produce a unified patient bill at the time of patient discharge plus inventory control, third party billing, and portions of the patient's medical record.

As in other types of facilities, computer power requirements are usually moderate at the central processor location and low at distributed input stations. For most installations found in hospitals, the total load at the central location will not exceed 45 kVA. Occasionally, large systems or multiple systems housed together may require up to 75 kVA.

At CRT or teletype input stations, power demand will not exceed 1 kVA.

While the quantity of power is important, the quality and reliability of the voltage supply are equally important. Use of isolating transformers is common, often including electrostatic shields. While there are exceptions, use of uninterruptible power supplies is not common. However, service as direct from the source as possible would be desirable.

Power demand from communication systems, as individual loads and as a whole, is low. Individual loads will not exceed 2 kVA usually, with most less than 1.5 kVA.

As in other commercial structures, there will be a large quantity of office equipment (typewriters, word processors, copiers) but power required will be low, on the order of 0.3 to 1.2 kVA per item. The exception will be large copy machines. These may be estimated at 3 to 6 kVA each.

2.4.3 Medical Equipment. Types of medical equipment employed in the several departments of health care facilities are discussed in Chapter 9.

Power distribution systems serving multiple X-ray machine installations require special attention. Designers should always be guided by the specific data furnished by vendors supplying equipment for the specific facility. However, an excellent planning guide is available as a NEMA standard (NEMA XR9-1984 [4]) and should be consulted.

Quality of voltage supplied is important to X-ray installations. Again, service as direct as possible from the source is desirable. Minimum transient disturbance and voltage drop are essential.

While momentary demand of X-ray installations will figure prominently in feeder and distribution equipment sizing, it need not be considered in calculating overall power demand imposed on the source, provided it is a part of a moderate size system. If the system requires 750 kVA or more, the momentary nature of X-ray operation will not add measurably to the overall demand. For small systems and for additions to existing facilities where service equipment is near capacity, some provision for X-ray demand may be advisable.

Clinical laboratories in hospitals require numerous branch circuits to serve the multitude of electrical devices but load density is usually low and individual equipment loads are low, most under 1 kVA. A few pieces of equipment in laboratories today perform multiple specialized tests. The loads for these will range between 3 and 8 kVA each. These same items often are sensitive to transient conditions on the power system and may require locally applied transient suppressors.

2.5 Overall Demand Factors. A tabulation of actual service entrance demand per gross square foot is presented in Tables 3 and 4 for a group of health care facilities. Data used in preparation of these tables was obtained from the Veteran's Administration and Hospital Corporation of America. Refer to footnotes accompanying the tables for the criteria on which these tables are based.

The tables show the type of facility, the gross floor area and number of beds for each, the geographic location and the major fuel type employed for HVAC systems in that facility. The derived factors may be used to estimate the anticipated demand for other facilities similar in size, location, and type of fuel. They also may be used to make initial estimates of service entrance capacity, switchgear size and space required for service entrance equipment. It is important to recognize, however, that they will be useful principally in the schematic design phase. As design proceeds through the preliminary and working drawing phases, these initial estimates should be modified by the actual conditions prevalent in the project.

Figures 1 and 2 present operating load data for a large general medical and surgical hospital located in the southeastern United States. It should be useful in visualizing changes in demand over time for a typical operating hospital. Candler General Hospital is a 305 bed facility, 402 000 gross ft^2, situated in Savannah, Georgia. The principal fuel employed for heating is natural gas with fuel oil standby. The chillers are centrifugal. Data for the charts was obtained by operating personnel during the cooling season, the peak period in this location.

2.6 Energy Management. To gain a better perspective of the impact of energy management on the nation's plan to meet future energy goals, an overall view of past, current and projected energy usage is necessary. Government and independent researchers have developed energy consumption projections to the year 2000 based on historical data on the total domestic energy usage over the past 81 years. Figure 3 is a graphic representation of usage from 1900 to 1981. Energy used in "quads" is plotted against years. A quad is 1 quadrillion Btu's (2.93 $\times$ 10^{11} kWh) or more conveniently the approximate amount of energy used by a city of 1 million people every three years. The distribution of usage by industrial, residential and commercial, and transportation is respectively three-eighths, three-eighths, and one-quarter of the total: 74 quads. An extrapolation of the historical data and a reasonable projection by the National Academy of Sciences to the year 2000 indicates consumption could be 175 quads. By incorporating the best

Table 3
Service Entrance Peak Demand (Veterans Administration)

Hospital	Floor Area Square Feet	Beds[*]	Degree Days[†] Cooling	Heating	Principal[‡] Fuel-HVAC	Watts Per Sq ft[§] Maximum	Average
V.A. Hospital #1	821 000	922	234	3536	NG/FO	4.5	3.5
V.A. Hospital #2	334 000	500	863	5713	NG/FO	5.2	3.9
V.A. Hospital #3	645 995	670	3488	1488	NG/FO	3.8	2.8
V.A. Hospital #4	681 000	600	1016	654	NG/FO	6.1	4.0
V.A. Hospital #5	503 500	697	3495	841	NG/FO	7.2	5.5
V.A. Hospital #6	800 000	1050	600	7400	NG/FO	5.9	4.2

[*] Total beds shown. Beds actually occupied could affect values shown for watts per square foot.

[†] Degree Days: Normals, Base 65 °F, based on 1941–70 period. From *Local Climatological Data Series*, 1974, NOAA.

[‡] NG/FO = Natural Gas/Fuel Oil; E = Electricity. Principal fuel is defined as that used for heating. In all cases, electricity was the fuel used for refrigeration.

[§] Watts per square foot based on measured values at service entrance during metering periods ranging from 9 to 17 days, during cooling season in all instances, 1981.

Table 4
Service Entrance Peak Demand (Hospital Corporation of America)

Hospital and Location	Floor Area Square Feet	Beds*	Degree Days† Cooling	Degree Days† Heating	Principal‡ Fuel–HVAC	Watts Per Sq ft§ Maximum
#1 — East	273 000	458	1353	3939	NG/FO	6.8
#2 — Southeast	278 000	250	2294	2240	NG/FO	6.3
#3 — Central	123 000	157			NG/FO	7.5
#4 — Central	36 365	62	2029	3227‖	E	13.7
#5 — Central	318 000	300	1107	4306	NG/FO	4.6
#6 — Southeast	182 000	225	3786	299‖	NG/FO	5.3
#7 — East	283 523	320	1030	4307	NG/FO	6.8
#8 — Southwest	135 396	150	2250	2621‖	NG/FO	6.6
#9 — West	190 000	97	927	5983	NG/FO	2.8
#10 — Southeast	161 000	170	3226	733‖	NG/FO	6.3
#11 — Southeast	157 639	214	2078	2146	NG/FO	7.3
#12 — Southeast	162 187	222	2143	2378‖	NG/FO	4.3
#13 — East	109 617	146	1030	4307‖	NG/FO	5.7
#14 — East	76 000	153	1030	4307‖	E	8.8
#15 — Southeast	135 150	190	1995	2547‖	NG/FO	5.9
#16 — Southwest	75 769	131	2587	2382‖	NG/FO	7.4
#17 — Central	75 769	128	1636	3505‖	NG/FO	6.3
#18 — Northwest	129 000	150	714	5833‖	NG/FO	4.4
#19 — Central	54 938	108	1694	3696‖	E	13.3
#20 — West	144 000	160	2814	1752	NG/FO	4.5
#21 — Southeast	149 000	123	2078	2146‖	NG/FO	4.5
#22 — Central	89 000	128	2029	3227‖	E	8.4
#23 — Central	128 500	150	1197	4729‖	NG/FO	6.2
#24 — West	135 169	170	927	5983‖	NG/FO	4.7
#25 — Southeast	80 000	124	1722	2975‖	NG/FO	6.2
#26 — Southeast	83 117	126	3226	733‖	NG/FO	8.5
#27 — Central	51 000	97	1569	3478	E	8.8
#28 — Southeast	66 528	120	2929	902‖	E	9.7
#29 — East	112 000	140	1394	3514	NG/FO	4.3
#30 — Central	202 000	223	1636	3505	NG/FO	4.8
#31 — Southeast	56 000	51	3786	299‖	NG/FO	7.4
#32 — West	47 434	50	927	5983‖	NG/E	7.0
#33 — Central	23 835	32	1694	3696‖	E	10.8
#34 — Southeast	105 000	95	2706	1465‖	NG/FO	8.3
#35 — West	48 575	60	3042	108‖	NG/E	7.7
#36 — Southwest	133 000	185	2587	2382‖	NG/FO	6.3
#37 — Central	42 879	66	1694	3696‖	E	15.7

* Total beds shown. Beds actually occupied could affect values shown for watts per square foot.

† Degree Days: Normals, Base 65 °F, based on 1941–70 period. From *Local Climatological Data Series*, 1974, NOAA.

‡ NG/FO = Natural Gas/Fuel Oil; E = Electricity. Principal fuel is defined as that used for heating. In all cases, electricity was the fuel used for refrigeration.

§ Watts per square foot based on measured values by utility company meter at service entrance, 1977.

‖ Data shown for nearest recorded location.

(Each facility was self-contained, in that refrigeration and air conditioning equipment loads are included in power demands shown.)

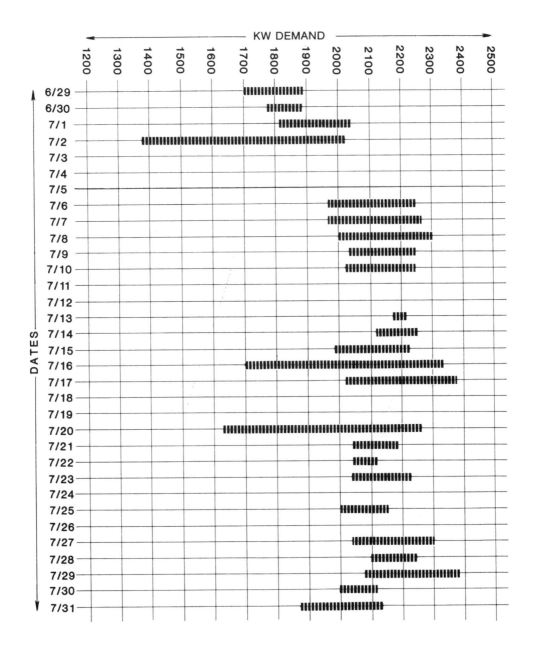

Fig 1
Load Profile
Candler General Hospital
6/29/81 - 7/31/81
kW Demand

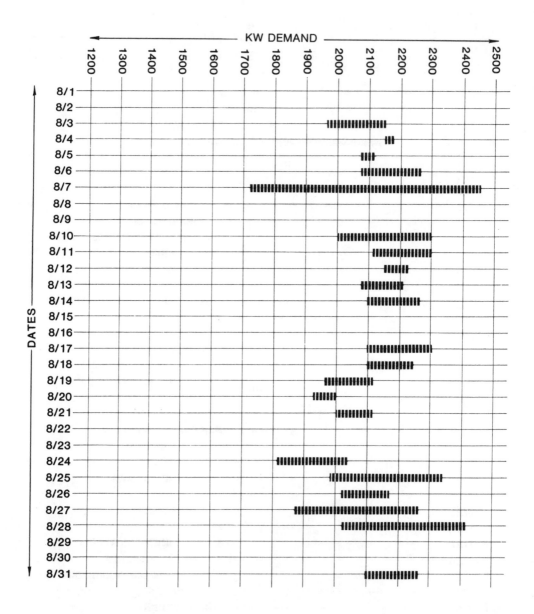

Fig 2
Load Profile
Candler General Hospital
8/1/82 – 8/31/82
kW Demand

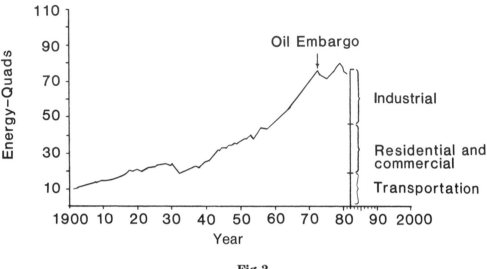

Fig 3
US Energy Consumption

estimates of the impact of "energy conservation" by Department of Energy (DOE) and other government and private agencies the 175 quad projection could be reduced by 65 quads to 110 quads, still 36 quads more per year than used in 1981. When one realizes the current level of usage is better than 15% beyond our domestic capabilities, including nuclear and renewable sources, the truth about the "energy crisis" is apparent.

Energy consumption in buildings totaled about 26 quads in 1981 which includes both residential and commercial sectors. Total energy consumption of hospitals was 1.1 quads. Assuming fixed percentages for estimating to the year 2000, 2.4 quads will be required without energy conservation measures and 1.5 quads with conservation, a reduction of approximately one third.

Energy management implies implementation of energy conservation measures and control over operating systems to minimize energy consumed. The designer has a responsibility to examine alternative design approaches and present these to the building owner with their tradeoffs. This arises not only from the need to conserve fuels but to control health care costs.

To develop an energy management program for any building, it is necessary first to know its types and usages of fuels or more commonly its energy balance.

The energy input to a hospital can arrive in a number of forms: electricity, natural gas, fuel oil, purchased steam, coal or other fuels. The size of the stream depends on the rate of fuel consumption and the Btu's of energy in that fuel. Oil and natural gas, of which the nation faces a limited supply, are important energy inputs in many hospitals. Even when they are not consumed directly, these non-renewable fossil fuels may have been used to produce other fuels. The total of all energy streams to a hospital is utilized for a number of functions. While the pattern in an individual hospital may vary, the largest single energy usage is usually the heating, ventilation and air conditioning (HVAC). Lighting represents the second most important use of energy in hospitals. Although the AIA/RC has tested small groups of hospitals to develop profiles for the development of Building Energy Performance Standards, the sampling was too small to establish target norms. Therefore, each hospital complex must be compared to itself to measure its progress in energy conservation.

2.6.1 Energy Economics. Energy codes promulgated since 1975 impose some mandatory requirements for energy conservation and suggest other voluntary opportunities that could be implemented. Incumbent on the building designer is the responsibility to investigate not only the energy conservation opportunities suggested, but also to evaluate nonrenewable fuel sources, energy recovery systems, operating system monitoring and controls, and maintenance management. Beyond the mandated requirements, most owners will require substantiation of the cost effectiveness of implementing energy conservation measures (ECM's).

Several methods exist for determining the cost effectiveness of alternative system designs. Common to all are two basic cost elements: (1) The cost to implement, or first cost, and (2) The net cost savings provided. Two of the methods are simple payback and life cycle costing.

(1) *Simple Payback.* The simplest method is the payback period. This method for determining the cost effectiveness of added ECM's is calculated by applying the following formula:

$$\text{Payback Period} = \frac{\text{First Cost}}{\text{Annual Savings - Annual Costs}}$$

The payback period is expressed in years. Annual savings are the first year's savings in fuel. Annual costs are the increased maintenance costs due to the measure. First cost is the total installed cost of the improvement.

Generally ignored in this method of analysis are the following:

(a) Cost of money—the annual interest on money borrowed

(b) Replacement cost—the cost to replace equipment

(c) Fuel inflation—the cost of fuel in future years

(d) Tax saving—the savings on purchase of equipment generated by federal tax incentives

(e) Depreciation.

Where the payback period is three years or less, this method is usually accurate enough to facilitate a decision.

(2) *Life Cycle Costing.* Life cycle costing is a means of evaluating the total cost of owning, operating, and maintaining a building or piece of equipment over its useful life. This method involves a systematic comparison of the estimated costs using a discount factor to relate future to present value.

The procedures required to prepare a life cycle cost analysis are:

(a) Establish nonfuel cost data, both initial investment and recurring cost

(b) Establish energy cost data for the time period chosen

(c) Determine the life cycle costs

(d) Determine net savings

(e) Calculate savings to investment ratio

(f) Perform certain sensitivity analyses

(g) Measure cost-effectiveness.

2.6.2 Utility Negotiations. In most cases, the selection of a power source will be determined by an analysis made by the design engineers and the utility engineers. Economics usually dictate selection and, with the exception of large high load factor complexes, the costs presently favor purchase of electricity for prime power requirements of most facilities. On-site total energy and cogeneration systems may appear more attractive in time as fuel availability and environmental restrictions raise utility costs. Standby electric generating equipment will be provided in hospitals to produce emergency power for critical loads upon failure of the prime source and may be used to reduce peak demand on the utility source.

The designer of hospital power systems plays an important role in selection of the distribution characteristic within the complex, the power source, and through his choices, long-term power costs. To make cost effective decisions for owners, the designer should have knowledge of utility rate structures metering and billing practices.

(1) *Electric Utility Rates.* Each electric utility has a series of rate schedules for supplying power to customers under various conditions. To arrive at the most economic choice for obtaining power, a comparison of these rates should be made. The following are factors that usually form the basis for establishing rates and evaluating them:

(a) Maximum demand in kilowatts or kilovolt-amperes

(b) Energy consumption in kilowatt-hours

(c) Adjustment for low power factor

(d) Voltages available

(e) Transformer or substation ownership

(f) Fuel cost adjustments

(g) Demand interval

(h) Minimum bill stipulations, including ratchet clauses

(i) Multiple-metering provisions

(j) Auxiliary or standby service charges

(k) Seasonal and time of day service rates

(l) Prompt payment savings

(m) Provisions for off-peak loads and interruptible loads.

Since the oil embargo of 1973, and as a direct consequence of the National Energy Act of 1978, a change in conventional electric utility rate practice is unfolding in a new concept called "rate reform." Essentially, "rate reform" usually incorporates various forms of:

1) Inverted rates

2) Flat rates

3) Lifeline rates

4) Marginal cost pricing

5) Long range incremental costing

6) Construction work in progress

7) Interruptible rates

8) Time of day pricing

9) Reduction in the number of declining blocks
10) Modification of fuel cost adjustments to be fuel rates
11) Deletion of electric heat discounts.

When comparing new "reform" rates to old rates, it is usually difficult to separate rate reform and rate increase. Each customer will be affected differently based on the type and schedule of operation and the extent of load management equipment existing or planned.

(2) *Utility Metering.* An understanding of utility metering practices is important for evaluating service arrangements. Practices vary depending upon local utility and regulatory body requirements. The design, usage, and load characteristic for a given application should be carefully weighed before selecting service voltage and metering characteristics. If large momentary demand, highly seasonal, or low power-factor loads are involved, billing penalties may be involved. On the other hand, high load-factor or high power-factor loads may merit a billing allowance or credit.

It is good practice to contact the electric utility supplying service early in the design. Late utility negotiations may result in increased costs and delays in service. A complete discussion of service, metering, and billing is always in order, no matter how preliminary. This should provide time for the consideration of various proposals and the selection of the one best suited to a given application.

(a) *Metering by Type of Premises.* Availability of a particular kind of metering and billing often depends upon the type of building and load. A single-occupancy building, such as a hospital, usually will be metered by the utility at the service entrance with a watt-hour demand meter. Should multiple services be required, and should they be permitted by the electric utility, watt-hour meter readings sometimes may be added to take advantage of lower rates, and demands may be totalized so the customer may benefit from diversity.

In some medical facilities, it may be desirable to sub-meter portions of the building. This could arise where physician offices, separately owned pharmacies or other concessionaires lease space within the project. Consent of the utility company should be obtained in such instances.

(b) *Metering by Service-Voltage Characteristics.* Metering of the incoming service may be located on the high-voltage or low-voltage side of the transformer, depending on the terms of the contract with the electric utility. When the meter is on the high side, the losses of the transformer will be charged to the customer. In some cases, the customer is given a discount to offset this loss.

(c) *Meter Location.* Subject to agreement with the utility, the meter may be installed indoors at the customer's secondary distribution point, in a suitable meter room, or in a separate control building which may also house primary switchgear and associated controls.

Outdoor installations include pole, exterior wall, and pad mounting. In general, utilities will require accessibility for meter readings and maintenance, and suitable meter protection.

(d) *Types of Metering.* Tabulated below are types of metering. Utility requirements govern the types available for a given project:

1) Master metering
2) Multiple metering
3) Primary metering
4) Secondary metering
5) Totalized metering
6) Impulse metering
7) Compensated metering
8) Submetering
9) Subtractive metering
10) Coincident demand
11) Telemetering
12) Power factor metering.

(3) *Utility Billing.* It is customary for utilities to meter and bill each customer individually. Utility rates usually consider fixed and variable cost requirements to provide services. Hence "rate schedules" generally take the form of a "block" rate, wherein incremental service costs usually vary as a function of customer usage. Electric service costs generally comprise two components, the demand charge and the energy charge. The demand charge is based upon the maximum rate of energy usage. The energy charge is based upon the total energy consumption. Many utilities have been granted permission to add variable cost factors to their rates. Examples include purchased fuel differential and real estate tax differential costs. Under these provisions, the utility may pass along increased costs; however, the utility must pass along decreased costs as well.

For hospital complexes, the primary metering and attendant billing forms are the following:

(a) *Conjunctional Billing.* Large institutional customers within the territory served by a given utility should explore the availability of conjunctional billing. This consists of adding the readings of two or more meters for purposes of a single billing. Due to the usual practice of decreasing rates for larger consumption, conjunctional billing may result in a lower energy usage billing than individual meters would produce. Conjunctional billing will generally result in a higher demand charge than a master or totalizing meter because the maximum demand readings on the individual meters are added. Since maximum demands seldom occur simultaneously, the arithmetic sum will be greater than the simultaneous sum, unless a provision is made for coincident demand measurement.

(b) *Power Factor Billing.* If the load to be served will result in a low power factor, an evaluation should be made to determine if power factor improvements can be justified to avoid penalties.

(c) *Flat Billing.* Some applications involve service to loads of a fixed characteristic. For such loads, the utility may offer no-meter or flat rate service. Billing is based upon time and load characteristics. Examples include area lighting and remote pumping stations.

(d) *Off-Peak Billing.* This is reduced rate billing for service utilized during off-peak periods such as water-heating loads. The utility monitors, and may control, off-peak usage through control equipment or special metering.

(e) *Standby Service Billing.* Also known as breakdown or auxiliary service, this service is applicable to utility customers whose electric requirements are not supplied entirely by the utility. In such cases, billing demand is determined either as a fixed percentage of the connected load or by meter, whichever is higher. This applies to loads which are electrically connected to some other source of supply but for which breakdown or auxiliary service is required.

(f) *Backup Service Billing.* This service is provided through more than one utility circuit, solely for a customer's convenience. The customer often bears the cost of establishing the additional circuit and associated facilities. Usually, each backup service is metered and billed separately.

(g) *Demand Billing.* Usually this represents a significant part of electric service billing and a good understanding of kilowatt demand metering and billing is important. An electric demand meter measures the rate of use of electric energy over a given period of time, usually 15 minute, 30 minute, or 1 hour time intervals. A demand register records the maximum rate over the preceding interval. The demand register is reset periodically when read for billing purposes.

(h) *Minimum Billing Demand.* A utility customer may be subject to minimum demand billing, generally consisting of (a) a fixed amount or (b) a fixed percenttage of the maximum demand established over a prior billing period. This type of charge may apply to customers with high instantaneous demands, customers whose operations are seasonal or those who have contracted for a specific service capacity. Equipment and service requirements should be reviewed carefully to reduce or avoid minimum billing demand charges.

Utility contracts also may include ratchet clauses which establish minimum demand charges based on maximum demand experienced in the previous contract period, e.g., one year's peak demand establishes next year's minimum demand. Designers should advise their clients to control peak demand for several reasons but especially where the utility contract includes a ratchet clause. Clients should be aware that a major decrease in demand may not be reflected in savings for up to 12 months, unless a modification to the ratchet clause is negotiated.

(i) *Load Factor Billing.* The ratio of average kilowatt demand to peak kilowatt demand during a given time period is referred to as the load factor. Many utilities offer a billing allowance or credit for high load factor usage, a qualification usually determined by evaluating how many hours during the billing period the metered peak demand was used. As an example of such credit, the utility may provide a reduced rate for the number of kilowatt hours that are in excess of the peak demand multiplied by a given number of hours (after 360 h for a 720 h month or a 50% load factor).

(j) *Interruptible Service.* A form of peak load shaving used by the utilities is interruptible service. Primarily available for large facilities with well defined loads that can be readily disconnected, the utility offers the customer a billing credit for being able to require a reduction of demand to a specified contract level during a curtailment period. Should the customer fail to reduce his measured demand during any curtailment period at least to the contract demand, severe financial penalties are imposed.

2.6.3 Alternative Sources. The designer has a responsibility to the client to investigate the potential for energy savings and recommend those with reasonable potential. The following are worthy of serious design investigation when their paybacks are within 15 years. Investment tax and energy tax credits will apply in many cases. Considering alternative forms of energy is a part of the total energy management scheme.

(1) *Wind.* Wind machines are recommended only in areas where there is at least 13 mph annual average windspeed. Even then they can be expected to run at a rated capacity only 22 to 38% of the time. Because of the large load in hospitals a significant first cost would be encountered and payback will be long, until power costs are high enough to justify their use.

(2) *Geothermal.* Geothermal steam deposits have proven reasonably economic sources of electrical production. but again the first costs are so great that its use is limited to central power plants, not site specific buildings.

(3) *On-Site Cogeneration.* On-site cogeneration is the simultaneous production of electric power at the point of use along with the production and use of the heat energy by-product of the electrical generation process. Its economic attraction is that the practice may be more efficient than utility produced power. The national average for system efficiency of utility produced power is 30%, whereas on-site cogeneration under ideal conditions can achieve a system efficiency in excess of 90%.

The National Urban Energy Cooperative Funding Corporation has compiled a list of methods of generating electricity on-site and their cost in 1980 dollars. See Table 5.

Cogeneration, using the energy where it is generated, produces greater efficiency by eliminating distribution and transmission losses. Its efficiency is increased still further by allowing energy to be used as near as possible to its original form,

Table 5
Methods of Generating Electricity On-Site

Cycle	Fuel	Total Plant Installed Cost ($/kW)
Gas turbine & waste heat boiler	Gas, #2 oil treated residual SNG (low Btu)	$350–400
Diesel engine & waste heat boiler	Gas, #2 oil treated residual Methane	$350–500
Steam boiler & turbine	Nuclear—any oil, coal wastes	$500–600
Combined cycle & waste heat boiler	Gas, #2 oil SNG	$350–450
Steam bottoming	Waste heat	$400–600
Organic bottoming	Waste heat	$400–700

reducing energy conversion losses. Also increasing the efficiency is the use of waste heat for domestic hot water, space heating and absorption cooling.

Generating equipment need not be large. Packaged units in the 500 to 800 kW range are available and have been installed in some hospitals for demand bottoming.

(4) *Solar Cells*. Solar photovoltaic electrical generation techniques and storage are changing as fast as computer technology has been in the past decade. The advancement of cell technology is bringing the cost down, the most recent breakthrough at $10/watt installed. Direct conversion to sunlight with no moving parts, low maintenance, no trained technicians and long life, result in these systems' being suitable to a wide range of applications.

Design considerations are solar radiation, the array, regulation, storage and load. Since few designers are trained to deal in all these areas it is advised that you contact the nearest DOE office and two or three manufacturers. If your facility is to be completed in the late 1980's it will be beneficial to consider this form of electrical energy as photovoltaics are expected to be cost competitive with other alternatives at that time.

(5) *Peak Demand Shaving*. Rather than an alternative method of generating one's own power, this is a technique that lowers the monthly demand charge by controlling or scheduling loads so as not to exceed a present limit. However, hospital loads are not as collapsible as others. Generating power from a standby power system is an alternative.

The many arguments, pro and con, for using the existing emergency generators boil down to a single question. Will the local building authorities allow it? If no, one may employ conventional load shedding only. If yes, an analysis of load which may be dropped will give enough information to estimate a simple payback. Further, it may be possible to use the same standby emergency generators as required by codes, without adding additional generators.

2.6.4 Design Considerations. Energy conservation and capital cost are frequently in conflict with one another. An energy management program should optimize the relationship. Achieving a balance requires consideration of the following topics during design.

(1) *Energy Value of Materials*. Construction materials and equipment possess energy value, built in from mine to construction site. Energy value is added during erection and installation.

Recognition of this restrains the designer to avoid overdesign. Careful analysis of initial loads to be imposed coupled with allowances for load growth are essential. At the same time, efficient materials and equipment may increase capital costs while lowering operating costs.

(2) *Lighting and Lighting Control*. As noted earlier in this chapter, lighting source choices and lighting control bear directly on energy utilization as well as system load. Principles of task lighting and equivalent sphere illumination are important design considerations for energy management.

(3) *Motors*. Selection of motors for efficient use of energy is essential. Induction motors are somewhat less efficient at partial load but their power factors are

considerably poorer. Motors should be chosen to operate in the upper portion of their load range.

(4) *Power Factor Maintenance.* Prediction of system power factor is difficult during design but more readily determinable in an operating system. Nonetheless, consideration should be given to application of capacitors at induction motors 50 horsepower and larger. In addition, application of capacitors to the system service entrance should be evaluated during design and provisions should be made to receive them without major renovation of service switchgear.

2.6.5 Energy Management Systems. Use of an Energy Management System (EMS) is one way to lower energy and demand costs and to conserve energy. Energy management is a technique for automatically controlling the demand and energy consumption of a facility to a lower and more economical level by shedding and cycling noncritical loads for brief periods of time.

Coordination among owner, architect, and engineers during schematic design may enable use of an Energy Management System for fire and security systems, communication systems and maintenance management.

An Energy Management System may be simple or complex in design and capability. Controls such as time clocks constitute a simple EMS where an on or off command is given to an item of equipment at predetermined times. Often these simple devices miss the more focused and expanded needs of the energy and maintenance managers. Computerized systems can replace much of the lost time expended by maintenance crews to verify operating status of boilers, fans, and other equipment. It can enable control of HVAC functions and lighting from a central processing unit, performing operations such as start-stop, load shedding, controlling air mixtures and duty cycling. These functions can be accomplished using mid-range energy controllers.

For maximum energy and manpower savings, the state of the art utilizes distributed architecture systems. Previous systems had all of the programmable intelligence in the CPU or an auxiliary storage device such as a disk. The remote panels were slaves implementing CPU instructions. They had no stand-alone intelligence. Today's systems have minicomputers and microprocessors spread throughout the system, including the field panels. The main computer is free to perform sophisticated energy management tasks, while delegating simpler tasks to the field panels. Each remote panel can be a stand-alone management center reporting to the central system and if the main CPU or a transmission link fails, the entire system is not disabled.

Options available today include color graphics on CRT's, routine operator input/output, conversational English communication, file editing and print-outs and fire and security functions.

(1) Systems for a large building, such as a hospital, should include the following:
   (a) Time program control
   (b) Optimum start/stop
   (c) Supply air and water supervisory control
   (d) Boiler/chiller plant optimization
   (e) Enthalpy control

    (f) Load shedding/demand limiting

    (g) Variable duty cycling

    (h) Supervisory feedback.

 (2) It should be possible to add such future developments as:

    (a) Use of light pens for system operation

    (b) Less expensive, higher power computers

    (c) End user programming

    (d) Direct digital control

    (e) Fiber optics transmission.

An important consideration in any system is the means by which communication among various pieces of equipment is accomplished. Options include hardwiring, telephone lines, wireless, and carrier current. This is particularly important if the energy management system is being designed for application in an existing facility.

The decisions that must be faced by one starting on the system design include answers to such questions as how much control does the owner want the system to have over electrical and HVAC systems? Should the control be distributed to the satellite field panels throughout the project? If the system is to control the emergency power generation, how extensive should the backup be and should the fail safe switchover be manual or automatic? What is the smallest item to be monitored or controlled by the system?

Much has been studied and written about the effect of these systems on the useful life of such items as fans and motor starters. There is no agreement on life expectancy or reduced service due to wearing of equipment from frequent modulating or start/stop cycles. Some energy management system manufacturers claim no appreciable change in equipment life due to energy management systems. It is advisable that the designer monitor the technical literature for conclusions of future studies on this subject.

Finally, a most important consideration in selecting EMS equipment is the service available from the manufacturer for diagnosis and repair of hardware, for modification of system and operating software, and for training of the owner's personnel in utilizing the system.

2.6.6 Energy Utilization Standards. A uniform standard for energy utilization in various types of facilities does not exist. Several nationally recognized building codes mandate performance for some building components. A number of states have written and adopted energy codes of their own. The Department of Energy developed Building Energy Performance Standards (BEPS) but failed to achieve a national consensus for their adoption. Until such time as a comprehensive standard is adopted, designers face the difficult task of establishing an appropriate Btu consumption for each facility, but the definition of what is appropriate will remain elusive.

Some good work toward standards has been done by the National Institute for Building Sciences, the American Institute of Architects Research Corporation and the American Society of Heating, Refrigerating, and Air Conditioning Engineers.

In the meantime, designers are obliged to consult legally adopted codes enforced in the jurisdiction where the facility will be constructed and to strive for the lowest energy consumption consistent with those codes and with the building owner's life-cycle-cost goals.

2.7 References

[1] ANSI/ASHRAE/IES 90A-1980, Energy Conservation in New Building Design.[13]

[2] ANSI/NFPA 70-1984, National Electrical Code.

[3] ANSI/NFPA 99-1984, Standard for Health Care Facilities.

[4] NEMA XR9-1984, Power Supply Guidelines for X-ray Machines.[14]

[5] CROOK, E.D. *Determination of Electrical Demand for V.A. Medical Buildings.* Washington, DC: Veteran's Administration, Office of Construction, 1982.

[6] HAROLD, R.M., et al. *Lighting Power Budget Determination by the Unit Power Density Procedure.* Illuminating Engineering Society (IES), Publication no EMS-6, 1979.

---

[13] This publication can be obtained from the Sales Department, American National Standards Institute, 1430 Broadway, New York, NY 10018, or from Publication Sales, American Society of Heating, Refrigerating, and Air Conditioning Engineers, 1791 Tullie Circle, NE, Atlanta, GA 30329.

[14] NEMA publications can be obtained from the National Electrical Manufacturers Association, 2101 L Street, NW, Washington, DC 20037.

3. Electrical Power Distribution Systems

3.1 General Discussion. As the medical profession grows increasingly more dependent upon complex electrical equipment and instrumentation for patient care, the design of electrical power distribution systems for health care facilities is becoming increasingly more complex. The proper selection of system components and arrangements is required to provide the health care facility with reliable, safe, and economical electrical power.

Total or partial loss of electric power in a health care facility can cause acute operational problems. Power loss to lighting systems in strategic areas makes it difficult or impossible to perform vital medical tasks, such as dispensing medicine, performing surgical procedures, or performing precise medical laboratory work. The loss of power to equipment such as tissue, bone, or blood bank refrigerators can leave the health care facility without the vital resources it needs. More severely, power loss to electrical equipment used for the preservation of life (heart pumps, medical vacuum pumps, dialysis machines, medical ventilators) can be fatal. Clearly, continuity of electrical power reliaility should be a major criteria in the design of the electrical distribution systems for health care facilities.

Safety is a particularly important design criteria in health care facilities because: (1) medical personnel frequently come into contact with electrical apparatus in their daily routines; (2) patients are vulnerable to electrical hazard and shock because of their weakened condition, drugs, anesthesia, and/or unconsciousness (electrical shocks which would not affect a healthy person could be fatal to someone in poor physical condition); (3) it is necessary for maintenance personnel in health care facilities to come in daily or weekly contact with electrical distribution equipment for routine maintenance or minor system additions and renovations.

The final basic design criteria is economy. Public pressure to reduce the cost of health care and the development of a more competitive market place for health care has intensified the need for more economical electrical designs. The designer must consider both the initial cost and the operating expense of the electrical system. Furthermore, the designer must build provisions into the electrical design which will enable economical future expansion to the system.

This chapter will further develop these basic design criteria as they relate to: System Planning, Electrical Power Systems, Voltage Considerations, Current Considerations, Grounding, Overcurrent Protection and Coordination, Electrical Equipment and Installation and System Arrangements.

3.2 System Planning. Systems planning is the first and probably the most important phase in the design of an electrical power distribution system for a health care facility. During this phase, preliminary design data is gathered by consulting with the administrators and staff of the health care facility, the local utility, and the local authorities having jurisdiction over electrical construction. All relevant national, state and local codes should also be reviewed. In addition, the architectural plans and existing site conditions should be examined from an electrical system perspective to determine potential problems.

The following sections will discuss some of the issues which should be addressed during the system planning phase of the design.

3.2.1 Consult with the Health Care Facility Administrator(s) and Staff. The first step in system planning is to obtain information on the specific needs of the facility such as:

(1) *The Facility Function.* The designer must become familiar with the specific functions to be performed in the facility. This information is needed in order to weigh the importance of reliability, quality of electrical power, safety, and economy. For example, the reliability that should be designed into a system serving a hospital which specializes in open heart surgery is not required in a hospital which only performs routine surgery. Or, a hospital which extensively utilizes computerized equipment would require a higher quality of electrical power than a hospital which does not use such equipment. The designer cannot possibly tailor his/her design to the specific functions of facility unless these functions are known.

(2) *Financial and Budget Information.* The designer must become familiar with the financial expectations of the the administrators before he/she can begin to develop an electrical system. The administrators may have developed a fixed budget (in dollars) or a variable budget (in dollars per square foot of facility). This budget must be considered in all phases of design in order to assure satisfaction. Any design, no matter how good, which is not economically feasible to the administrators is of questionable value.

(3) *Administrator Preferences on Systems or Equipment.* The administrator or the medical staff may have preferences on the types of systems or equipment to be installed in their building. The reasons for these preferences are many and varied. Whatever the reason, the designer should keep these preferences in mind throughout the system design. If the designer feels that these preferences are unjustified or ill conceived, he/she should discuss his/her feelings and reach an understanding.

(4) *The Skill of Maintenance Personnel.* The skill of the facilities maintenance personnel is an important design consideration. For example, if the maintenance personnel for a particular facility does not include skilled electricians, the designer may consider specifying a system which requires little maintenance over a system which requires much more maintenance.

(5) *Future Expansion of the Facility.* The administrator of the facility will usually have plans for the future of the facility. They will depend on the administrator's financial position and expectations of the future socioeconomic conditions in the relevant service area. These plans could be in the form of rough ideas or be well-documented. It is essential that these plans be analyzed and well incorporated into the electrical system design.

3.2.2 Consult with the Project Architect. Another vital step in system planning is to consult with the project architect and review his/her preliminary schematics from an electrical system perspective. The architect needs the electrical designer's input early in order to correct potential problems due to building limitations and electrical requirements such as:

(1) Inadequate electrical equipment room sizes.

(2) Space omitted in certain areas for electrical equipment.

(3) Electrical rooms which are located so that accessibility to electrical equipment and devices is greatly limited.

(4) Wet areas located near electrical rooms that could be potentially hazardous.

ANSI/NFPA 70-1984 (Article 384-2) [15][15] requires that an electrical-equipment room must be within a dedicated space. Piping, ductwork or any architectural appurtenances, which do not serve that room space and only that room, are not permitted to penetrate the walls of electrical space. Accordingly, the designer should work closely with the architect to ensure proper placement of electrical spaces. One common problem is the location of toilet rooms or mechanical equipment rooms directly over electrical spaces.

3.2.3 Determine the Basic Loads and Demand Data. The designer should begin to tabulate preliminary load data. The preliminary architectural floor plans can be used effectively by superimposing load data on them. The floor plans should show major equipment loads, block loads based on square footage, and any future loads or buildings which the power system should be designed to accommodate.

In the initial stages of planning, exact load data will seldom be known. However, the designer can estimate probable loads based on existing similar health care facilities. Helpful data is listed in Chapter 2 of this standard and ANSI/IEEE Std 241-1983 (Chapters 2 and 16) [8]. The sum of the electrical ratings of each piece of equipment will provide a total connected load. Since some equipment will operate at less than full load and some intermittently, the resultant demand on the power source is less than the connected load. Standard definitions for these load combinations have been devised and defined in Chapter 2 of this standard, IEEE Std 141-1976 (Chapter 2) [17], and ANSI/NFPA 70-1984 (Article 220) [15].

3.2.4 Consult with the Local Electric Power Company. The designer must discuss the proposed health care facility with the local utility to determine their specific requirements and limitations. The power company will be interested in the size of the load, the power factor, and any unusual demand. The designer should be concerned with the following issues:

---

[15] The numbers in brackets correspond to those in the references at the end of this chapter.

(1) Are there any limitations on the size of load the utility can service?

(2) Will there be any user development charge for supplying power to the facility?

(3) What type of service does the utility plan to provide?

    (a) Single phase (two or three wire)

    (b) Three phase (three or four wire)

    (c) Voltage

    (d) One circuit

    (e) Two circuits

    (f) Overhead or underground

    (g) Termination details

    (h) Space requirements

(4) What components of the electrical service will the owner be required to furnish?

    (a) Primary conduit

    (b) Primary trenching and backfill

    (c) Primary cables

    (d) Primary protectors

    (e) Transformers

    (f) Transformer vault

    (g) Concrete pads

    (h) Metering or metering conduit

(5) What are the utility's billing rates and structure?

    (a) Are there penalties for poor power factor?

    (b) Are there penalties for multiple services and/or meters?

    (c) Is it economical to purchase power at primary voltage level rather than a lower voltage level?

(6) How reliable will the power source be? (Obtain a copy of the utility's outage record for the past year.)

(7) What will be the expected maximum and minimum voltage at their power supply? (Will voltage regulating equipment be required?)

(8) Can internal generation, if it exists in the proposed system, be operated in parallel with the utility?

(9) What will be the maximum short circuit current available, including future expectations from their power supply?

(10) What are their protective device coordination requirements?

Even though the utility is not required to follow any codes in providing an electrical service, the designer should stress the utility's ethical responsibility to provide the health care facility with a safe, reliable, grounded service. The degree of reliability will depend on the function of the health care facility. Section 3.9 of this chapter will discuss various recommended electric service arrangements for different types of health care facilities.

3.2.5 Consult with the Local Authorities Having Jurisdiction Over New Electrical Construction. The designer should become acquainted with the local authorities having jurisdiction over electrical construction and discuss their interpretations of all relevant codes. The designer should become familiar with these interpretations during the system planning stage in order to minimize later conflicts with these authorities. The local authorities can also provide input on any local natural phenomena which may effect the electrical design such as the presence of frequent violent electrical storms, seismic conditions, ot a corrosive environment.

3.2.6 Summary. This section discussed the System Planning and some of the issues which should be addressed during this phase of design. It is important that all information gathered be well-documented to enable ease of reference throughout the project. The designer should continually update this planning information as changes or new developments occur.

Once the System Planning phase is complete, the designer will have the necessary information to begin the actual design of the electrical system for the health care facility.

3.3 Electrical Power Systems. As previously stated, power systems for health care facilities require a high degree of safety and reliability. Some areas of health care facilities require electrical design similar to that documented in ANSI/IEEE Std 241-1983 [8]. However, most areas will require additional considerations as dictated by: (1) numerous governing codes and standards; (2) the use of complex and electrically sensitive medical equipment; and (3) most importantly, the fact that patients and medical personnel *must* be guarded against electrical hazards. Where flammable anesthetics are used, extreme care should be exercised to prevent fire and explosion. These areas are deemed hazardous, and the designer should refer to ANSI/NFPA Std 70-1984 (Articles 500-503) [15], ANSI/NFPA 99-1984 (Chapters 3 and 4) [16] and any other national and local codes that may be applicable. In certain areas, such as in operating rooms, special attention has to be given to power distribution. For example, general purpose overhead lighting fixtures are usually powered from the normal grounded distribution system, provided the fixtures cannot be touched by personnel during the course of surgical procedures. However, surgical fixtures that may be adjusted during surgery, outlets for electrical surgical instruments, monitoring equipment, portable X-ray, etc, should be powered though an isolation transformer with a line-isolation monitor as outlined in Chapter 6. Refer to Chapter 4 of this standard for power distribution requirements in other specific areas.

3.3.1 Power Sources. Generally, the normal power source(s) is furnished by the electric utility company and the required alternate power source by an on-site power source, such as a generator set or battery system, depending on type of health care facility involved. However, when the normal source consists of an on-site power generator(s), the alternate power source required can be either another power generator unit(s) or the electric utility. Battery system or systems can be applied as principal alternate power sources for nursing homes, residential custodial care facilities, and other health care facilities provided they meet the conditions outlined in ANSI/NFPA 99-1984 [16]. A generator set is required as the alternate power source for hospitals. Additional data pertaining to generator units and batteries can be found in Chapter 5 of this publication, as well as

ANSI/NFPA 70-1984 (Articles 517 and 700) [15], ANSI/NFPA 99-1984 (Chapter 8) [16], and ANSI/IEEE Std 446-1980 [9].

3.3.2 Distribution Circuits. Distribution systems for the health care facilities are basically divided into two categories: the *Normal Electrical* System (Nonessential) and the Essential Electrical System. Both systems are supplied by the normal power source; however, the essential electrical system is transferred to an alternate power supply whenever the normal power source experiences a power failure.

(1) *Nonessential Electrical Systems.* The nonessential electrical system consists of distribution equipment and circuits that supply electrical power from the normal power supply to loads which are not deemed essential to life safety or the effective operation of the health care facility.

(2) *Essential Electrical System.* The essential electrical system consists of the alternate power supply or supplies, transfer equipment, distribution equipment, and the circuits required to assure continuity of electrical service to those loads deemed as essential to life safety, critical patient care, and the effective operation of the health care facility.

For hospitals, the essential electrical system is subdivided into two systems — the *Emergency System* and the *Equipment System.*

The *Emergency System* is comprised of two branches defined as the *Life Safety Branch* and the *Critical Branch.* These consist of distribution equipment and circuitry, including automatic transfer devices required to enable emergency loads to be transferred from normal to emergency power sources. To increase the reliability of the system, each circuit is required to be installed separately from each other and all other circuits. ANSI/NFPA Stds 99-1984 [16] and ANSI/NFPA 70-1984 [15] also require that this system be designed to permit automatic restoration of electrical power within 10 seconds of power interruption and define the electrical loads to be served by the Life Safety Branch and Critical Branch. Article 517-63(a)(9) of ANSI/NFPA 70-1984 [15] allows the designer to install "other equipment and devices necessary for the effective operation of the hospital" on the critical branch of the emergency system. This gives the designer some degree of flexibility in tailoring the design to the specific needs of the hospital. The designer should use his/her experience, hospital staff input, and good engineering judgment in applying this article to the design.

The *Equipment System* consists primarily of three phase distribution equipment and circuits, including delayed automatic or manual transfer devices to serve equipment loads essential to the effective operation of the facility as defined by ANSI/NFPA 99-1984 (Chapter 8) [16].

In addition to these essential systems, the Joint Commission on Accreditation of Hospitals requires that if a hospital has a fire pump it shall be connected to the essential system.

For nursing homes and residential custodial care facilities which provide patient or resident care requiring electromechanical sustenance and/or offers surgical treatment requiring general anesthesia, the Essential Electrical System is subdivided into two systems — the Emergency System and Critical System. The

Emergency System is limited to those loads defined in the Life Safety Branch for hospitals in addition to providing sufficient illumination to exit ways in dining and recreation areas. Emergency circuits are required to be installed separately and independently of nonemergency circuits and equipment. The NFPA Standards require that this branch be designed to permit automatic restoration of electrical power within 10 seconds of power interruption. The *Critical System* is limited to certain critical receptacles, task illumination, and equipment necessary for the effective operation of the facility.

For other health care facilities excluding hospitals, nursing homes, and residential custodial care facilities discussed where the facility administers inhalation anesthetics or requires electro-mechanical life support devices, the Essential Electrical System consists of one system supplying a limited amount of lighting and power considered essential for life safety and orderly cessation of procedure whenever normal electrical service is interrupted for any reason. The type of system selected should be appropriate for the medical procedures performed in the facility.

Additional design data for distribution circuits can be found in ANSI/NFPA 70-1984 [15] and ANSI/NFPA 99-1984 (Chapters 8 and 9) [16]. ANSI/NFPA 99-1984 (Appendix C-8-1) [16] discusses various electrical power distribution system arrangements for health care facilities. Refer to that section for wiring diagrams illustrating the normal and essential electrical systems and their interconnection.

3.4 Voltage Considerations. The proper selection and regulation of utilization voltages throughout a health care facility is extremely important because of the extensive use of medical equipment which is voltage sensitive and available in many different voltage ratings. This equipment may be used for diagnostic or life sustaining functions; therefore, it is essential that the integrity of the equipment not be jeopardized by misapplied or poorly regulated voltage. The dynamic characteristics of the system should be recognized and the proper principles of voltage control applied so that satisfactory voltage will be supplied to all utilization equipment under all conditions of operation.

The reader is referred to IEEE Std 141-1976 (Chapter 3) [17] and ANSI/IEEE Std 241-1983 (Chapter 3) [8] for a general discussion of voltage. The reader should be familiar with voltage terminology (such as voltage spread, drop, regulation, unbalance, dips and fliches, transients, and harmonics) in order to obtain a full understanding of this important topic.

3.4.1 Select System Voltages. The voltage levels selected will depend on the utility voltage available, the size of the health care facility, the loads served, expansion requirements, the building layout, voltage regulation requirements, and cost. The system should be capable of providing proper voltage to all equipment under all operating conditions.

Typically, a health care facility will be supplied power at a medium voltage level from the utility and step it down to either 480Y/277 V or 208Y/120 V for utilization. 480 or 208 V is used to feed mechanical equipment (chillers, fans, pumps, etc), medical equipment (radiology, medical air pumps, etc), and other support equipment such as laboratory equipment and kitchen equipment. 120 V is the predominant utilization voltage and is used to supply receptacle and lighting loads throughout the hospital. 277 V can be used to supply some equipment loads and/or lighting loads. The use of 277 V lighting in lieu of 120 V in large health care facilities is a major design decision and deserves careful consideration. The application of 277 V lighting in hospitals differs from other commercial facilities because of the requirement for the four divisions of the electrical system (normal, critical branch, life safety branch, and the equipment system). Applying 277 V lighting results in having both 120/208 V and 277/480 V panels for all these systems on each floor or in each electrical room. There are no rules of thumb on when to apply 277 V lighting. Each individual application should be analyzed to determine its feasibility.

3.4.2 Nominal Voltage. Once the nominal utilization voltages have been selected, the voltage of all medical equipment to be installed in the facility should be carefully checked to assure proper application. If the equipment is not available in the system voltage, then "buck"/"boost" transformers should be used to supply rated voltage to the equipment. One common misapplication is the use of nominally rated 230 V motors installed on a 208 V system.

Radiology equipment is available in a variety of single phase and three phase voltages. It is necessary to know the exact voltage requirements and tolerances of the equipment from the manufacturer's data in order to properly plan for its installation. A common misapplication is the use of single phase, 240 V rated equipment on 208 V systems. Another common problem occurs in the application of 380 V European manufactured radiology equipment in the United States. This equipment will require a dedicated transformer when applied on 480 or 208 V systems.

3.4.3 Voltage Variation and Disturbances. Variations in the sinusoidal voltage waveform can be caused by many different types of power system disturbances. Transient overvoltages and surges are caused by lightning, capacitor switching, fault switching, arcing grounds, brush-type motors, or switching of inductive loads, such as motors and radiology equipment. Voltage sags and dips are caused by utility faults, motor starting or improper grounding. Momentary total loss of voltage is the result of utility switching operations, utility circuit breaker reclosing, surge arrester operation, or equipment failure.

There is a variety of voltage protection, regulating, and conditioning equipment available on the market. Surge arresters, voltage relays, transient voltage suppressors, shielded isolation transformers, voltage regulators, power conditioners, uninterruptible power supplies, or combinations of this equipment can be applied to solve voltage variation problems. The choice of which equipment to apply depends on the nature of the voltage variations and the characteristics of the equipment to be protected.

Surge arresters, voltage relays, and transient voltage suppressors are designed to remove overvoltages from the power system for protection of distribution and utilization equipment. Shielded isolation transformers will provide a clean, noise-free ground. However, they are generally ineffective in rejecting transients, although there is some attenuation. Voltage regulators or constant voltage transformers are designed to tightly control output voltage regardless of variations of input voltage. The range of input voltage for which the output voltage will remain regulated is generally +10% to -20% or +15% to -15%. In addition to input voltage range, other considerations in applying a voltage regulator are: regulator load sensitivity, load compatibility, energy efficiency, and electrical isolation. Power conditioners generally combine regulation, isolation and/or transient suppression into one package. Uninterruptible power supplies provide a clean, constant frequency sinusoidal voltage with standby capacity for power failure and short outages.

The first step toward solving a voltage variation problem is to properly diagnose exactly what the problem is. Applying various voltage regulating, protection, or conditioning equipment available without knowing *exactly* what the problem is and what is causing it will probably not solve the problem and may even amplify the problem. A high accuracy powerline analyzer is a most effective tool in diagnosing voltage problems. The electrical service or a portion of the electrical system can be observed over a period of time and voltage variations recorded including magnitude, duration of the variation, and the time it occurred. This data can then be matched with medical equipment operational problem logs or reports to determine the exact problem.

Variations in the voltage in a health care facility will normally be noticed first in the operation or output of radiology, laboratory, and computerized equipment.

Radiology machines draw very high momentary currents during an exposure. Therefore, a low impedance source is necessary to assure that the voltage drop is within acceptable limits, usually three to five percent. The X-ray tube will experience loss of life and equipment malfunction if proper voltage regulation is not maintained.

Voltage regulators applied on radiology equipment feeders may not improve regulation because the pulse width of the equipment may be less than the response time of the regulator.

Voltage fluctuations and dips caused by motor starting within hospital should be maintained within the limits dictated by radiology and computerized apparatus. This is normally accomplished by providing reduced voltage starters on large motors located throughout the hospital. The designer should carefully study the application of these starters on each motor to minimize system voltage drops at reasonable costs.

3.5 Current Considerations. The full load and overload current requirements in a health care power system are determined by the load equipment. However, the short circuit current requirements are determined by the power sources principally and to a lesser degree by the load equipment.

The current flow during a fault at any point in a system is limited by the impedance of circuits and equipment from source or sources to the point of fault and is not directly related to the load on the system. However, additions to the system which increase its capacity to handle a growing load while not affecting the normal load at some existing parts of the system may drastically increase the fault currents.

In some health care facilities, the fault current contribution can differ in magnitude and decay rate between the normal and alternate power sources. This can occur when:

(1) the normal power source is from a public utility having a high fault current capability and the common service point is removed by several transformations and transmission circuits from the utility generation sources;

(2) the alternate power supply consists of a relatively small on site generator or generators and relatively short distribution circuits between the alternate power supply and essential electrical power circuitry.

Thus, for a fault occurring within the essential electrical power system, the fault current magnitude from the normal power source would be relatively large and have a slow decay rate. In fact, for all practical purposes, the decay rate of the alternating current rms portion of the total fault current could be considered negligible while for the same fault conditions the fault current magnitude from the alternate power source would be relatively small and have a fast decay rate. These factors should be taken into account when rating and setting protective devices since the essential electrical system can be fed power from either source.

The nature and calculations of short-circuit currents *must* be understood to correctly apply protective equipment, choose adequately rated system operating equipment, choose protective devices to determine degree of coordination achieved, and calculate the voltage dips of impact loads such as motor starting, etc. The reader is referred to IEEE Std 141-1976 (Chapter 5) [17] and ANSI/IEEE Std 241-1983 (Chapter 9) [8] to obtain information on the fundamentals and procedures of fault current calculations.

3.6 Grounding. The word "grounding" is commonly used in electrical power system work to cover both "equipment grounding" and "system grounding." These and other terms used when discussing this topic are defined in ANSI/NFPA Std 70-1984 [15] and ANSI/IEEE Std 142-1982 [7]. Familiarity with these definitions will result in a better understanding of grounding principles.

In health care facilities, both the system and equipment are grounded. In addition, special grounding requirements must be applied to those subsystems and equipment involved in patient care areas, operating rooms, anesthetizing locations, and special environments as presented in Chapter 6 of this publication, ANSI/NFPA 70-1984 (Article 517) [15] and ANSI/NFPA 99-1984 (Chapters 8 and 9) [16].

3.6.1 Equipment Grounding. Equipment grounding is the interconnection and grounding of nonelectrical conducting material that either encloses or is adjacent to electrical power conducting components. Its purpose is to prevent electrical shock hazards and provide freedom from fire hazards due to electrical discharges. To attain this end, the grounding conductor circuit must be designed and properly installed to present a sufficiently low impedance path and an adequate ground-fault-current carrying capability both in magnitude and duration.

For ac systems, the return ground current will flow through the lowest impedance path, not the lowest resistance path as for dc systems. The lowest impedance path will be a path closest to the power conductors, such as a ground conductor installed with the power conductors or the metal raceway enclosing the power conductors (that is, metal housing of cables, conduit, housing of busway). Furthermore, to maintain a low impedance ground current return circuit, junctions and terminations should be properly installed. Metal joints should make good contact to avoid sparking during fault conditions. Adequate connections between equipment ground buses and/or housings and metal raceways have to be provided. In addition, the ground return circuit components, ground conductor junctions, terminations, etc, have to have a sufficient ground fault current carrying capability to avoid dangers of thermal distress for all types of fault escalations and durations permitted by the overcurrent protection system.

3.6.2 System Grounding. The term "System Grounding" relates to what type of grounding will be applied to the electrical system. The basic reasons for system grounding are the following:

(1) To limit the differences of electrical potential between all uninsulated conducting objects in a local area.

(2) To provide for isolation of faulty equipment and circuits where a fault occurs.

(3) To limit overvoltages appearing on the system under various fault conditions.

In ungrounded systems, a fault condition can, in certain instances, lead to system resonance that causes an overvoltage to be imposed on the system. This overvoltage can be sufficient in magnitude to create severe shock hazard condtions to which patients and health care facility personnel are exposed, as well as cause electrical equipment failure due to insulation breakdown. Furthermore, equipment appearing to have survived the overvoltage will most probably have lost a good portion of its useful life. Thus, it is recommended that system grounding be employed for all health care facilities.

There are several methods available to ground a system such as line grounding, mid-phase grounding, neutral grounding, etc. The preferred method for health care facilities is neutral grounding, since the system neutral is generally readily available. This will avoid the special system operating precautions required when employing the other grounding methods as outlined in ANSI/IEEE Std 142-1982 [7].

(a) *Selection of System Grounding Points.* It is necessary to ground at each voltage level to achieve the advantages of neutral grounding in all parts of the system. Each voltage level may be grounded at the neutral lead of a generator, power transformer bank, or neutral deriving grounding transformer provided they meet the requirements of ANSI/NFPA 70-1984 (Article 250-5) [15].

When there are two or more major source bus sections, each section should have at least one grounded neutral point since the bus-tie circuit may be open. If there are two or more power sources per bus section, there should be provision for grounding at least two sources on each section.

(b) *Neutral Circuit Arrangements.* When the method of grounding and the grounding point have been selected for a particular power system, the next question to consider is how many source generator or transformer neutrals, or both, will be used for grounding, and whether 1) each neutral will be connected independently to ground, or 2) a neutral bus with single ground connection will be established.

(c) *Medium Voltage Source Neutral(s).* The medium voltage portion of the power system, when existing for health care facilities, is usually a three phase, three wire system where the neutral is not used as a circuit conductor. Thus the source, generator and/or transformer neutrals can be effectively grounded or resistance grounded. The latter method, where the system neutral is connected in series with a resistor to ground, is preferred specifically where no direct exposure to lighting exists. This method has the following advantages and disadvantages.

1) *Advantages:*

a) Reduce burning damage in ground faulted electric equipment such as switchgear, cables, motors, generators, etc.

b) Reduce thermal and mechanical stress in circuits and apparatus carrying fault current.

c) Reduce electric shock hazard to personnel caused by stray ground fault currents in the ground return path.

2) *Disadvantages:*

a) Line to neutral voltage rated surge arresters are not applicable, line to line voltage rated units need to be applied thus sacrificing some degree of overvoltage protection.

b) Added cost of the resistor and possible additional cost of relaying.

When one or two sources are involved, the use of individual neutral resistors is preferable to the use of a common resistor. When more than two sources are involved, however, the ground current is increased each time a source is added and may be raised to levels that are undesirably high. Each resistor must be rated for sufficient current to ensure satisfactory relaying when operating independently. Consequently, the total ground current with several resistors will be several times the minimum required for effective relaying. A solution to this problem is to consider the use of only one resistor as outlined in ANSI/IEEE Std 142-1982 (Section 1.6.6) [7].

(d) *Low Voltage Source Neutral(s).* The low voltage system for health care facilities is usually a three-phase, four-wire system where the neutral is used as a circuit conductor. Thus, the service source neutral should be effectively grounded to permit neutral loading as well as meet the requirements of ANSI/NFPA 70-1984 (Article 250-5) [15].

Where the power supply consists of services that are dual fed in a common enclosure or grouped together in separate enclosures and employ a secondary tie, the common neutral conductor can be effectively grounded at one point. Where the power supply for the health care facility consists of a normal and ac alternate power supply, at least one of the power supplies—usually normal—is considered the service and its neutral(s) should be effectively grounded. If the normal and ac alternate power supply are not electrically connected, then both power supply neutrals can be effectively grounded.

The type of system grounding that is employed, and the arrangement of system and equipment grounding conductors, will affect the service continuity. Grounding conductors and connections must be arranged so that objectionable stray neutral currents will not exist and ground fault currents will flow in low impedance, predictable paths that will protect personnel from electrical shock and assure proper operation of the circuit protective equipment.

Where phase-to-neutral loads must be served, systems are required to be solidly grounded. However, 600 V and 480 V systems may be high resistance grounded or ungrounded where a grounded circuit conductor is not used to supply phase-to-neutral loads. High resistance grounded systems may provide a higher degree of service continuity than solidly grounded systems. Ungrounded systems are not recommended since they may be subjected to overvoltage stress due to resonance conditions occurring during a ground fault condition.

When the ac alternate power supply (generator(s) or separate utility service) and its wiring system are electrically interconnected with the normal power supply, either by the neutral or phase conductors, or both, then the alternate power supply, per ANSI/NFPA 70-1984 (Article 250-5(d)) [15] is not a separately derived system, and thus its neutral is not permitted to be grounded. Only the normal power supply neutral is permitted to be effectively grounded as shown in Fig 4. This is to prevent objectionable neutral load currents from flowing in the system ground conductors. Note that the equipment grounding conductor defined as "EGC" in Fig 4 is still required; thus, the generator neutral must be insulated from the machine frame.

When the ac alternate power supply (generator(s) or separate utility service) and its wiring system are not electrically interconnected with the normal power supply wiring system either by the neutral or phase conductors, or both, then the alternate power supply, as in ANSI/NFPA 70-1984 (Article 259-5(d)) [15], is a separately derived system and its neutral is grounded at the alternate power supply in addition to the neutral(s) of the normal power supply. Figure 5 depicts a system where the neutral and phase conductors between the alternate and normal power supply wiring systems are not electrically interconnected by the use of a four pole or three pole with neutral contacts transfer device. Thus, the on-site generator is defined as a separately derived system and its neutral is effectively grounded. Since the neutral conductor is isolated between power systems, grounding of the generator neutral will not provide a path for objectionable neutral load currents to flow in the system ground conductors.

The choice of whether or not to switch the neutral should be balanced against cost of applying a transfer device capable of switching all power conductors versus a transfer device capable of switching only the phase conductors and necessary additional ground fault monitoring equipment, if required.

Some application problems that need attention when considering to switch or not to switch the neutral are as follows:

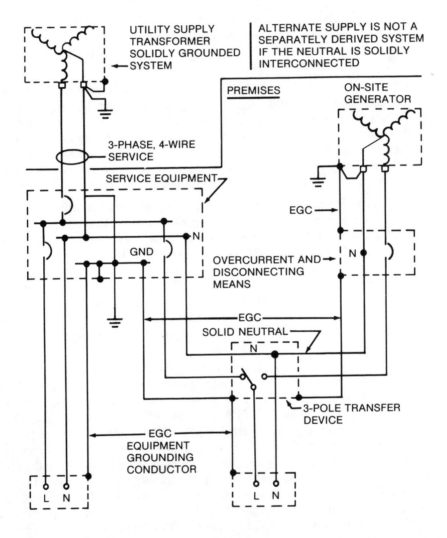

Fig 4
Solidly Interconnected Neutral Conductor
Grounded at Service Equipment

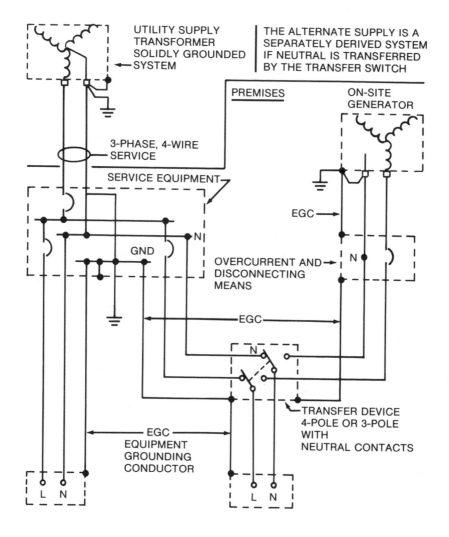

Fig 5
Transferred Neutral Conductor Grounded at Service Equipment
and at Source of Alternate Power Supply

1) Generally, the transfer device is located as close to the load as possible to provide maximum service continuity. Thus, the distance of the neutral conductor between the normal power source, transfer device and emergency generator set could be substantial. Should the normal power supply be interrupted then to avoid the load from being transferred to an ungrounded emergency power supply, a direct neutral tie between the normal and emergency system should exist for a system not switching the neutral. This requirement would be needed for a system having a switching neutral capability.

2) A power system design whereby the neutral is not switched requires additional current sensor monitoring to prevent nuisance tripping of the normal power source protector for a ground fault occurring when the load is being powered from the emergency power source.

The choice of whether grounding or not to ground the ac emergency power supply at its source will not affect the ability to provide proper ground fault relaying. However, it should be noted that ground fault protection applicable to radial power systems are not necessarily applicable for multi-source systems as outlined in Section 3.6.

The reader is referred to IEEE Std 141-1976 (Chapter 6) [17], IEEE Std 142-1982 [7], ANSI/IEEE Std 241-1983 (Chapter 4) [8], and ANSI/NFPA 70-1984 (Article 250) [15] for further information on system grounding.

3.7 System Protection and Coordination. The system and equipment protective devices guard the health care facility power system from the ever present threat of damage caused by overcurrents and transient overvoltages that can result in equipment loss, system failure, and hazards to patients and personnel. To achieve this protective function, protective equipment such as surge arresters, surge capacitors, reactors, and circuit interrupting devices are applied. All protective equipment should be applied within their ratings of voltage, frequency, and current. In addition, the location or site where they are to be applied needs to be taken into account—such as altitude, seismic, temperature, etc. The various standards provide a guide or list to which the circuit interruption devices should conform, as to description, rating application and limits, and derating factors if required. These requirements are documented in IEEE Std 141-1976 (Chapter 4) [17], ANSI/IEEE Std 241-1983 (Chapter 9) [8], and various ANSI, NEMA, and IEEE standards listed in Section 3.10.

3.7.1 Protection. Protection in an electric system is a form of insurance. The protective features built into a system are inactive until called upon to clear a fault or some other unplanned or unintentional disturbance. It can be credited with reducing the extent and duration of the power interruptions, the hazards of property damage, and personnel injury.

It would be neither practical nor economical to build a fault-proof power system. Consequently, modern systems are designed to provide reasonable insulation, clearances, etc, to avoid faults from occurring. However, even with the best design possible, materials deteriorate and the likelihood of faults increases with age. Every system is subject to short circuits and ground faults. A knowledge of the effect of faults on system voltages and currents is necessary to design suitable protection as defined in IEEE Std 141-1976 (Chapter 4) [17] and ANSI/IEEE Std 241-1983 (Chapter 9) [8].

3.7.2 Current Sensing Protectors. The current sensing detectors in protectors must detect three phase, phase to phase, double phase to ground as well as single phase to ground short circuits. The current magnitude of those faults involving ground depends to a large extent on the method of system grounding — the magnitude of ground impedance, and, in low voltage systems, the arcing fault impedance.

(1) *Protection Requirements.* The design of a protective system involves two separate although interrelated steps:

(a) The selection of the proper device to do the task;

(b) Selecting the correct protector ampere rating or setting for the devices so they will operate selectively with other devices to disconnect that portion of the system in trouble and with as little effect on the remainder of the system as possible.

Protective devices should be selected to be insensitive to normal operating conditions such as full load current, permissible overload current and starting or inrush currents, but be chosen so that pickup currents and operating times are short. Further, the devices should be coordinated so that the protective device closest to the fault opens before upstream devices open. Determining the ratings and settings for protective devices requires familiarity with the NEC requirements for the protection of cables, motors, and transformers and with ANSI/IEEE C57.12.00-1980 [14] for transformer magnetizing inrush current and transformer thermal and magnetic stress damage limits. Determining the setting for the overcurrent protective device in a power system can be a formidable task that is often said to require as much art as technical skill. Continuity of health care facility electrical service requires that interrupting equipment operates selectively as stated in ANSI/NFPA 99-1984 (Chapter 8) [16] and ANSI/NFPA 70-1984 (Article 517) [15]. As total selectivity and maximum safety to personnel are sometimes competing objectives, a total short circuit, coordination and component protection study should be performed. This study first determines the available short circuit current at each panel and each component throughout the system. Then coordination curves are drawn to determine whether or not the overcurrent devices are selectively coordinated at the various available fault currents. Then the component withstand ratings are checked to see if NEC Section 110-10 is met. This method of analysis is useful when designing the protection for a new power system, when analyzing protection and coordination conditions in an existing system, or as a valuable maintenance reference when checking the calibration of protective devices. The coordination curves provide a permanent record of the time current operating relationship of the entire protection system. Usually, the coordination plot is made on log-log graph paper with current as the abscissa, X-axis, or horizontal axis and time in seconds as the ordinate, Y-axis, or vertical axis. A choice of the most suitable current and time settings is made for the device to provide the best possible protection, safety to personnel and electric equipment, and also to function selectively with other protective devices to disconnect the faulted equipment with as little disturbance as possible to the rest of the system. Details and examples of a coordination study for various system equipment and operating conditions are documented in IEEE Std 141-1976 (Chapter 4) [17] and ANSI/IEEE Std 241-1983 (Chapter 9) [8].

(2) As a summary, an orderly approach to performing a protective device coordination study is as follows:

(a) Construction one line diagram of system.

(b) Recorded on one line diagram pertinent data:

1) distribution equipment ratings

2) load equipment ratings

3) impedance data

(c) Perform calculations to determine short circuit currents.

(d) Determine equipment operating and protection rating boundaries as defined by ANSI/NFPA 70-1984 [15], equipment nameplates, ICEA (Insulated Cable Engineers Association) texts or handbooks, manufacturers' bulletins, etc. List results on one line diagram.

(e) Determine the protective device ratings required to meet the system voltage, frequency, continuous current and short circuit duty, as well as any unusual conditions due to site application such as altitude, seismic, temperature, etc. Also, take into account any UL, NEC, or local code requirements. List the ratings chosen on the one line diagram.

(f) Choose a tentative protection device full load rating based on load conditions. List choice on one line diagram.

(g) Obtain characteristic time current curves of all protective device detectors involved in the system under study.

(h) Develop time current plots to determine device settings and be able to analyze degree of coordination and selectivity achieved.

3.7.3 Ground Fault Protection. Phase overcurrent devices settings are determined by the load requirements principally. They are set to be insensitive to full load and inrush currents as well as provide selectivity between downstream and upstream devices. Accordingly, the phase overcurrent device cannot distinguish between normal load currents and low magnitude ground fault short circuit currents of the same magnitude. Therefore, ground fault detection is added to supplement the phase overcurrent devices to provide proper protection.

To provide a high degree of reliability, health care facilities are required by ANSI/NFPA 70-1984 (Article 517) [15] and ANSI/NFPA 99-1984 (Chapters 8 and 9) [16] to have a normal emergency power supply. For those health care facilities, the application of ground fault protection requires additional attention.

(1) *Equipment Selection.* When choosing ground fault protective devices, the system ground currents and system wiring configuration have to be considered.

(2) Several types of ground currents can exist in any power system:

(a) Insulation leakage current from appliances, portable cleaning equipment and/or tools, etc. Normally, the magnitude of this current is very low (in the order of microamperes in small systems to several amperes in extensive systems).

(b) Bolted fault ground current commonly caused by improper connections or metallic objects wedged between phase and ground. For this type fault, the current magnitude may be equal to or less than the three phase fault current.

(c) Arcing fault ground current commonly caused by broken phase conductors touching earth, insulation failure, loose connections, construction accidents, rodents, dirt, debris, etc. The current magnitude may be very low in relation to the three phase fault current.

(d) Lightning discharge through a surge arrester. The magnitude of current could be quite large depending on the energy in the lightning stroke.

(e) Static charge.

(f) Capacitor charging current, etc.

(3) Solutions to equipping the electrical system to handle or prevent these currents are varied, such as:

(a) Insulation leakage — higher order of insulation and monitoring for same at low level and removing power promptly. Refer to Chapter 6, which further discusses monitoring equipment utilized in health care facilities.

(b) Lightning discharges, static charges apply properly rated grounding conductors and grids.

(4) For the bolted and/or arcing fault, the solution involves a two-pronged approach.

(a) First, minimize the probability of fault initiation by:

1) Careful attention to system design and to the settings of protective devices.

2) Selecting equipment that is isolated by compartments within grounded metal enclosures.

3) Selecting equipment with drawout, rack-out or stab-in features, thereby reducing the necessity of working on energized components.

4) Providing insulated bus. This alternative should be considered to prevent the occurrence of ground faults — especially on the line side of mains where the utility does not provide ground fault protection.

5) Proper installation practices and supervision.

6) Protecting equipment from unusual operating or environmental conditions.

7) Insisting on a thorough clean-up immediately before initial energization of equipment.

8) Executing regular and thorough maintenance procedures.

9) Maintaining daily good housekeeping practices.

(b) Second, sense and remove the defective circuit quickly so that damage will be minimized.

(5) The system designer should balance economics against cost of equipment damage to arrive at a practical ground fault protection system, keeping in mind that the extent of equipment damage can increase the extent of power service loss, thus increasing risk to patients and ensuing liabilities.

There is no single solution for all power systems; each should be analyzed individually. In this analysis, the important factors to be considered are:

(a) *Power System Selection.*

1) The type ground fault detection scheme applied is a function of voltage level and system arrangement. Most health care facility applications are low voltage with a radial arrangement which is the easiest to analyze and lends itself to a straightforward protection system design. The problem becomes more difficult and involved with secondary selective and spot network circuit arrangements.

(b) *Neutral Circuit.*

1) A three-phase, three-wire or three-phase, four-wire power system with a radial neutral presents few problems.

2) For a power system neutral that is used as a load conductor and looped or continuous between alternate power sources and grounded only at the sources or grounded downstream, extreme care should be taken in applying ground fault protection. Every circuit should be checked for stray returning neutral and/or ground fault currents that could cause the ground fault unit to be desensitized, misoperate, or not operate at all. A simple method to check the application is to draw a one line diagram of the power system and superimpose assumed neutral loads and ground faults. Then, trace the current flow to determine the effects on the ground fault units. Keep in mind that the return current flow tends to seek the lowest impedance path. A given path, although initially the lowest impedance path, may not remain so as the magnitude of current increases. It might be determined that the neutral conductors, because of their interties, present such good paths for stray returning currents that the only solution to providing ground fault protection is to use ground differential or ground summation schemes.

(c) *Ground Return Path.* The ground return path should be designed to present a low impedance path and provide adequate ground fault current carrying capability to hold the voltage gradients along its path to less than shock hazard threshold values. This design will also permit sensitive detection of ground fault currents.

(d) *Reliability Desired.* In the normal sense of reliability, radial systems are quite reliable for general use. However, life support and high value continuity uses deserve the redundancy offered by the higher order systems. The system designer must face the increased engineering analysis that accompanies the higher levels, including continuity of service, reduction in false outages, and the improved level of equipment protection, all balanced against cost.

(6) *Ground Fault Detection Schemes.* The ground fault current can be monitored either as it flows out to the fault or on its return to the neutral point of the source transformer or generator. When monitoring the outgoing fault current, the currents in all power conductors are monitored either individually or collectively. When monitoring the return fault current only, the ground return conductor is monitored. Caution is required to assure that the returning ground fault current bypasses the outgoing monitoring current transformer but does not bypass the current transformer monitoring the return ground fault current.

The ground fault relay pickup level is adjustable and may be equipped with an adjustable time delay feature. Operation of the relay activates a trip mechanism on the interrupting device. Selectivity is achieved through a time delay and/or current setting or blocking function. Zone selectivity can be achieved by using a differential or blocking scheme.

(7) *Medium Voltage Systems.* As previously discussed in Section 3.6.2(c), medium voltage systems for health care facilities are generally three-phase, three-wire systems with the neutrals solidly grounded or resistance grounded. When the neutral is solidly grounded, the ground fault current magnitude is relatively high and a residual connected ground fault relay is usually applied. This residually connected ground fault relay, shown in Fig 6, monitors the outgoing ground fault current.

When the neutral is resistance grounded, the ground fault current magnitude is relatively low—1200 A or less—and a ground sensor connected ground fault relay is usually applied. This ground sensor relay, shown in Fig 7, monitors the outgoing ground fault current.

The ground sensor relay shown in Fig 8 monitors the returning ground fault current.

(8) *Low Voltage Systems.* As previously discussed in 3.6.2(d), low voltage systems for health care facilities are generally three-phase, four-wire systems. The normal power source neutral is effectively grounded. When required, the ac alternate power source neutral may or may not be effectively grounded at the alternate source. The ground fault schemes applicable will depend on how the ac alternate power supply is grounded.

Fig 6
Residually Connected Ground Fault Relay

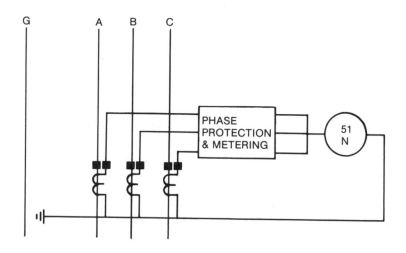

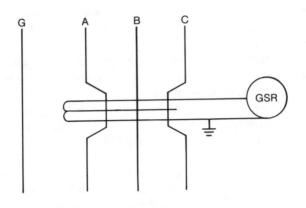

Fig 7
Ground Sensor Ground Fault Relay

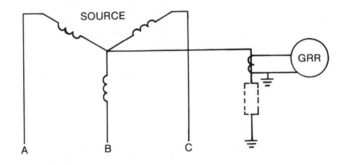

Fig 8
Ground Sensor Ground Fault Relay with Ground Resistor

For feeder circuits having no neutral conductor requirements (three-phase, three-wire loads) or for three-phase, four-wire loads where the neutral conductors are not electrically interconnected between power sources on the load side of the feeder breaker, residually connected, ground sensor, or integral ground fault relays (Figs 9, 10, and 11) are applicable for the feeder breakers.

For feeder circuits with neutral conductor requirements where the neutral conductors are electrically interconnected between power sources on the load side of the feeder breaker, ground fault summation schemes will be applicable. Figure 12 is an example of such a circuit.

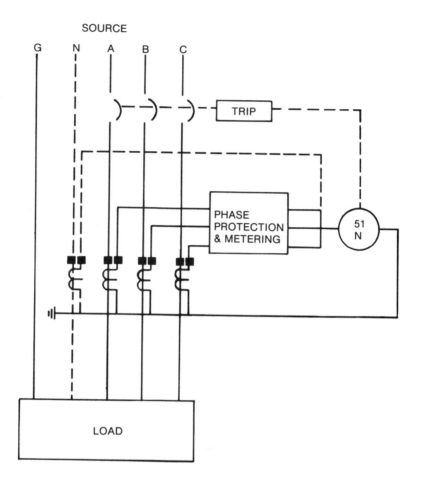

**Fig 9
Residually Connected Ground Fault Relay
with Shunt Trip Circuit Breaker**

For power systems having no neutral conductor requirements (three-phase, three-wire systems) or when the required neutral conductors for the system are radial down to the loads (no neutral interties exist, except through ground connections at the sources), residually connected, ground sensor, or integral ground fault relays (Figs 8, 9, and 10) are applicable for main and tie breakers.

For power systems having a neutral conductor intertie or several interties between power sources within the system standard ground fault relaying will not function properly for the main, tie, or feeders feeding loads whose power source can be obtained from the normal or emergency power supply. Summation schemes

Fig 10
Ground Sensor Fault Relay

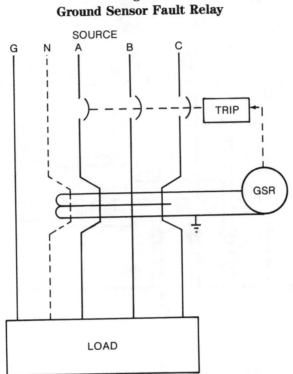

Fig 11
Integral Ground Fault Relay

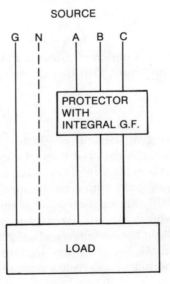

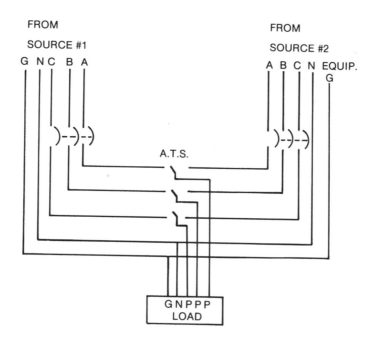

Fig 12
Dual Source Electrically Interconnected

will be required for these circuits. As an example, referring to Fig 13, the ground fault current return path from the transferrable load to the on-site generator is through the equipment grounding conductor to the transfer switch to the service equipment, hence through the main bonding jumper in the service equipment and the neutral conductor from the service equipment to the generator. When a fault occurs as shown at the load equipment, the ground fault current following the return path previously described will flow through the current sensor, and if sufficient in magnitude, it will activate the ground fault relay, thus tripping the main service disconnect even though the ground fault is on a circuit supplied by the generator. To avoid this outage, a summation scheme should be applied in preference to the ground return scheme presently applied.

Many summation schemes are applicable and when taking into account all system connection possibilities, it becomes impractical to list all possible schemes and their modifications. However, a typical ground fault relaying system is shown (Figs 14 and 15) for a health care facility power system that consists of normal and alternate power supplies. The power systems shown in Fig 11 has an electrical power conductor interconnection between power supplies. Note the summation ground fault relaying scheme required for the power system shown in Fig 14. In both Fig 14 and Fig 15, ground fault relay R2 is optional.

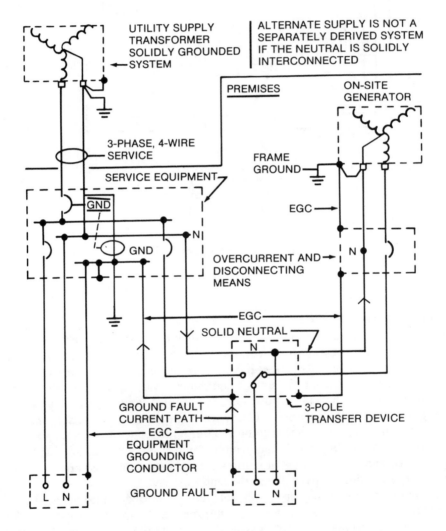

Fig 13
Ground Fault Current Return Path to Alternate Supply,
Neutral Conductor Grounded at Service Equipment Only

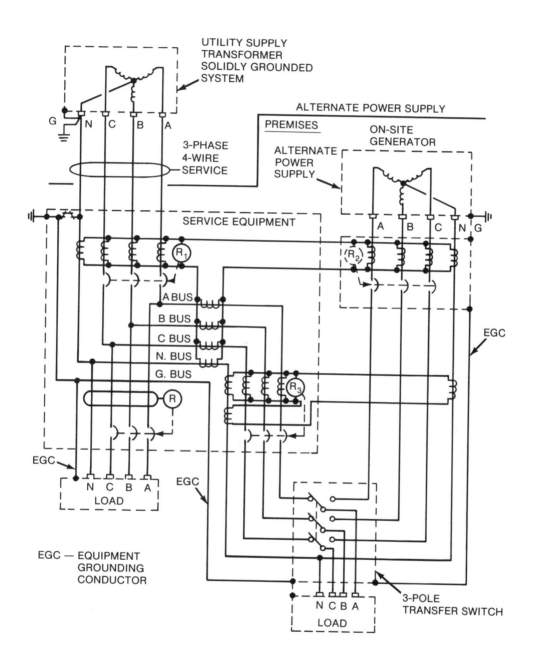

Fig 14
Ground Fault Scheme for a Normal and Alternate Power Supply Having
an Electrical Power Conductor (Neutral) Interconnection Between Supplies

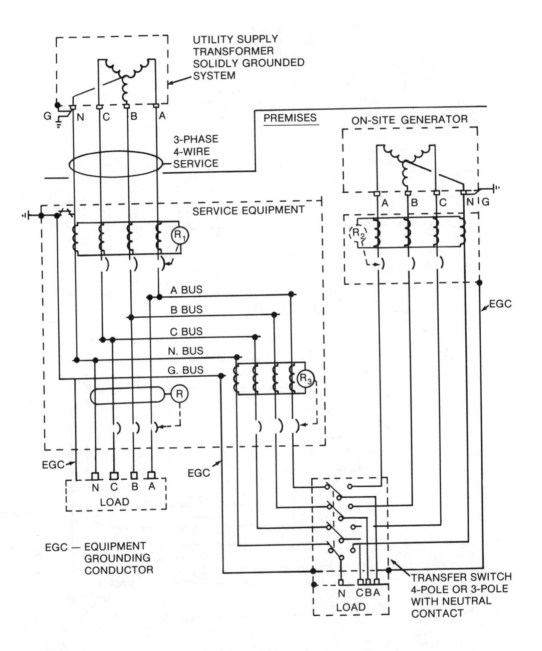

Fig 15
Ground Fault Scheme for a Normal and Alternate Power Supply
with No Electrical Power Conductor Interconnection Between Supplies

3.8 Electrical Equipment and Installation. Electrical power distribution equipment is described in depth in IEEE Std 141-1976 [17], and ANSI/IEEE Std 241-1983 [8] is extensively used in hospital power systems. However, when used in health care facilities, there are simply different criteria involved in the choice of equipment. Some of the factors influencing the engineers' choice of equipment are: reliability protection and coordination requirements, how rapidly vital service can be replaced following an outage, initial cost including installation, maintenance facilities, maintenance cost, availability, and cost of space. When the engineer is weighing the importance of each factor, he/she must bear in mind that not just revenues or production will be lost should the system fail, but possibly human lives. The system should therefore provide the most continuous power possible (within economic feasibiity) to patients and procedures that require electrical power.

All the components used in the electrical system for health care facilities should have adequate ratings and be installed in a proper manner to provide a reliable and safe electrical system. Careful consideration during the design and installation should be given to the location of the electrical components to minimize exposure to hazards such as lightning, storm, floods, earthquakes, or hazards created by adjoining structures or activities. Ample room around electrical components should be provided to permit task requirements, installation, maintenance, testing, operating, etc, to be performed in a safe manner.

Proper labeling of a permanent type should be applied to all components so that it is obvious where power is initiated and terminated. Equipment such as switchgear, switchboards, motor control centers, panelboards, automatic transfer switches, etc, should have engraved plastic nameplates which designate purpose and loads served, including location, applied on incoming sections, tie sections, and feeder sections. All cables, busway and bus should be identified as to phase represented to assist in maintaining proper phase sequence.

Upon completing installation and before energizing, the electrical components should be thoroughly cleaned. A visual inspection should be performed to assure that all components are installed properly, protective devices are set properly, and all of the above is ready for test procedure. All components including protective devices and circuitry, control circuitry, etc, should be tested to assure proper operation before energization.

In selecting and installing the electrical distribution components for the essential electrical system, high priority should be given to achieving maximum continuity of the electrical supply to the load. To achieve this high reliability desired, the components (distribution circuitry, electrical equipment, etc) for the essential electrical system should be installed so that they are physically separate from the nonessential power system components. Furthermore, as in ANSI/NFPA 99-1984 (Chapters 8 and 9) [16], each branch of the emergency system should be installed so as to be physically separate and independent of each other and all other wiring. An exception is allowed only where the electrical components require two separate services, such as in a transfer switch. This redundance requires separate panelboards and raceways for the emergency system.

The following sections discuss the equipment commonly applied in health care facilities. Considerations mentioned here are those of specific concern in a health care facility. The in-depth considerations as outlined in IEEE Std 142-1982 [7] and ANSI/IEEE Std 241-1983 [8] should be understood to assist in choosing proper equipment.

3.8.1 Transformers. Transformers in a hospital are usually used to change from a supply or distribution voltage to a utilization voltage. In today's energy conscious environment, considerable attention is focused on transformer operating cost. While this is an important factor when selecting a transformer, consideration should also be given to initial cost, reliability, sound level, thermal life, overload capability, installation costs, size, weight, availability of application and servicing resources. Contrary to popular belief, a lower temperature rise transformer may have higher operating costs than a higher temperature rise unit. Transformer operating costs are a function of transformer losses and transformer loading. The operating cost of each transformer for the application under consideration must be calculated to determine which is the most economical. Commonly available size transformers should be used so that replacement time will be minimized in the event of transformer failure. In addition to operating cost considerations, the voltage spread due to transformer impedance should also be taken into account.

3.8.2 Switchgear, Switchboards and Motor Control Centers. This equipment should be located as close as possible to their loads to shorten cable runs and minimize voltage drop. They should not be located near electronic monitoring equipment to avoid electromagnetic interference. If this is unavoidable, proper care should be taken to shield the electronic equipment. Adequate clearances and ventilation should be planned for present equipment and possible future expansions.

Adequate metering equipment should be incorporated in the switchgear, switchboard, or motor control center to permit proper monitoring of the current and voltage conditions of the power system.

3.8.3 Protective Devices. Overcurrent protective devices should be chosen to provide complete coordination of the system. If a fault or overload occurs, it is important to isolate the affected circuit while maintaining power to the other circuits.

Circuit interrupting devices have two basic elements that provide a detecting function and a switching function. They may generally be divided into four categories: circuit breakers equipped with protective relays or direct acting trips, contactors equipped with overload relays, transfer switches equipped with voltage sensing relays, and switches equipped with fuses.

(1) When applied within their ratings, the switching devices are generally capable of performing the following:

(a) *Contactors and Transfer Switches.* Repetitively closing, carrying and interrupting normal load currents; interrupting overload currents; withstanding but not interrupting any abnormal currents resulting from short circuits.

(b) *Switches.* Closing; carrying and interrupting load current; and when properly coordinated with a fuse, withstanding but not interrupting any abnormal current resulting from overloads and short circuits. The fuse provides detection and interrupting feature for overloads and short circuits.

(c) *Circuit Breakers.* Closing; carrying and interrupting load current; withstanding and interrupting overload and short circuit currents.

Of these devices, only circuit breakers and fused switches are generally applied as overcurrent protective devices that interrupt overload and short circuit currents. Transfer switches are applied to transfer loads from one source of power to another by monitoring power source voltage. Contactors are applied as load powering devices such as motor starters, etc.

(2) There are basically three types of detectors used with the protective devices: fuses, relays, and direct acting trips.

(a) Fuses detect and interrupt the abnormal current in one nonadjustable element. They are thermal type devices which are sensitive to ambient temperature and the current flowing through them. The continuous current ratings are based in open air, and when applied in equipment, need to be derated to account for increased ambient temperature. Normally, an 80% derating factor is applied. These single-phase devices (three required for a three-phase circuit) are generally applied with switches and breakers.

(b) Protection relays are designed to be responsive to electrical quantities which change during normal and abnormal conditions. The basic quantities that may change are: current, voltage, phase-angle, and frequency. Protective relays are designed to be responsive to one or more of these quantities instantaneously or at a time rate dependent on magnitude. Generally, they are field adjustable, have a wide operating ambient temperature range, and drawout construction. They can be attained with special features such as sensitivity to directional quantities only, etc. Relays, although not limited to, are normally applied in conjunction with high and medium voltage circuit breakers. Upon closure, their contacts generally energize the trip circuit of the circuit breaker which opens all breaker poles.

(c) Direct acting trips are responsive to current either instantaneously or at a time rate dependent on the current magnitude. They are mounted inside low voltage circuit breakers in a series with the breaker poles, and when activated, mechanically toggle the breaker trip mechanism which opens all breaker poles. They are either of a thermal, electromagnetic, electromechanical, or static design. As for fuses, the thermal type requires a derating factor consideration. Some units are ambient compensated. The electromagnetic, electromechanical, or static types are generally field adjustable.

Ground fault detection in medium voltage systems is generally accomplished by electromagnetic overcurrent relays and standard window or bar type current transformers. Generally, in low voltage systems, static relays and mated current sensors, whether integral or external to the protective device, provide the ground fault protection.

A word of caution—ground fault detection requires additional attention as outlined in 3.7.3(6) if nuisance power outage is to be avoided.

The operating characteristics of the protective devices are plotted on log-log scale transparencies. Generally, the vertical or Y axis represents time in seconds and the horizontal or X axis represents current in amperes or per unit setting. Typical time current characteristics can be seen in Fig 16 for an inverse time overcurrent relay. Figure 17 shows the typical time characteristic; from left to right of low voltage protectors: current limiting fuse, molded case breaker equipped with a nonadjustable thermal instantaneous detector, molded case breaker equipped with a nonadjustable thermal and adjustable instantaneous detector, molded case or insulated case circuit breaker equipped with an adjustable static trip, and power circuit breaker equipped with an adjustable static trip.

For further protective device description and application, the reader is referred to IEEE Std 141-1976 (Chapter 4) [17], ANSI/IEEE Std 241-1983 (Chapter 9) [8], manufacturers' publications, and engineering handbooks listed under references and bibliography at the end of this chapter.

3.8.4 Transfer Switches—Automatic and Manual. Transfer switches are applied to transfer from one power service to another to maintain electric power service to the emergency power system and designated equipment. Due to their important function in the health care facility power system, they are required to be approved for emergency electrical service, have adequate capacity for the loads being served as well as properly located and installed to provide reliable service. Furthermore, they must have adequate withstandability ratings to prevent contact welding due to load, overload, or short circuit currents.

Automatic transfer switches are required to be electrically operated and mechanically latched to prevent change of state, open or close, whenever control power is unavailable for operation. This is to permit the transfer and retransfer of the load automatically when required. Manual or nonautomatic transfer switches are required to have a mechanical latching feature. Other requirements such as switch position indication, interlocking, voltage sensing, time delay, etc, are outlined in ANSI/NFPA 99-1984 (Chapter 8) [16] and ANSI/NFPA 70-1984 [15].

To permit ease of maintenance, consideration should be given to providing bypass isolation switches; however, cost should be balanced with ease of maintenance, since temporary bypasses can usually be made.

For additional information on transfer switches, refer to Chapter 5 of this publication.

3.8.5 Generators. Generally, in health care facilities, on-site generators are applied as an alternate power source for the essential electrical system whenever normal power is not available. The generator and its prime mover should be selected to meet the load requirements of the essential electrical system. Factors to be considered in this selection include:

(1) Type prime mover which will determine the fuel storage requirements, if any.

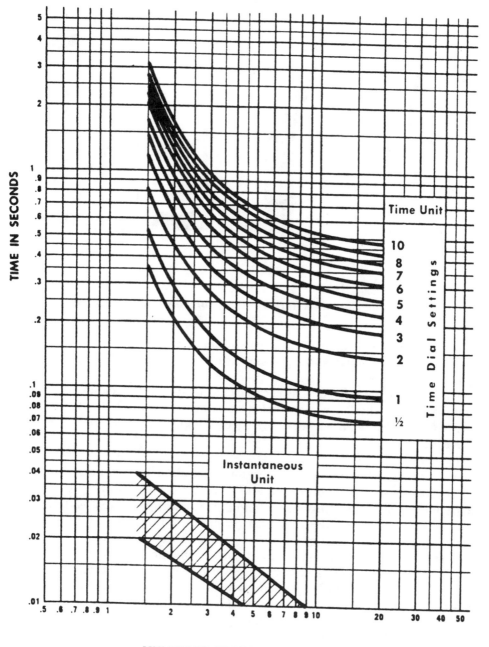

**Fig 16
Time-Current Characteristics of a Typical Inverse-Time Overcurrent Relay**

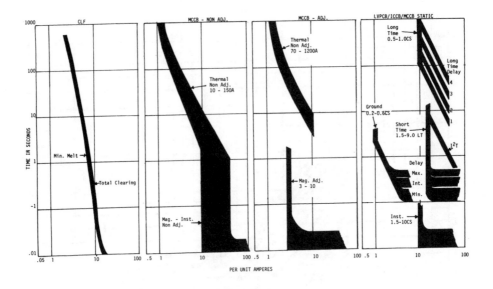

Fig 17
Typical Time-Current Characteristics for Low-Voltage Protection

(2) Adequate rating capability of prime mover as well as generator to serve the load at the proper voltage and frequency as well as current, full load and inrush requirements.

(3) Installation factors such as location, adequate space, ventilation, cooling, foundation, noise when operating, fuel storage, etc.

(4) Maintenance requirements—degree of complexity, spare parts required, and storage, etc.

(5) Overall cost.

For additional information on generator application in health care facilities, refer to Chapter 5 of this publication and ANSI/IEEE Std 446-1980 [9].

3.8.6 Wire, Cable and Busway. In addition to meeting general code requirements as noted in ANSI/NFPA 70-1984 (Chapters 1 through 4) [15], wire and cable installed in areas classified as hazardous must meet certain installation requirements. Class 1, Division 1, areas such as flammable anesthetizing areas shall have wire and cable installed in approved rigid metal raceways utilizing threaded connections and be properly sealed. All boxes, fittings and joints for connection to rigid metal raceways shall be explosion proof. Above hazardous locations, wire and cable are to be installed in metal raceways. Type M1 cable or type MC cable which employs a continuous gas and vaportight metallic sheath is permitted to be used above a hazardous location busway, wire, and cable installed in rigid raceways. Wiring supplying the primary of isolation transformers are restricted to having no more than 600 V between conductors. Furthermore, the conductors shall have a dielectric constant of 3.5 or less and be color coded as in ANSI/NFPA 70-1984 (Article 517) [15]. Caution is required when installing the conductors in the isolation secondary circuits. The method should not increase the conductor dielectric constant.

3.8.7 Panelboards. Power panelboards should be located as close to the load as possible. Receptacle and lighting panelboards should be located on the same floor as the loads they serve. Sufficient number of lighting and receptacle panelboards should be applied to maintain approximately 75 feet between panelboard and load, thus providing proper voltage levels. Panelboards should be located in a convenient area for ease of operation and have sufficient number of spare circuits to accommodate future expansion. Good design would provide a low ground path for all panelboards ground bus and housings back to the source of power to limit shock hazards and provide a low impedance path for ground fault currents in a grounded system.

3.8.8 Isolated Power Supplies. Isolated power supplies consist of an isolating transformer, motor-generated set, or batteries, a line isolation monitor and its ungrounded circuit conductors. The reader is referred to Chapter 6 of this publication for further discussion on this very important topic.

3.9 System Arrangements. In the design and installation of the electrical power system, careful attention should be devoted to selecting the proper electrical system arrangement to provide a reliable power system.

A power service consisting of two or more separate dedicated utility service feeders fed from separate distribution buses provide a higher degree of reliability than one utility service feeder. Furthermore, the reliability is enhanced if each service feeder is installed separately so that a fault in one feeder circuit will not affect the other feeder. This type installation will most probably permit serving a higher equipment system load during need, thus improving the effectiveness of patient care and safety.

Distribution system arrangements should be designed and installed to minimize interruptions to the electrical systems due to internal failures by use of adequately rated equipment. Among the factors to be considered as outlined in ANSI/NFPA 99-1984 [16] are:

(1) Abnormal currents: current sensing devices, phase and ground, should be selected to minimize the extent of interruption to the electrical system due to abnormal current caused by overloads or overcurrents.

(2) Abnormal voltages such as single phasing of three phase utilization equipment, switching and/or lightning surges, voltage reductions, etc.

(3) Capability of achieving the fastest possible restoration of any given circuit after clearing a fault.

(4) Effects of further changes such as increased loading and/or supply capacity.

(5) Stability and power capability of the prime mover during and after abnormal conditions.

(6) Sequence reconnecting of loads to avoid large current in rushes that could trip overcurrent devices or overload the generator(s) in the alternate power supply.

Feeder and branch circuits should be adequately rated to power their electrical loads and sufficient in number to allow load dispersement that will minimize the effect of a feeder or branch circuit outage.

A good portion of the electrical distribution system is installed in electrical closets. The space requirements and location of these closets should be identified early in the preliminary phases of a health care facility development. The ideal location for electrical closets is in the center core of the facility or in the middle of large wings so that branch circuits can be run in many directions, but not exceed 75 ft in length. Electrical closets on adjacent floors should be aligned so that electrical power circuit risers can be installed without bends or inaccessible taps. The closets should be large enough to accommodate the electrical panels and transformers and permit space for access and maintainability. Closets containing dry transformers should be ventilated to prevent heat buildup. Sprinkler heads should not be located in electrical closets since their operation could cause loss of normal and emergency power service. However, where local jurisdictions insist upon installing sprinkler heads in electrical closets, the highest permissible temperature head should be considered for installation.

Health care facilities frequently have motors with high inrush fed from the same power source that supplies voltage sensitive equipment. Precautions should be taken to prevent these inrush currents from adversely affecting the voltage sensitive equipment. A method is to provide a separate feeder for powering the voltage sensitive equipment. It is not unusual for systems to be installed with motor feeders separated from the general lighting and power feeders in a double ended switchgear or switchboard or segmented bus arrangement in order to reduce the effects of motor starting on other electrical loads. It is important that elevator motors, specifically for hydraulic elevators, be installed with proper NEMA code letter, as in ANSI/NFPA 70-1984 (Article 430, Table 430-7(b)) [15], which specifies the maximum inrush current permitted and proper starting method, that is full voltage or reduced voltage starting. Generally, the only other motors in a health care facility which might cause voltage dip problems are large chiller motors. However, due to their infrequent starting once or twice a day, they seldom present a problem. The electric power supply for radiology should be installed to provide a low voltage spread, usually three percent or less to prevent malfunction on the X-ray equipment as well as other voltage sensitive equipment.

3.9.1 Radial System Arrangement. For small facilities, small nursing homes and residential custodial care facilities, a single service entrance panelboard or switchboard and a small generator can be the major components of the electrical system (Fig 18). These facilities usually have several normal panelboards fed from the nonessential overcurrent device. If motor loads are to be energized by the generator, their restoration under emergency conditions can be delayed by using a time delay relay in the automatic transfer switch (refer to Chapter 5) or by adding a time delay relay in the motor starter which is energized by auxiliary contacts within the transfer switch as shown in Fig 19.

Where there will be significant emergency power requirements, several transfer switches may be used to increase reliability. The transfer switches used for the

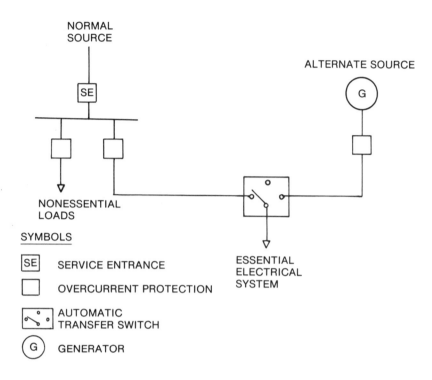

Fig 18
Major Components of the Electrical System

equipment system can be adjusted to transfer sequentially, thus minimizing generator inrush requirements. However, the transfer switches used in the emergency system must transfer within 10 seconds.

ANSI/NFPA 70-1984 (Article 517) [15] requires that the emergency system be automatically transferred to an alternate power source following an interruption of the normal source. However, equipment such as elevators, heating units, or heating and ventilating fans may be manually transferred following a power outage. Where trained personnel are available on a 24-hour basis, manual transfer switching of certain equipment loads may be a less expensive method of applying emergency power than automatic switching. Manual switching also allows equipment to be energized as generator loading permits. ANSI/NFPA 99-1984 (Chapter 8) [16] and ANSI/NFPA 70-1984 (Article 517.64) [15] specify where manual switching is permissible.

As health care facilities become larger, additional feeders for nonessential loads and essential electrical systems will be required. The essential electrical system will thus require several transfer switches, some of which could be nonautomatic. Using several smaller transfer switches in lieu of a large switch will contribute to system stability and reliability, but at an increased cost. Further reliability can be obtained by placing the transfer switches as close to the ultimate load as possible.

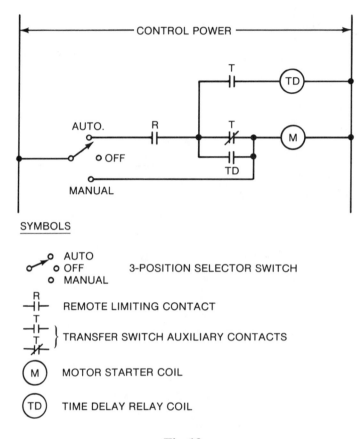

SYMBOLS

Fig 19
Time Delay Relay in Transfer Switch of Motor Starter

For example, Fig 20 shows two schemes for distributing power through vertical risers. When an outage occurs in the normal power supply of either scheme, the transfer switches will direct an alternate power supply to the essential electrical system power panels. However, if a specific normal feeder outage occurs, only Scheme A can sense the specific outage and restore power to the affected panel via the alternate power supply. Scheme A is more reliable than Scheme B, but is a more costly arrangement. Loss of normal power is sensed at the transfer device to initiate startup of the emergency power unit via auxiliary contacts. When adequate emergency power is available, it is sensed to cause switching to the alternate power source. Finally, restoration of normal power causes the transfer devices or switches to return to the normal power source while initiating a shutdown of the emergency power unit. Note that time requirements between switching events are documented in ANSI/NFPA 99-1984 (Chapter 8) [16].

3.9.2 Double Ended System Arrangement. A double ended substation should be considered where transformation will exceed 750 kVA.

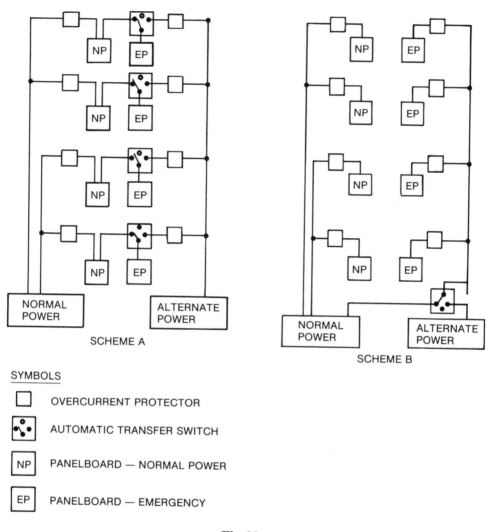

SCHEME A

SCHEME B

SYMBOLS

⬜ OVERCURRENT PROTECTOR

⬛ AUTOMATIC TRANSFER SWITCH

NP PANELBOARD — NORMAL POWER

EP PANELBOARD — EMERGENCY

Fig 20
Two Schemes for Distributing Power Through Vertical Risers

For example, Fig 21 utilizes a normally open tie protector which is interlocked with the main protectors (fused switch or circuit breaker) so that all three protectors cannot be closed simultaneously. Upon loss of a single transformer or its feeder, the tie protector can be manually closed and load added to the remaining transformer. Additional benefits of the double ended substation are lower fault currents than with a single transformer and the ability to separate motor loads from lighting and X-ray loads that require a higher degree of voltage regulation.

If the double ended substation scheme uses a normally open electrically operated tie protector that will automatically close upon loss of either incoming

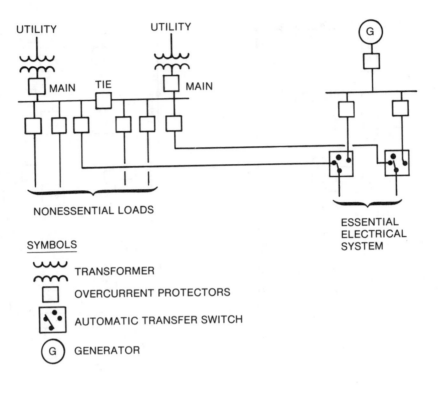

UTILITY   UTILITY

MAIN   TIE   MAIN

NONESSENTIAL LOADS

ESSENTIAL
ELECTRICAL
SYSTEM

SYMBOLS

TRANSFORMER

OVERCURRENT PROTECTORS

AUTOMATIC TRANSFER SWITCH

G   GENERATOR

Fig 21
Normally Open Tie Protector Interlocked With the Main Protectors

feeder, then additional control and protective relaying must be added to prevent the bus tie protector from closing when a main protector has tripped due to overload or short circuit conditions.

In rare instances, a utility may permit a double ended substation to be operated with a closed tie and main protectors. The advantages of using a double ended substation with mains and tie normally closed are greater reliability, better voltage regulation, and flickerless transfer upon loss of one power source. The disadvantages are greater complexity, greater fault current, and greater cost. The greater complexity requires that the design engineer coordinate and specify the required additional protection to assure proper operation.

3.9.3 Network System Arrangement. A network service consists of two or more transformers with their secondaries bussed together through network protectors as shown in Fig 22.

The advantages of network service are high reliability, no service interruption when one feeder is removed from service, and good voltage regulation. The disadvantages are high cost, high fault currents, and inability to expand the network service without increasing the interrupting ratings and sizes of existing components.

In metropolitan areas, an electric service powered from an existing utility owned network may be available. The utility's network in urban areas consists of many network transformers with their secondaries tied into a grid of secondary cables covering a large area. This network usually allows one primary feeder to be removed from service at any time, or two primary feeders to be removed from service during lightly loaded periods without causing undue low voltage on the secondary grid. Where demand is over 500 kVA, utilities may opt for a "spot network" consisting of two to four network transformers in close proximity with their secondaries bussed together, but not connected to the general urban area network.

The network service is considered the most reliable, but most expensive type of electrical service. Life cycle costs may be reduced somewhat by having the hospital own and maintain the network transformers rather than the utility in order to qualify for a primary service discount.

Fig 22
Network Service

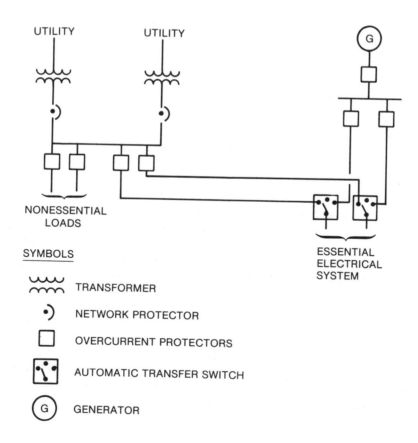

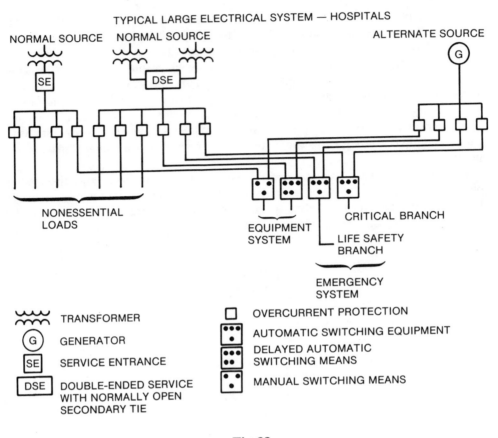

Fig 23
Adequately Rated Substation

In recent years, the trend has been away from network and closed tie substations and towards open tie substations with automatic transfer of essential circuits to on-site generation when required. This trend is due to the higher cost and complexity of the closed tie and network system, plus the fact that essential hospital load can be served by on-site generation during normal power failures.

3.9.4 High-Voltage System Arrangements. The most commonly used high-voltage systems for hospitals are the loop and the primary selective systems. Both of these systems allow a single cable section or feeder to be removed from service without a prolonged outage. The use of performed separable connectors in manholes and at transformers can expedite the isolation of a faulted cable section. Also, fault current detectors can be attached to cable in manholes to aid in locating cable faults. More detailed descriptions of the loop and selective primary systems can be obtained from IEEE Std 141-1976 (Chapter 1) [17].

3.9.5 Existing System Arrangement. Where extensive new load is added to a hospital having an existing substation, it is almost always more convenient to add a new transformer than to change the older substation provided it is still adequately rated as shown in Fig 23. This might provide an excellent way to introduce 480 V distribution if the older substation is rated at a lower voltage.

3.9.6 Metering Arrangement. The designer of an electrical system using several primary transformers should attempt to obtain totalized metering from the utility since this will result in lower monthly electrical costs. Because electrical rates usually price each additional block of power less expensive than the previous block, a single meter will record the expensive blocks of power only once each month.

However, most utilities will only permit totalized metering if the hospital purchases all power at a single point and single voltage. If the power is purchased at the primary voltage level with the hospital owning and maintaining its own primary system, not only can a single meter be utilized, but the hospital may be eligible for a lower electrical rate or discount. The design engineer should evaluate these savings versus the cost of purchasing and maintaining a high voltage distribution system, when deciding on the character of electrical service.

3.10 Standard References

The following standard publications were used as references in preparing this chapter:

[1] ANSI C37.16-1980, Recommendations for Low-Voltage Power Circuit Breakers and AC Power Circuit Protectors, Preferred Ratings, Related Requirements and Application.[16]

[2] ANSI C57.12.10-1977, Requirements for Transformers 230 000 Volts and Below 833/958 Through 8333/10 417 kVA Single Phase, and 750/862 Through 60 000/ 80 000/100 000 kVA, Three Phase.

[3] ANSI C57.12.20-1981, Requirements for Overhead-Type Distribution Transformers 67 000 Volts and Below, 500 kVA and Smaller.

[4] ANSI C57.12.21-1980, Requirements for Pad-Mounted Compartmental-Type Self-Cooled Single-Phase Distribution Transformers with High-Voltage Bushings.

[5] ANSI C84.1-1982, Voltage Ratings for Electric Power Systems and Equipment (60 Hz).

[6] ANSI C97.1-1972 (R1978), American National Standard for Low-Voltage Cartridge Fuses 600 Volts or Less.

[7] ANSI/IEEE Std 142-1982, IEEE Recommended Practice for Grounding of Industrial and Commercial Power Systems.

[8] ANSI/IEEE Std 241-1983, IEEE Recommended Practice for Electric Power Systems in Commercial Buildings.

---

[16] ANSI publications can be obtained form the Sales Department, American National Standards Institute, 1430 Broadway, New York, NY 10018.

[9] ANSI/IEEE Std 446-1980, IEEE Recommended Practice Emergency and Stand-by Power for Industrial and Commercial Applications.

[10] ANSI/IEEE C37.010-1979, Application Guide for AC High-Voltage Circuit Breakers Rated on a Symmetrical Current Basis.[17]

[11] ANSI/IEEE C37.5-1979, Guide for Calculation of Fault Currents for Application of AC High-Voltage Circuit Breakers Rated on a Total Current Basis.

[12] ANSI/IEEE C37.13-1981, Low-Voltage AC Power Circuit Breakers Used in Enclosures.

[13] ANSI/IEEE C37.41-1981, Design Tests for High-Voltage Fuses, Distribution Enclosed Single-Pole Air Switches, Fuse Disconnecting Switches, and Accessories.

[14] ANSI/IEEE C57.12.00-1980, General Requirements for Liquid-Immersed Distribution, Power, and Regulating Transformers.

[15] ANSI/NFPA 70-1984, National Electrical Code.

[16] ANSI/NFPA 99-1984, Standard for Health Care Facilities.

[17] IEEE Std 141-1976, IEEE Recommended Practice for Electric Power Distribution for Industrial Plants.

[18] IEEE Std 242-1975, IEEE Recommended Practice for Protection and Coordination of Industrial and Commercial Power Systems.

[19] NEMA AB1-1975, Molded Case Circuit Breakers.

[20] NEMA SG2-1981, High-Voltage Fuses.

3.11 Bibliography

BEEMAN, D.L., editor. *Industrial Power Systems Handbook.* New York: McGraw-Hill, 1955.

FISCHER, M.J. *Designing Electrical Systems for Hospitals.* Vol 5 of *Techniques of Electrical Construction and Design.* New York: McGraw-Hill, 1979.

MASON, C.R. *The Art and Science of Protective Relaying.* New York: John Wiley & Sons, 1956.

---

[17] ANSI/IEEE publications can be obtained from the address listed in footnote 16 or from the Sales Department, IEEE Service Center, 445 Hoes Lane, Piscataway, NJ 08854.

4. Planning for Patient Care

4.1 General Discussion. Electrical power is of ever-increasing importance in the planning and design of health care facilities and hospitals. Because of this, it is important that the electrical engineer designing a hospital locate the correct device in the correct location. This arrangement should optimize patient care, as electrical power can dictate the patient's comfort and even affect life-and-death situations.

This chapter is divided into two sections. The first discusses the typical wiring devices utilized in a hospital, while the second discusses some suggested "good practice" in laying out patient areas. The devices described in the first section are shown in the second section.

4.2 Wiring Devices

4.2.1 General. In general, hospitals have two sources of power available, normal and emergency. It is vital that the wiring devices on emergency power be easily identified. This reduces the time wasted locating receptacles to power life-support equipment when even seconds are critical. There are two ways to identify devices: (1) by a distinctive color, such as red, or (2) by labeling. Marking with a distinctive color is not only easier and less costly than labeling but can prevent confusion later. For instance, when painters remove the lettered emergency and normal cover-plates, there is no longer a distinction between devices. Also, since receptacles in critical care areas must have panelboard and circuit number labels, the device cover-plates tend to become cluttered. The distinctive color is also easily spread into other portions of the emergency systems (such as lighting control) to maintain uniformity. Consideration should be given to using lighted emergency power receptacles in any patient areas that do not have emergency lighting, thus making the receptacle easier to find in the near-darkness of a power outage.

Devices in a hospital need to be mounted for easy use by staff and patients. Since a large number of hospital patients spend time in wheelchairs, special attention should be given to "handicapped" requirements. These requirements are typical of occupational therapy areas (Aids to Daily Living—A.D.L.) and are described in 4.3.9(2). It is to the advantage of all patients and staff, if all receptacles are mounted 24 in (610 mm) above the floor (see 4.3 and 4.3.9(2)(b)). This mounting height will reduce the fatigue caused when staff members must repeatedly bend down to connect or disconnect a plug.

4.2.2 Hospital-Grade Receptacles—High Abuse. *Application.* In accordance with the National Electrical Code (NEC), hospital-grade receptacles are listed as suitable for use in Health Care Facilities. Health care facilities are defined in ANSI/NFPA 70-1984 (Article 517) [2][18] as: "Buildings or parts of buildings that contain, but are not limited to, hospitals, nursing homes, extended-care facilities, clinics, and medical and dental offices, whether fixed or mobile."

The receptacles and plugs should be UL-listed "Hospital Grade" (ANSI/UL 498-1980 [4]). The "Hospital Grade" receptacle meets UL test criteria for mechanical strength as well as superior electrical characteristics. Among these criteria, and perhaps of primary importance to the health care facility, are stringent minimum retention and ground resistance specifications. While it is true that some "Spec Grade" receptacles are of high quality and fully equal to those UL-listed as "Hospital Grade," no formalized standards exist for a "Spec Grade" receptacle. Consequently, it is very difficult to control the desired quality level and minimum standards when a project or purchase specification lists "Spec Grade" as its only requirements.

Parallel blade devices should be mounted ground pin or neutral blade up. In this configuration any metal which drops between the plug and the wall will most likely contact a nonenergized blade.

When only one receptacle is connected to a 20 A circuit, it must be a 20 A receptacle. If all the receptacles specified are 20 A, it is easier for the maintenance department to stock and store.

The use of 15 A receptacles in any area of the hospital limits the use. Housekeeping equipment is used in *all* areas and buffers usually draw more than 15 A.

4.2.3 Hospital-Grade Isolated Ground Receptacle. *Application.* These receptacles are used where separation of the device ground and the building ground is desired. This is normally when digital electronic equipment is used, including computer cash registers, computer peripherals, and digital processing equipment. Transient voltages on the ground system can cause operational malfunction in digital circuits.

4.2.4 Hospital-Grade Safety Receptacles. *Application.* Safety receptacles prevent contact with an energized contact in the receptacle unless a grounding-type plug is inserted. These receptacles, sometimes referred to as tamperproof receptacles, should be used exclusively in pediatric and psychiatric locations. When selecting safety receptacles, the specifier should be careful not to permit the type which makes and breaks contacts to be used where life support equipment may be needed. It is always best to specify tamperproof hardware with all safety receptacles as well as in pediatric and psychiatric locations.

4.2.5 Hospital-Grade Ground Fault Circuit Interrupter Receptacles and Ground Fault Circuit Interrupter Circuit Breakers. *Application.* Ground fault

---

[18] The numbers in brackets correspond to those in the references at the end of this chapter.

circuit interruption (GFCI) protection can be provided by either GFCI breakers or GFCI receptacles. GFCI protection is used in wet locations, where protection from electrical shock is desired. GFCI receptacles and breakers should be used only where interruption of power is acceptable. If the interruption of power is not acceptable, for example, in areas where life support equipment may be used, an isolated power system should be used.

4.2.6 Anesthetizing Location Receptacles. *Application.* Receptacles for use in anesthetizing locations are manufactured as both hazardous area and non-hazardous area devices. This permits use in all anesthetizing locations. This type of receptacle assures electrical power and ground connection due to the spring loaded rejection feature. Being of Power-Lok® construction, they resist unintended removal. Local code requirements should be checked when using this type of receptacle.

While it may be permissible to use straight blade hospital grade devices in non-hazardous anesthetizing locations, this may not be a "safe" policy. Some, but not all Power-Lok twist-lock plugs being sealed to the cord with a sealing compound, can be washed without worrying about a short. Due to the sealing compound and construction, these plugs are expensive and can only be used once. Straight blade plugs, however, are not normally sealed to keep water out. This may present a problem with sterilization.

4.2.7 Mobile X-ray Plugs and Receptacles. *Application.* X-ray plugs and receptacles should be noninterchangeable with any other equipment plugs. This prevents high-impulse loads on branches and feeders which were not designed for such service. X-ray devices come in 50 A and 60 A models which are designed to be used on isolated power. A 50 A plug can be connected to either a 50 A or 60 A receptacle, while a 60 A plug can only be connected to a 60 A receptacle. When locating these receptacles, the force required to insert the plug must be considered. These receptacles have a spring-eject type feature which guarantees that the plug will be fully inserted. Because of the insertion pressure required, they should be mounted at 30 in (735 mm) minimum. If used in an anesthetizing location these plugs should be similar to those in 4.2.6. Other acceptable devices are pin and sleeve, normal twist-lock, and straight blade. The hospital should be contacted for their preferences.

4.2.8 High-Abuse Wallplates. *Typical Specification — Wallplates.* Wallplates should be of high-abuse construction, manufactured of high impact plastic, stainless steel (type 304 minimum), or anodized aluminum. Configurations should match wiring devices. If plastic plates are used, plate color should match device color. All plates should hold up under frequent cleaning with hospital cleaning chemicals.

These wallplates should be suitable for use in accordance with Federal, State, County, Municipal and Local Codes, including ANSI/NFPA 70-1984 [2], as required by OSHA. In addition, they should be suitable for use in health care facilities. The use of rigid metal plates should be carefully examined because once they are bent by carts they will snag and tear clothes, and cut arms, fingers, and legs. The major drawback to nylon plates is that they warp and bend when installed in other than ideal conditions. Metal plates are rigid and therefore do not suffer from this problem. However, a superior product is the new high-impact plastic wallplates.

4.2.9 Headwall Units. The use of prefabricated patient care units (headwall units) is now so prevalent as to be almost standard in both renovation and retrofit projects, as well as new construction projects. Headwall units can and are used in all patient care areas of the hospital. It should be pointed out that the term "headwall" is general and applies to many units which are not even remotely similar to "Walls" (that is, see Fig 30).

Headwalls normally contain electrical power distribution systems. While headwall units do contain some mechanical equipment and could be considered architectural, they are considered more of an electrical device than anything else and, consequently, they are typically specified by the electrical engineer.

(1) *Considerations.* Several basic reasons for using headwall units are: future flexibility, serviceability, shortened construction schedule, superior appearance, expenditure deferral, cost savings, etc. Perhaps the reason for the rapid rise in popularity of headwall units is that the advantages of using them can be appreciated by the nurse, patient, administrator, maintenance department, architect, engineer, and contractor.

Nursing personnel will find the pre-planned component locations accessible and convenient, resulting in fast, efficient patient service, thereby maximizing the patient's comfort. Hospital maintenance personnel find the quality headwall both durable and easily serviced. Hospital administrators find that they can defer the cost of the headwall along with all of the equipment it contains until just shortly before the hospital is scheduled to open. Architects and engineers find that both design and coordination of services is greatly simplified for both new or remodeling construction.

Contractors find that their jobsite labor costs are significantly reduced and their coordination of service problems at the patient location also can be greatly reduced.

(2) *Selection.* While the selection and specification of headwall units is far simpler than locating and specifying the individual services within the structural wall, time, thought and some study must be done in order to assure that everyone's needs as well as the needs of the area served are satisfied. Whenever possible, the medical team responsible for that area of the hospital to be served by the headwall in question should be consulted as to quantity, location, and type of equipment required to serve the patients in that area. After a design has been selected, it is helpful to review the choice through the use of a full size mock-up or full size drawing. Confirming locations and dimensions in this fashion can eliminate some undesirable surprises after the unit is installed. The architect should be consulted on color selection.

Due at least in part to the widespread acceptance of the headwall concept, many styles of headwalls are available for the specifier's choice. Oftentimes, several types are available from a single manufacturer. The style or type selected will often be dictated by the medical team requirements. Figure 24 illustrates what is commonly referred to as a short wall designed for use in a general care patient area. This construction is generally used where space is at a premium and the area below the wall is required for placement of a bedside table or similar equipment. As shown in Fig 25, the junction boxes for the various services are located within the wall. A wall mounting bracket becomes the top of the wall and a suitable termination point for services before the wall is in place. Note the drawing of the wall in Fig 26, which shows the junction box located as an integral part of the wall mounting bracket above the ceiling. This section can be scheduled to arrive at the jobsite during the rough-in stages and becomes the termination point for the services. Either method is acceptable; the important thing is to have a method of terminating services without having to install the headwall unit. Figure 27 is an illustration of a full single section general care wall. This type of

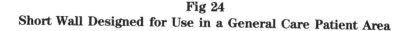

Fig 24
Short Wall Designed for Use in a General Care Patient Area

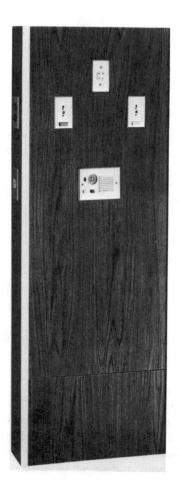

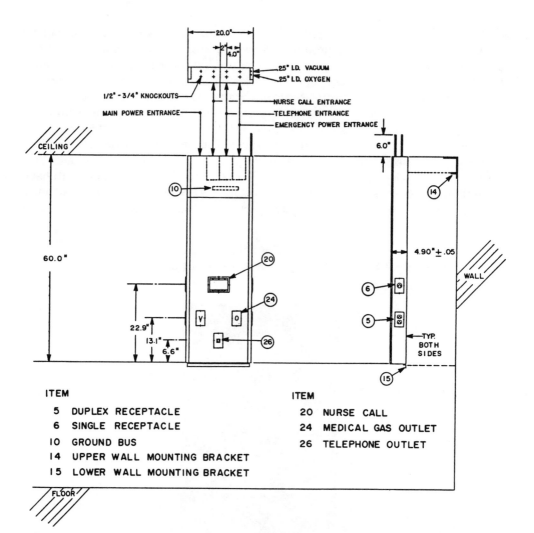

Fig 25
Junction Boxes Located Within the Wall

unit, as well as the single section short wall, can be designed either for a single bed or two patient bed location.

The headwall, by necessity, contains considerably more equipment when it is designed to serve an intensive care or coronary care patient. Figures 28 and 29 illustrate a three-section and a single-section wall, both of which are designed to serve an ICU/CCU environment. The three-section wall allows the luxury of dividing the equipment on both sides of the patient. Better segregation of medical gases and electrical receptacles is maintained. If a single-section wall is used for an ICU/CCU area for economical reasons, it is recommended that at least one

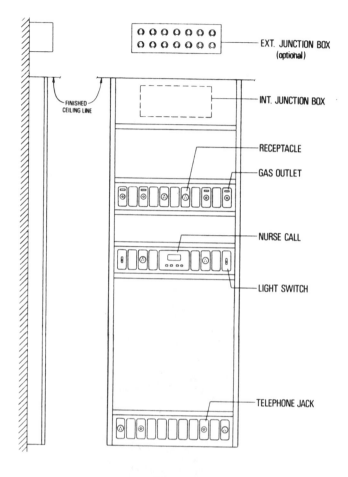

Fig 26
Junction Box Located As Integral Part of Wall Mounting Bracket Above Ceiling

duplex receptacle be placed on the side of the bed opposite the headwall unit. This should also be considered in general care areas. Another difference between the walls shown in Fig 28 and Fig 29 is that the unit in Fig 28 uses both vertical and horizontal placement of the equipment, whereas the unit in Fig 29 is an illustration of the unit using horizontal placement only. Each of the design methods has its benefits and advocates. It is an area in which personal preference often plays an important role. It should be pointed out that many times manufacturers will make both design versions to meet the individual requirements of their customers.

One other popular variation of the ICU/CCU wall, although it is not illustrated here, should be noted, that is, the use of a single-section module on each side of the bed without the use of a center section. This variation provides the advantages of greater equipment placement flexibility at somewhat less expense than the full three-section wall.

The unit illustrated in Fig 30 would perhaps more appropriately be called a neonatal service console, rather than a headwall unit. However, it does fall under this general category and units of this type are being used extensively. The unit pictured here is intended for a neonatal intensive care area and can be used as an island unit or installed against a structure wall. It often provides storage facilities and work areas as well as the normal electrical and mechanical patient services. Variations of this unit have also been used in adult intensive care areas.

Figures 31 and 32 show another variation of the headwall which has recently been finding great favor among hospitals. These are free standing service columns which offer the advantage of greater access to the patient. The head of the

Fig 27
Full Single Section General Care Wall

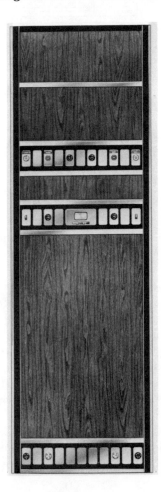

patient bed is generally located two to three ft from the closest wall, thereby allowing medical personnel an immediate access to that area behind the patient's head. These service columns do require more floor space per patient than the flat column concept in order to fully utilize all the advantages that they offer. Careful consideration should also be given to traffic patterns as well as patient visibility.

It can readily be seen that firm recommendations on the selection of headwall units are not practical due to the many variables from project to project. Consideration should be given to medical team practices and preferences, available space, hospital specialties, and hospital budget.

(3) *Medical Gas Services.* The specification for medical headwall units should clearly state the type and style of desired medical gas outlet. The outlets can be furnished by the headwall manufacturer, or the mechanical contractor can be requested to furnish these devices to the headwall manufacturer. The former is the most desirable since it allows the headwall manufacturer to coordinate delivery times directly with the manufacturer. Additionally, there is often more than one mounting method available within a given style of outlet, and allowing the

Fig 28
Both Vertical and Horizontal Placement of Equipment

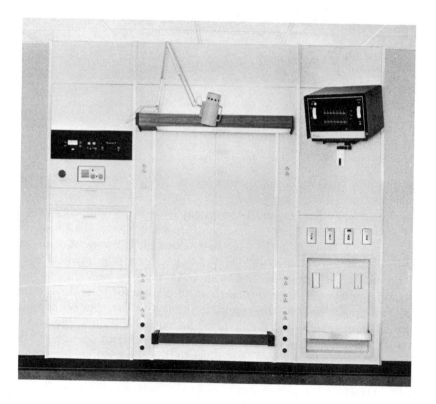

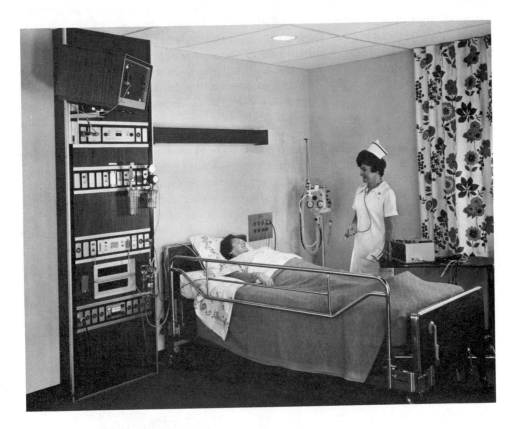

Fig 29
Unit Using Horizontal Placement of Equipment

headwall manufacturer to do his own ordering diminishes many of the coordination problems that could otherwise be encountered.

The medical gas outlets are most commonly located on one side of the patient even within an intensive care environment. However, there are times when the medical team will request outlets on both sides of the patient, and this is of course possible when multisection headwalls are used. The medical gas outlets should be maintained within the headwall and the piping brought out to an area which would be convenient for the mechanical contractor to make the final connections. This is generally at the top of the unit and the connections are made above the lay-in ceiling. Where the medical gas outlets are all located on the side of the patient, a single pipe for each service is extended to the top of the headwall. An approximately 6 in stub is allowed for final connection. Where gas outlets are furnished on each side of the patient in a multisection wall, it is not practical to manifold the piping from both sides within the headwall. The specification should clearly show that the contractor will have to make the final connections to each set of gas outlets external to the headwall.

It is important that the headwall manufacturer install and test the mechanical gas outlets and associated piping in accordance with the specification in ANSI/NFPA 56F-1983 [1]. It should be pointed out that this testing does not excuse the mechanical contractor from doing a final system test which would include the piping and outlets contained within the medical headwall unit. These test requirements are also contained within ANSI/NFPA 56F-1983 [1].

The spacing of medical gas outlets is critical since in use they will have collection containers and pressure regulating devices extending both above and below the outlet. There will also be tubing running between these devices and the patient. Coordination with the hospital team responsible for these services to determine the exact size of the equipment to be used is essential. The general rule for spacings is to leave a minimum of 4.5 in, centerline to centerline, between outlets horizontally, and 12 to 14 in between outlets vertically. While these are the general minimums, the specific use to which the outlets will be placed and the equipment they will accommodate will sometimes allow some reduction in these numbers; however, careful consultation with the hospital personnel and the gas equipment manufacturer before such reductions are undertaken is required.

The accepted manifold pipe sizing is shown Table 6.

Generally, some type of storage facility in the headwall or hanging facility is required for vacuum collection receptacles. Reusable bottles, disposable bottles, and disposable plastic bags are all used for this purpose. While a hospital may use only one of these types of receptacles, at the moment there is no assurance that they will not expand their usage to other types. Therefore, vacuum bottle slides should be furnished as an absolute minimum, and if it is known that bottles will be used, the convenience of a vacuum bottle storage tray or tub is recommended. The vacuum bottle tub provides an easily cleaned and protected location for vacuum bottles, and even allows for storage of an empty bottle for immediate use. As an alternative to the bottle tub, a long (36 in) vacuum bottle slide may be incorporated.

(4) *Electrical Services.* The headwall unit can, and usually does, contain all of the electrical services required to serve the patient. The minimum services required are described in other appropriate sections of this chapter. Equipment which can

Table 6
Medical Gas Manifold Pipe Size

Outlets	Gas Service Type		
	O_2	Air	Vacuum
1	¼″ ID	¼″ ID	¼″ ID
2	¼″ ID	¼″ ID	½″ ID
3	¼″ ID	¼″ ID	¾″ ID
4	¼″ ID	¼″ ID	¾″ ID

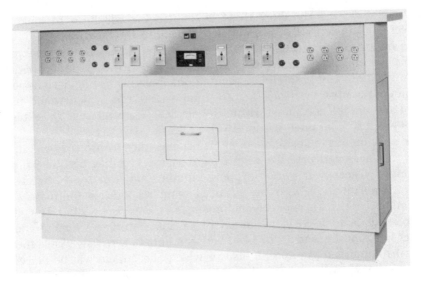

Fig 30
Neonatal Service Console

be accommodated within the headwall would include patient and general lighting, examination lighting, power receptacles, ground jacks, isolated and grounded electrical distribution systems, clocks and timers, portable X-ray outlets, night lighting, low voltage electrical lighting systems, emergency electrical services, etc.

Typically, a general care wall would contain four duplex receptacles per patient. Intensive care walls would contain six to nine duplex receptacles per patient.

Normal lighting in a headwall unit would consist of an overbed fluorescent fixture providing two (2) 30 W lamps for up lighting or general illumination, and one (1) 30 W lamp for patient reading light or bed light use. At a minimum the down light should be controllable by the patient. A night light should be provided and should be located below the bed level so as to minimize patient disturbance. Low level chart lights are best provided within the fluorescent overbed fixture. These lighting specifications are applicable to both general care and intensive care areas. For additional information on patient area lighting, see Chapter 7.

Examination lights are generally required in all areas and they are available in a large range of styles and prices. They can, for instance, be high intensity lighting units mounted in the ceiling over the bed and controlled by switching in the headwall unit. The most universally accepted are of the adjustable arm type, which are attached to the headwall or the overbed light fixture. General care areas require only an incandescent type exam light, which can also double as an over-the-shoulder reading light. Intensive care usually calls for some type of high intensity lighting with a better color balance. The extended arm type of lighting can create some obstruction problems and, therefore, location of these lights should be given careful thought so as to preclude interference with other equipment.

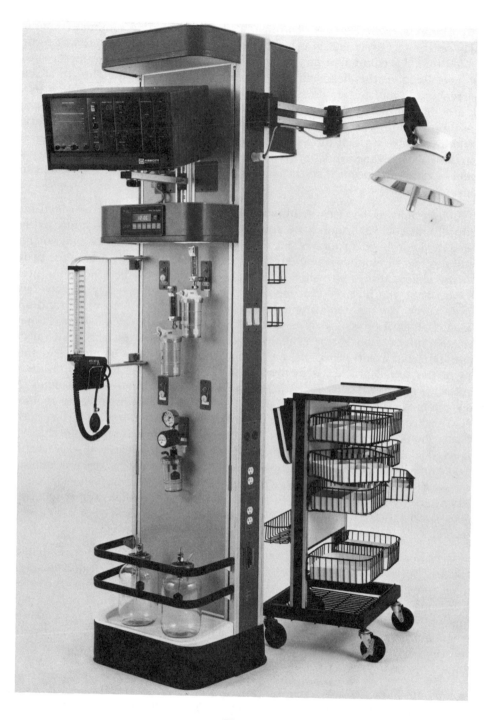

Fig 31
Free Standing Service Column

(5) *Communication Services.* The headwall should contain minimal communication services as described in other areas of this chapter. However, it is recommended that this equipment not be furnished by the headwall manufacturer. For best coordination, the headwall should contain provisions for the nurse call, emergency call, and telephone services. These provisions should include a backbox of sufficient size to accept the equipment and raceways from that backbox to an appropriate junction box located at the top of the headwall. Installation should be possible without disassembly of the headwall other than that necessary to expose the entrance junction box at the top of the headwall. Conduit size should be carefully specified so that it will accommodate the necessary cable and connectors.

(6) *Miscellaneous Services.* A number of services which can be provided in a headwall unit could fall under the category of miscellaneous. Almost any patient service item can be incorporated into a medical headwall. Some we find so commonly used as to be almost standard. For example, physiological monitor provisions are almost always furnished on a headwall intended to be used in an intensive care area. the physiological monitor is commonly supplied by the headwall manufacturer. The manufacturer must be furnished with the correct brand and catalog number of physiological monitor which the hospital intends to use. Sometimes this information is not available until after shipment of the headwalls is required. In that event, provisions for the monitor bracket can be made and shipment of the actual bracket is delayed until the hospital has made its choice of monitor. One duplex power receptacle should be located immediately behind the bracket for convenient connection of the equipment. The physiological monitor outlet (electronic signal) is handled in the same manner as nurse call. That is, the box size should be specified (generally a two gang electrical box) and this box connected to an entrance compartment at the top of the headwall with its own raceway or conduit. If a patient physiological outlet provision is desired, another box near the patient level is provided and connected to the physiological outlet junction box by separate conduit. Care should be taken again in specifying the correct size conduit so that it will accommodate the necessary cable and connectors.

Services not so commonly found are hyperthermia provisions and renal dialysis provisions. In the case of hyperthermia, the headwall unit may contain the necessary plumbing and a portable hyperthermia unit can be plugged into the headwall by quick disconnects. In other cases, the entire hyperthermia unit may be permanently housed within the headwall. The provisions provided in the headwall for renal dialysis would be the correct electrical services as well as pressure water connections and drain connections. These connection points would again be of the quick disconnect variety.

Various mechanical devices can be provided in or on the headwall unit. As an example, sphygmomanometers of various types can be furnished by the headwall manufacturer, or provisions for mounting same can be specified. Mechanical rail systems for hanging medical instrumentation can be supplied by many of the

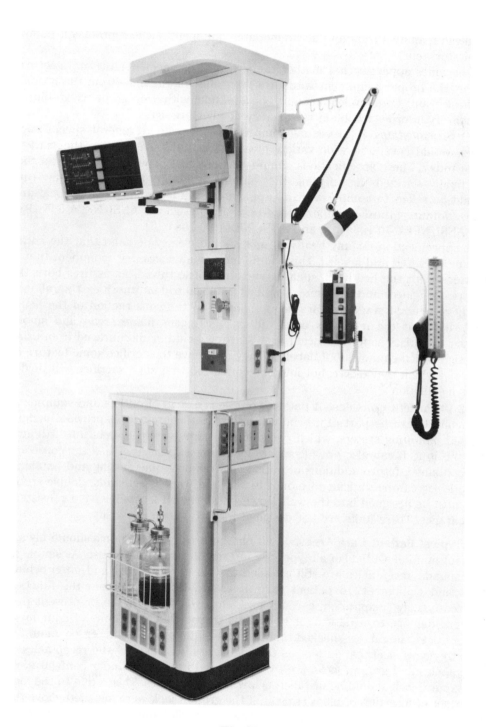

Fig 32
Free Standing Service Column

headwall manufacturers and accommodate equipment such as profusion pumps, respirators, etc.

It becomes apparent that neither the electrical engineer nor the architect can specify the proper equipment without a great deal of guidance from the hospital medical team. Communication and coordination with this group is absolutely mandatory in order to obtain satisfactory headwall design.

(7) *Specifications.* It is virtually impossible to write a general specification which would cover the wide variety of headwall units available in the marketplace today. These specifications should be tailored to the specific designs that are finally selected. In selecting the equipment within a headwall unit, care should be taken to comply with all applicable standards. Aside from local and state standards, those of importance to hospital design are ANSI/NFPA 56F-1983 [1], ANSI/NFPA 70-1984 [2], and ANSI/NFPA 99-1984 [3].

The specification for any headwall unit should clearly demand that the entire unit be UL listed and labeled. This should include all accessory equipment that is provided with the headwall, such as vacuum bottle tubs. This assures both the electrical engineer and the user, as well as the local code authorities, that all currently recognized standards are being followed in the construction of the headwall, and that the materials used will pass stringent flamespread and smoke emission regulations for this occupancy. Clients should be discouraged from using a design which cannot be UL labeled. They may have to sacrifice some feature or material which they desire, but must be convinced that such sacrifice will yield a safer installation.

4.2.10 Patient Consoles. A patient console is a strip of outlets and equipment. The console can be part of a headwall unit or self-contained. It provides a rigid, aligned mounting system, which consolidates many varied outlets into a homogeneous unit. It can also provide spaces for future expansion. When the console is self-contained, future additions of outlets will require some cutting and patching. This device can be difficult to mount in the headwall—steel studs, double studs, etc, must be designed into the wall. However, all the outlets will have a consistent appearance. These units are not designed for easy future flexibility.

4.3 Typical Patient Care Areas. In all patient areas, several items should always be kept in mind. Outlets of all types are installed for someone to use. As simple as this sounds, receptacles are still installed too close to the floor and often behind beds and equipment. In patient care areas, the ability to obtain the function desired quickly (respiration, cardiac level, etc.) could save a life or prevent permanent damage to a patient. It is for this reason that elevations of equipment and outlets should be checked. Medical gas outlets should never be mounted directly above electrical outlets, as the regulators will obstruct the receptacles. If receptacles and ground jacks are to be mounted in an over-under configuration, the ground jack should be installed below the receptacles. This is due to the logical order of insertion of plugs (that is, if the ground jack were installed above the receptacle, once the ground cable is connected it will hamper the insertion of the power plug since the hanging cable obstructs the receptacle). Receptacles should be mounted between 24 in (588 mm) and 48 in (1176 mm) above the floor, to make them accessible to a visitor or to a patient in a wheelchair and also to lessen the fatigue on staff members who must constantly bend over to connect and disconnect equipment (see 4.3.9(2)(b)). Any area which uses life support devices should have an alternate power system available that can be reached with a 50 ft (14.7 m) extension cord. Consideration should be given to making the entire area a dual power source area, having one alternate (emergency or normal) power receptacle at each bed. Outlets should always be located so that cords connected to them provide the minimum amount of hindrance to the staff.

Each vacuum outlet needs space not only for a regulator on the outlet but also for a vacuum collection bottle either on the outlet, on a slide, in a rack, or on the floor. If patients from one area can overflow into another, these overflow beds should be designed to the most stringent requirements. As an example, if general care beds are sometimes used as acute care beds they should be designed as acute care beds.

4.3.1 Patient Rooms

(1) *Light Care Bed Locations.* Patients in these areas are normally ambulatory, hospitalized for diagnostic testing, physical therapy, or for post-operative and pre-operative observation. They could be undergoing ultrasound, thermography, or radiological examinations. This class of patient requires little nursing care. However, as the age of the patient increases, the care required could approach that of acute care. In some facilities these spaces are listed as hospice or long-term care.

(a) *Medical Gases.* One vacuum outlet between two beds is required for oral suction or sump drains (drains placed in an incision to drain fluid while under slight vacuum). One oxygen outlet at each bed is required for oxygen therapy or Intermittent Positive Pressure Breathing (IPPB). IPPB can be administered pre- and post-operatively.

(b) *Electrical Power Outlets.* An electrical outlet located on the headwall or headwall column is required for each of the following:

1) electric bed
2) portable suction
3) treatment use (for example, K-pad)
4) EKG machine for inpatient test or for an additional K-pad
5) television set
6) patient equipment, shaver, etc.
7) respiratory therapy equipment

When K-pads (hospital heating pads) are used to treat phlebitis, normally both arms or both legs are treated. In the case of an obese person two K-pads may be required for each leg. K-pads are also used to treat blood clots and ulcer patients.

(c) *Communications.* A system should be available at each bedside for both patient and staff to summon help.

(2) *Acute Care Bed Locations.* Acute care represents about 80–85% of the inpatients in a hospital. These patients usually rely on machines of some type and require more nursing care than the light care patient. They may have stomach disorders or require oxygen treatment or suction bags. Post-operative patients, accident victims and people with medical disorders can usually be found in acute

care beds. The vast majority of hospitals being built today are acute care hospitals since more procedures every year are being done at clinics and on an outpatient basis.

(a) *Medical Gases.* Two vacuum outlets should be provided at each bed. One vacuum outlet is for oral suction, while the other is for a sump drain. Increasingly, surgeons are using two sump drains on one patient; this requires both vacuum outlets. One oxygen outlet should be provided at each bed as most acute care patients require either oxygen or oxygen-related therapy. It is suggested that one medical air outlet be provided for the respiratory therapy equipment.

(b) *Electrical Power Outlets.* A typical acute care patient may be a postoperative surgical patient, who is classified stable. His electrical requirements include outlets for:

1) electric bed

2) chest pump

3) portable suction

4) K-pad

5) IVAC machine (used to monitor intravenous solution drips)

6) patient appliance (shaver) or other portable suction (that is, if the patient has two sump drains); this could also be used for monitoring or test equipment

7) television set

8) respiratory therapy equipment

Depending on the intensity of the care offered in the area, emergency power is recommended for at least one duplex outlet. These should be in the headwall. It is recommended that six outlets (three duplex receptacles) be installed.

(c) *Communications.* A system should be available at each bedside for both patient and staff to summon help.

4.3.2 Coronary Care Areas. Coronary care patients vary from electrically susceptible critical list patients to patients ready for release. Depending on the size and operating procedures of the hospital, noncritical patients may be transferred to stepdown and later to acute care.

(1) *Medical Gases.* Each patient bed should be equipped with two vacuum outlets for suction. Also, each bed should have three oxygen outlets and one medical air outlet for respiratory care. Each oxygen outlet can supply approximately 10 liters per minute, while a patient on 100% oxygen can breathe 30 liters per minute.

(2) *Electrical Power Outlets.* The NEC permits the use of single phase grounded power circuits for this area. There are some states that still require the use of ungrounded, isolated power. Where this is the case, specifications for isolation systems are the same as those found in Chapter 6 for use in flammable anesthetizing areas. It is recognized that isolation systems do contribute to overall electrical safety and continuity of power in the event of a line to ground fault.

Eight electrical outlets or 4 duplex outlets should be provided, as cardiac patients can use many pieces of electrical equipment at one time, including

(a) heating water in respirator

(b) suction for nasal gastric tube

(c) swan ganz line

(d) chest pump

(e) electrical bed (if the patient is transferred to the unit from another part of the hospital in "distress" the bed is not usually switched until his condition is stable)

(f) rotating tourniquet

(g) IVAC machine (used to monitor intravenous solution)

(h) respiratory therapy equipment

The lights over the bed should have both a high and a low level.

Each bed shall have at least one dedicated outlet. Emergency power shall be supplied for use with a respirator in coronary care. Circuit breakers should be near the bed and clearly labeled. Consideration should be given to placing a circuit breaker panel in the room.

(3) *Communications.* A system should be available at each bed for both patient and staff to summon help. In these coronary care beds, special consideration should be given to the increased chance of cardiac arrest. Also, a cardiac arrest alarm should be provided with an automatic trip from the monitor and an elapsed time clock to start upon cardiac arrest.

4.3.3 Intensive Care Areas. The intensive care bed may be used for:

Surgical post-op patients

Artificial ventilation of patients

Treating for shock

Cardiac monitoring of post-op

Pacemaking

Peritoneal or haemodialysis

Biochemical correction of severe metabolic disorders

Facilities for portable X-ray use should always be provided. The ICU isolation room can be used to perform tracheotomy or haemodialysis. ICU special patient treatments may include:

Maximum care (breathing and tetanus insufficiency)

Hyperbaric oxygen treatment

Induced hypothermy (−12 °C)

(1) *Medical Gases.* Three vacuum outlets, two oxygen outlets, and one medical air outlet for respiratory care should be provided at each bed. The vacuum outlets are most often used for post-operative patient drains.

(2) *Electrical Power Outlets.* The NEC permits the use of single phase grounded power circuits for this area. There are some states that still require the use of ungrounded, isolated power. Where this is the case, specifications for isolation systems are the same as those found in Chapter 6 for use in flammable anesthetizing areas. It is recognized that isolation systems do contribute to overall electrical safety and continuity of power in the event of a line to ground fault.

At least eight outlets or four duplex electrical outlets should be provided, as cardiac patients can use a lot of electrical equipment at one time, including:

(a) heating water in respirator

(b) suction for nasal gastric tube

(c) swan ganz line

(d) chest pump

(e) electrical bed (if the patient is transferred to the unit from another part of the hospital in "distress," the patient is not usually moved from the electric bed until his condition is stable

(f) rotating tourniquet

(g) IVAC machine (used to monitor intravenous solution)

(h) respiratory therapy equipment

The lights over the bed should have both a high and a low level.

Each bed must have at least one dedicated outlet. Emergency power must be supplied for use of respirator in intensive care. Circuit breakers should be near the bed and clearly labeled. Consideration should be given to placing a circuit breaker panel in the room.

(3) *Communications.* A choice should be available for music or quiet in the bed, quiet for ulcer patients, music to calm or entertain other patients. A nurse call system should be available at each bed for both patient and staff to summon help. Also, a cardiac arrest alarm should be provided with an automatic trip from the monitor and an elapsed time clock to start upon cardiac arrest.

4.3.4 Emergency Suites. An emergency department may consist of trauma, treatment, and minor operating and exam rooms, where a variety of medical procedures takes place. These procedures range from treating accident victims to delivering babies and to typical outpatient work during off-hours. A minor operating room (OR) should be treated as a small surgery room. One class above the minor OR is the trauma room where somewhat similar operations take place without the inhalation anesthetic. General anesthetics are not normally used in emergency room. Both these rooms can involve invasive procedures, and special care should be used as these patients can be electrically susceptible. In some hospitals, babies will be delivered in an OB/GYN room on an emergency basis. This is most apt to happen when a hospital closes its maternity wing or when it is near a poverty-stricken urban area and does not have a maternity wing. The rooms in any emergency department must be analyzed by the governing body of the hospital as to their probable use. The patient holding rooms should be treated as acute care beds as these are used to watch developments. Typically, various emergency department rooms should be designed like the same type of room as found elsewhere in the hospital (that is, a cardiac room is much like a CCU treatment room). Some emergency suites have surgery rooms while others have a less intense treatment philosophy. The hospital must be contacted for the usage.

4.3.5 Surgical Room. There are many types of surgical procedures, each with its own set of criteria. The most important point in surgery room layout is how the room will function. Description of function, typical procedures and traffic patterns can be obtained from the hospital planner(s) who planned the suite. Care should be exercised in equipment layout to prevent obstruction to traffic in the surgery room.

(1) *Medical Gases.* Medical gases need to be determined by both the medical procedures to be performed and the surgical staff operating procedures.

(2) *Electric Power Outlets.* Emergency isolated power is required. Due to the large quantities of equipment used in surgery, 16 electrical outlets (8 duplexes, if straight blade devices are used) are recommended. These outlets should be located primarily in the ceiling-mounted service columns. Provisions should also be made for X-ray power or fluoroscopy machine.

4.3.6 Pediatrics. The pediatrics area is used to treat juveniles. It is important not to alienate any children by sending them to other areas. The pediatrics area should be at least as well equipped as a general care area.

(1) *Pediatric Patient Room.* These rooms should be designed similar to general care rooms, with some rooms equipped similar to acute care rooms and intensive care rooms.

(a) *Medical Gases.* The following medical gas outlets should be provided: one vacuum outlet and one oxygen outlet between each two beds.

(b) *Electrical Power Outlets.* Four electrical outlets or two duplex outlets per bed are recommended. All outlets should be safety-type with tamperproof screws.

(c) *Communications.* Similar to other areas.

(2) *Playrooms.*

(a) *Medical Gases.* For emergency use, playrooms should have one vacuum outlet and one oxygen outlet.

(b) *Electrical Power Outlets.* All electrical outlets should be safety-type with tamperproof screws.

(c) *Communication.* Both staff communication and emergency-help call should be provided.

(3) *Pediatric* (Critical Care). These beds are similar to ICU and CCU: one critical care bed per 20 regular pediatrics beds is suggested, with three oxygen outlets and two vacuum outlets. These beds should be located in the pediatrics wing, once again to prevent alienation of children. The medical gases, electrical power outlets and communications equipment installed in these areas should be similar to those in 4.3.3, except that they should be tamperproof.

4.3.7 Nurseries

(1) *General Nurseries.* These nurseries are where normal newborns are housed. The baby normally sleeps in a bassinet. Nursing care is minimal, while observation is important.

(a) *Medical Gases.* Each bassinet should be equipped with one oxygen and one vacuum outlet. This arrangement permits typical care if minor complications develop.

(b) *Electrical Power Outlets.* Two duplex electrical outlets should be located at each bassinet, one on each side. These should be supplied from emergency power. Normal power should be located outside the bassinet area but within reach of a 50 ft cord as in 4.3.7(3)(b). We suggest that one normal power duplex receptacle be placed in each room.

(c) *Communications.* Each bassinet should be equipped with a staff help/call station, to summon help from the nursing station. At a minimum, place a staff help/call station between the bassinets. In nurseries with limited nighttime staffing, each nursery should be equipped with an emergency help/call system to an adjoining department such as labor-delivery.

(2) *Special Care Nurseries.* Newborns requiring specialized care are kept in the special care nursery. These are babies who have developed complications. The isolette is larger than a typical bassinet, therefore outlet spacing and height should be checked.

(a) *Medical Gases.* Due to the length of care anticipated, each incubator or isolette location should be equipped with two vacuum outlets, two oxygen outlets, and two medical compressed air outlets.

(b) *Electrical Power Outlets.* Due to the increased care in this area, each isolette should be provided with at least 12 electrical outlets or 6 duplex outlets. One should be a dedicated outlet for the incubator or isolette. All outlets again should be on emergency power. Normal power should be located outside the isolette area but within reach of a 50 ft cord as in 4.3.7(3)(b). We suggest that one normal power duplex receptacle be placed in each room.

(c) *Communications.* Communication requirements are the same as in general care nurseries (4.3.7(1)(c)).

(3) *Neonatal Nursery.* Premature babies can be housed in a neonatal or a special care nursery. A large percentage of the babies requiring special care are premature. Premature babies are kept in incubators or isolettes.

(a) *Medical Gases.* Medical gas requirements are the same as in special care nurseries (4.3.7(2)(a)).

(b) *Electrical Power Outlets.* Each incubator should be provided with 12 electrical outlets or 6 duplex outlets and a dedicated incubator outlet, all powered by emergency power. Normal power should be available outside the isolette area within reach of a 50 ft extension cord. We suggest that one normal power duplex receptacle be placed in each room. This will provide power in the event of a failure in the emergency power distribution system.

(c) *Communications.* Communication requirements are the same as in general care nurseries (4.3.7(1)(c)).

4.3.8 Psychiatric Care Areas. Psychiatric care areas are occupied by basically two types of patients, sedate and violent.

(1) *Patient Room* (Sedate). Sedate patients are normally treated in open-type dormitory housing. These rooms are very much like semi-private dormitory rooms. Four electrical outlets (two duplex receptacles) should be provided per bed (one duplex receptacle to each side of bed). All receptacles should be safety-type receptacles with tamperproof screws. Medical gases and communication systems are not usually necessary.

(2) *Patient Care* (Violent). Patients in this category range from physically violent to suicidal. These rooms should therefore be designed to provide as little danger as possible to both the staff and the patients. The staff usually continuously monitors these patients.

(a) *Medical Gases.* For the treatment of medical or emergency cases, one vacuum outlet and one oxygen outlet should be provided. These should be protected and securely concealed when not required, in a locked cabinet or shallow locked closet.

(b) *Electrical Power Outlets.* Three duplex outlets should be provided. These also should be protected and securely concealed when not required, for example, in a shallow locked closet. The general configuration should be similar to acute care beds (4.3.1(2)(b)).

(c) *Communication.* Audio monitoring should be provided via a concealed speaker microphone. Provisions should also be made for staff to summon help.

4.3.9 Rehabilitation Areas

(1) *Drug and Alcohol Abuse.* Patient rooms are similar to dormitory-type psychiatric patient rooms (sedate). Also, there should be detoxification rooms for medical treatment and observation of newly admitted patients. These should be similar to those for violent psychiatric patients, and equipped for medical treatment. See 4.3.8(1) and 4.3.8(2) for the requirements of these rooms.

(2) *Occupational Therapy or Aids to Daily Living—A.D.L.* This area is occupied mostly by patients with new handicaps. Special care should be taken to make their transition back into society a smooth one.

(a) *Light Switches.* Light switches should be located between 36 in (915 mm) to 42 in (1070 mm) above the floor. For convenience, no more than two switches should be located on a single plate. Switch action should be simple and positive. While large area "decorative" type rocker switches permit easier operation by forearm, elbow, etc., normal high quality toggle type switches are not impossible to operate. Normal toggle switches should have full-sized handles for this operation.

Care should be taken to locate all controls (switches), outlets, thermostats, etc.) away from corners and to avoid placing controls over counters, since these locations are particularly inconvenient for persons using wheelchairs.

(b) *Electrical Power Outlets.* In general, electrical outlets are placed at least 24 in (610 mm) above the floor. In areas designed specifically for use by disabled persons, 24 to 32 in (610 to 815 mm) high outlets are recommended.

(c) *Telephones.* Telephone dials, handsets, and coin slots should be located within 48 in (1220 mm) of the floor. Wherever possible, push-button type instruments are recommended over conventional rotary dial sets. Handsets should be on 36 in (915 mm) or longer cords.

4.4 References

[1] ANSI/NFPA 56F-1983, Standard for Nonflammable Medical Gas Systems.

[2] ANSI/NFPA 70-1984, National Electrical Code.

[3] ANSI/NFPA 99-1984, Standard for Health Care Facilities.

[4] ANSI/UL 498-1980, Safety Standard for Attachment Plugs and Receptacles.[19]

---

[19] ANSI/UL publicatios are available from the Sales Department, American National Standards Institute, 1430 Broadway, New York, NY 10018 or from Publication Stock, Underwriters Laboratories, Inc, 333 Pfingsten Rd, Northbrook, IL 60020.

5. Emergency Power Systems

5.1 General Discussion. Emergency power systems are required for all health care facilities. The basic requirements are defined in various local, state and federal codes. Organizations, such as the Joint Commission on Accreditation of Hospitals, also have standards requiring adherence.

This section describes requirements and equipment which are recommended for health care facility emergency power systems and their operation. Suggested methods for system design, installation, testing and maintenance are also included.

The main components of emergency power systems are the generator sets, automatic transfer switches, engine generator controls, engine cranking batteries, and battery charger. Additional equipment may include synchronizing and paralleling equipment for multigenerator set installations, utility peak demand reduction controls, elevator emergency power selector systems and bypass/isolation switches for automatic transfer switches, and uninterruptible power supplies.

5.1.1 Codes and Standards. The following codes and standards offer guidance and mandatory requirements for the design of essential electrical systems in hospitals and other health care facilities.

(1) ANSI/ASME A17.1-1984, Elevators, Escalators, and Moving Walks.[20]

(2) ANSI/NFPA 20-1983, Standard for the Installation of Centrifugal Fire Pumps.

(3) ANSI/NFPA 56F-1983, Standard for Nonflammable Medical Gas Systems.

(4) ANSI/NFPA 70-1984, National Electrical Code

(5) ANSI/NFPA 71-1982, Standard for the Installation, Maintenance and Use of Central Station Signaling Systems.

(6) ANSI/NFPA 72A-1985, Standard for the Installation, Maintenance and Use of Local Protective Signaling Systems.

---

[20] This publication is available from the Sales Department, American National Standards Institute, 1430 Broadway, New York, NY 10018 or from the Order Department, American Society of Mechanical Engineers, 22 Law Drive, Fairfield, NJ 07007.

(7) ANSI/NFPA 72B-1979, Standard for the Installation, Maintenance and Use of Auxiliary Protective Signaling Systems.

(8) ANSI/NFPA 72C-1982, Standard for the Installation, Maintenance and Use of Remote Station Protective Signaling Systems.

(9) ANSI/NFPA 72D-1979, Standard for the Installation, Maintenance and Use of Proprietary Protective Signaling Systems.

(10) ANSI/NFPA 72E-1984, Standard on Automatic Fire Detectors.

(11) ANSI/NFPA 75-1981, Standard for the Protection of Electronic Computer/ Data Processing Equipment.

(12) ANSI/NFPA 99-1984, Standard for Health Care Facilities.

(13) ANSI/NFPA 101-1985, Code for Safety to Life from Fire in Buildings and Structures.

(14) ANSI/NFPA 418-1979, Standard on Roof-top Heliport Construction and Protection.

5.1.1.1 Applicability of Codes and Standards. The codes and standards listed above have been, generally, uniformly adopted by enforcing authorities throughout the United States. It is incumbent upon the designer to ascertain which standards are mandatory within the jurisdiction wherein his project is located. In addition, many municipalities and government agencies have adopted either different or more stringent requirements for the design of essential electrical systems. As an example, all of the military services have adopted standards which, in some cases, differ materially from the codes and standards referenced above. Before undertaking the design of any health care facility, it is always prudent to determine exactly what parameters are required by the Code Enforcing Authority (Authority Having Jurisdiction) in order to avoid unnecessary redesign.

5.1.1.2 Interpretation. In case of questions by the designer as to the intent of any of the listed codes and standards, each document contains a paragraph which outlines the procedures required to obtain an official interpretation. In many cases, an unofficial interpretation may be obtained through informal correspondence with the appropriate committee chairman.

5.2 Generator Sets. An engine driven generator set with on-site fuel supply is the predominant type of emergency power source in hospital and health care facilities. Gas turbine driven sets have not found much usage up to the present time because their starting time normally exceeds the 10 s "on line" requirement. However, turbine manufacturers have recognized this problem and some sets are becoming available with improved starting times. For a discussion on gas turbines refer to ANSI/IEEE 446-1980 [1].[21] Capacities of the engine driven type sets range from approximately 5 kW (6.25 kVA) to 1200 kW (1500 kVA). Gasoline engines are normally used in the lower ranges while diesel engines are used almost exclusively for capacities of 100 kW (125 kVA) or more. Code exceptions sometimes permit the use of off-site fuel supplies for natural gas and LP gas

---

[21] The numbers in brackets correspond to those in the references at the end of this chapter.

driven engines when there is a low probability of both the outside electrical utility and off-site gas line failing simultaneously. Gas driven sets are generally available in sizes similar to diesel.

5.2.1 Location. The preferred location for a standby generator set is the ground floor of the facility. Careful consideration must be given to the location of the standby generator set in order to minimize interruptions caused by natural forces common to the area (for example, storms, floods, earthquakes or hazards created by adjoining structures or activities). Basement locations are to be avoided when they are subject to flooding. It is also more difficult to conduct combustion air, cooling air, and exhaust gases away from engines located in basements. If engine generator sets are installed above ground level, additional vibration isolation between the generator set and the floor is frequently required to prevent structural damage to the building. Standby generator sets may be added to existing buildings in a small separate enclosure. Controls and transfer switches are usually located inside the main building.

5.2.2 Mounting. Two cardinal rules for installing standby generator sets are:

(1) Do *not* attach a generator set directly to a concrete floor. It will crack the structure and transmit unacceptable vibration.

(2) Do *not* directly attach any rigid system, that is, exhaust, remote radiator cooling, to an engine on vibration isolators. The relative motion will eventually fatigue and crack the attachment.

5.2.3 Vibration Isolation. A sheet of fiberglass or waffle rubber mounting pads between the generator set base and the floor may provide adequate vibration isolation where optimum isolation is not required.

Spring type vibration isolators are available. These are also placed between the generator set base and the floor. Spring type vibration isolators have different load ratings. Select the correct number of properly sized isolators to support the total generator set (including water and oil) weight. Locate the isolators so that no isolator is overloaded. Spring type vibration isolators typically have an efficiency of 95 percent or better. This means that less than 5 percent of the vibration of a generator set will be transmitted to the floor.

When spring type vibration isolators are used, the generator set rocks around the crankshaft-generator shaft axis during start-up and shut-down. There is also some rocking during single step load changes of 50 percent or more of generator capacity. Use flexible connections in all external lines connected to the generator set. This includes electrical conduit, exhaust pipe and fuel lines as a minimum. It may also include coolant lines to a remote radiator, lube oil makeup and drain lines and engine air intake connections.

Additional generator set mass gives additional vibration isolation. The generator set mass may be increased by attaching an inertia block weighing one or more times the generator set package weight. With greater mass, the vibration energy has less effect. Spring isolators are then placed between the inertia block and the supporting structure to further reduce transmitted vibration (see Fig 33). This arrangement is frequently used when generator sets are installed on floors above ground level. If the generator set package is mounted to an inertia block supported by earth, it may be isolated from the floor of the building by pouring a rubber gasket between the two surfaces (see Fig 34). Table 7 lists the load bearing capability of various materials. Lining the inertia block excavation with tamped sand or gravel will minimize the vibration transmitted through the earth to nearby equipment.

Installations should be coordinated with and reviewed by the responsible structural engineer on the project.

Fig 33
Steel-Concrete Inertia Spring Mounts

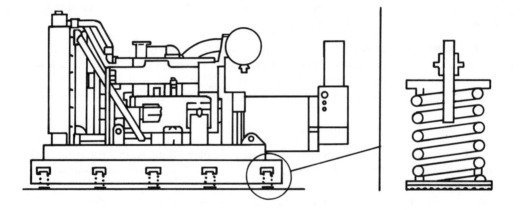

Fig 34
Poured Rubber Gasket Between Two Surfaces

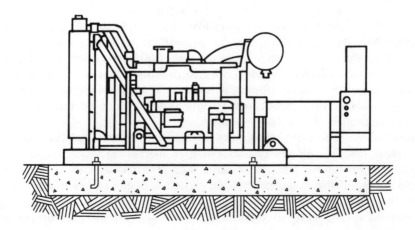

Table 7
Load-Bearing Capabilities of Various Materials

Nature of Bearing Material	Safe Bearing Capacity (lb/ft^2)
Hard rock—granite, etc	50 000–200 000
Medium rock—shale, etc	20 000– 30 000
Hardpan	16 000– 20 000
Soft rock	10 000– 20 000
Compacted sand and gravel	10 000– 12 000
Hard clay	8 000– 10 000
Gravel and coarse sand	8 000– 10 000
Loose, medium and coarse sand, compacted fine sand	6 000– 8 000
Medium clay	4 000– 8 000
Loose fine sand	2 000– 4 000
Soft clay	2 000

5.2.4 Exhaust System. In order to produce rated power, the exhaust system restriction at the engine must not exceed the engine manufacturer's recommendations. In addition, the exhaust system components must not impose undue stress on the engine exhaust outlet connection. Weight, inertia, relative motion of components, and thermal growth from temperature change all contribute to stress on the engine exhaust outlet. The exhaust system should also prevent water from entering the turbocharger or the engine proper. Common sources of water are rain, snow, and condensation of exhaust gas. As a final consideration, the exhaust gas should be directed so that it does not have an adverse effect on the air cleaner, the cooling system, the generator set ambient temperature, or the operator.

If an engine must work against excessive back pressure in the exhaust system, the usable engine power is reduced. Also, the air-fuel ratio is reduced because of incomplete scavenging of the cylinders, the fuel economy is reduced, and exhaust temperatures increase.

The exhaust back pressure imposed in a given engine installation depends on the size of the exhaust pipe, the number and type of bends, and fittings, and the silencer selection. Tight bends usually contribute the most to high exhaust back pressure. Back pressure is proportional to the fifth power of pipe diameter. Therefore, a small increase in exhaust pipe diameter dramatically reduces system back pressure. The engine manufacturer can normally provide the exhaust gas flow and temperature. The pressure developed in the pipe can be determined from Fig 35. The exhaust silencer manufacturer can provide the pressure drop through the silencer for a given flow and temperature. The pressure developed in the pipe and elbows plus the pressure drop through the silencer gives the back pressure at the engine.

Provisions should be made for relative movement between the exhaust piping and the engine so that no damaging stresses will be imposed on the exhaust system components because of engine mounting flexibility or thermal growth.

Fig 35
Back Pressure Nomograph

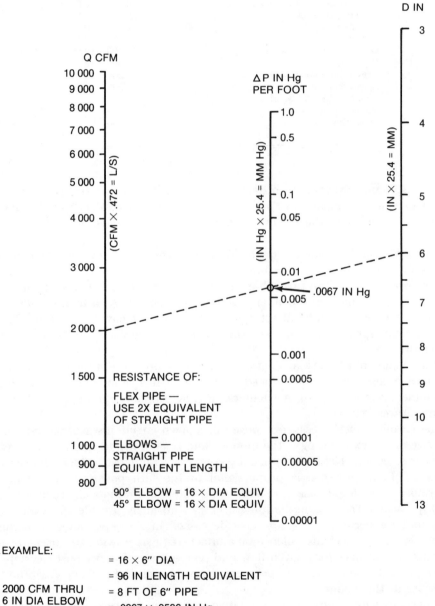

A 50 ft length of pipe expands over 3 in when the temperature is raised from 70 °F to 800 °F. The most common method of obtaining flexibiity is through the use of flexible piping (spiral or bellow type). Flexible sections are required in the piping between any components where either relative motion or thermal growth will subject the components to excessive stresses. The optimum location for the flexible section is within 4 ft of the engine exhaust outlet. For proper installation, the flexible pipe should not be used to form pipe bends or compensate for misalignment.

Black iron schedule 40 pipe is most commonly used for permanent installation where the weight is not a factor.

There are many ways to obtain the desired flexibility while still adequately supporting the piping and other components in the system. To reduce the loading imposed on the exhaust manifold or turbocharger, it is necessary to support long lengths of piping from the surrounding structure. However, flexibility should still be maintained through the design of the support and the use of flexible connections. The weight of all external engine exhaust piping should be supported so as not to impose any dead weight loads on the engine exhaust outlet connection.

Rain and snow should not enter the exhaust outlet opening. Counterbalanced flapper type rain caps are used in many installations. Conical and other ventilating covers are not widely used since they produce a relatively high exhaust pressure or are not suitable for operation in the prevailing exhaust temperature. Exhaust outlets which point upward are preferred since they do not direct the exhaust noise toward adjacent structures. Where the noise in a specific direction is not a problem, horizontal exhaust outlets may be used. Cutting the end of the pipe at a 45-degree angle with the top extended is normally adequate to prevent the entrance of rain and snow. If horizontal exhaust pipes are used, care should be taken so that the exhaust gas will not be drawn back into the engine room with the ventilation air. Care should also be taken in the location of the exhaust outlet point so that exhaust gas will not be drawn into any of the outside air intakes.

From an aesthetic point of view, care should be given to the location of the exhaust outlet point and the tendency over a period of time for exhaust gas carbon deposits to accumulate on any nearby structures.

Water is formed in the combustion of gas, gasoline or diesel fuel. Therefore, a condensate trap and drain valve should be installed in the exhaust system. The condensate trap should be as close to the engine as practical.

In multiengine installations, special consideration should be given when manifolding or joining the exhaust runs from two or more engines into one common exhaust run. Engines will have a lower back pressure if each exhaust enters the exhaust flow at an angle toward the flow rather than opposing the flow (refer to Fig 36).

If all engines are not run at the same time, the exhaust gas from the operating engines can condense in the engine which is not running. This may cause a hydraulic lock in the stopped engine. Check valves in the exhaust lines have not solved this problem and in general are unsatisfactory in exhaust systems.

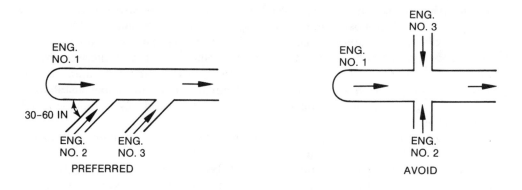

Fig 36
Exhaust Pipe Manifolding Plan View

5.2.5 Air Supply. A generator set requires air for combustion and cooling. Even when remote radiator or heat exhanger cooling systems are used, air flow is required to remove the heat produced by the generator as well as the heat radiated by the engine and exhaust system.

Generators are normally rated for operation in a 104 °F (40 °C) ambient temperature. If the air intake is to be higher than 104 °F, some reduction of the output rating is required. The engine manufacturer can give the engine combustion air requirements at rated load and will define the maximum air restriction permissible and the recommended air intake temperature range. The engine air intake system should be able to supply clean combustion air to the engine without excessive restriction and within the manufacturer's temperature range. Dirt is the basic cause of wear in an engine. The effectiveness of the air cleaner and air piping system has a significant impact on engine life and maintenance costs. Dry type air cleaners filter the air through a replaceable pleated paper element. The efficiency of a dry type air filter is normally greater than 99.9% at any air flow. Dry type air cleaners do become plugged and provide excessive air restriction when dirty. Oil bath air filters have an efficiency greater than 98% at rated air flow. This efficiency decreases to approximately 95% at 15% of rated flow. Oil pullover into the engine is possible at excessive air flows. However, oil bath air filters do not become plugged or offer excessive air restriction at rated air flow. Dry type air filters are preferred for standby generator sets.

Most standby generator sets for hospitals have an engine mounted air cleaner which meets the engine requirements for adequate clean air.

When a generator set mounted radiator and fan are used, the fan drives the room air throughout the radiator and out of the building. Under load, the air from the radiator is normally at 150 to 185 °F (65 to 85 °C). If the air flow were reversed, the room temperature would approach 150 to 185 °F which is much too hot for the engine, the generator or any people in the room. When the fan is blowing radiator air out of the room, there must be an adequate area for air to enter the room. If the radiator fan delivery is known, this area can be calculated to give a maximum air intake velocity. An air intake velocity of up to 20 mi/h (30 ft/s or 9 m/s) is frequently acceptable. If the fan delivery is unknown, an air intake area equal to 1½ times the radiator core area is frequently used as a rule of thumb.

The air intake area is preferably located to the rear of the generator set. Fresh air then flows around and through the generator, then past the engine and through the fan and radiator. Frequently the intake air must enter at the top or sides of the room. In such cases, air flow outside the room should be checked to make sure that radiator and engine exhaust are not drawn back into the room with the intake air.

Many standby generator sets do not have a fan and radiator in the engine room. A remote mounted radiator or heat exchanger is frequently used. Installations without a radiator fan require auxiliary room ventilation to remove the heat from the room. Installations with a radiator fan in the generator set room normally have adequate room air flow and the following calculations are unnecessary.

The heat produced by the generator and radiated by the engine at rated load is approximately 35% of the kW rating of the generator. This percentage can be 5% higher for units under 100 kW and 5% lower for units over 500 kW. Uninsulated exhaust pipes and mufflers within the generator set room add to the heat which must be removed by the auxiliary ventilation system.

The auxiliary air flow required is determined by the heat to be removed and the acceptable temperature rise in the room. Many engines begin to have a significant loss of power when combustion intake air temperature exceeds 120 °F (49 °C). Maximum ambient air temperatures vary widely. A 100 °F ambient covers most of the more populous regions of the world. The difference or acceptable temperature rise is 20 °F (11 °C). The specific heat of air at constant pressure (Cp = .24 Btu/lb-°F) is essentially constant for air over a range of 80 to 130 °F (27 to 54 °C). The density of air changes with barometric pressure as well as altitude. At standard conditions, air density is .075372 lb/ft^3 at 500 ft altitude. Multiplying the specific heat by the density at 500 ft gives a heat coefficient of .018089 Btu/ft^3 °F. For general use, this may be rounded to .018 Btu/ft^3 °F. From this, the air flow in cfm is equal to the rate of heat rejection divided by the heat coefficient and the acceptable temperature rise.

$$C = \frac{Q}{0.018 \cdot T}$$

(Eq 1)

where

C = air flow in ft^3/min

Q = heat rejection in Btu/min

T = acceptable temperature rise in °F

One kW is the equivalent of 3412 Btu/hr or 58.87 Btu/min. Substituting this in Eq 1 yields:

$$C = \frac{kW \cdot 10^3}{0.305 \cdot T} \qquad\qquad \text{(Eq 2)}$$

where

  C = air flow in ft^3/min

kW = heat rejection to room in kilowatts

  T = acceptable temperature rise in °F

Example: A 250 kW generator set is to be installed in a hospital basement. The radiator and fan are remotely mounted on the roof of the building. The maximum outdoor design temperature is 105 °F. It is desired to limit the engine room temperature to 120 °F.

The temperature rise in the room (ΔT) is 120 °F – 105 °F = 15 °F.

The heat produced in the room at rated output will be approximately 35 percent of rated output or .35 · 250 kW = 87.5 kW. From Eq 2 the air flow is:

$$C = \frac{87.5 \cdot 10^3}{0.305 \cdot 15} \quad \text{or } 19\,126 \text{ ft}^3/\text{min}$$

5.2.6 Cooling. Almost all standby generator sets 50 kW and larger use liquid cooled engines. The cooling air flow requirements for air cooled engines should be obtained from the engine manufacturer.

Liquid cooled engines usually have a generator set mounted radiator and engine drive fan. The selection of radiator core, fan, shroud, guards, fan drive ratio, etc, is made to provide adequate cooling of the engine. However, this selection is based on a free flow of cool (normally 100 °F or less) air to the radiator core and a free flow of air away from the core. The quantity of air required is normally listed by the manufacturer or generator set assembler.

The arrangement of the power room and the facilities availability (that is, raw water) normally dictate whether a radiator or heat exchanger is used for a liquid cooled engine. If there is a choice, a generator set mounted radiator is normally preferred. It is independent of an external source of water and there is normally an adequate supply of combustion and generator cooling air. With a set mounted radiator, there are no coolant flex connections, long coolant lines or coolant shutoff valves, all of which are potential trouble sources.

Remote radiators do provide a means of removing fan noise to a noncritical location. Heat exchangers are not a noise source and also do not require power from the engine for a fan. A heat exchanger cooled unit can normally deliver three to five percent more power from the generator.

The combination of a heat exchanger feeding a remote radiator should be avoided if at all possible. Such a system has all of the disadvantages of each system at approximately four times the cost. Since the cooling capacity of both the heat exchanger and radiator depend on the temperature difference of the cooling media, both the radiator and the heat exchanger must be approximately doubled in size.

Ducting may be required to take the hot air from the radiator to the outside. The ductwork must be smooth and free from obstructions, seams, fins, leaks, or sudden bends. If louvers or grills are added to the exit, then the frontal area must be increased accordingly in a smooth transition to the larger opening size. If bends in the duct are unavoidable, then turning vanes may be required to reduce pressure loss.

A heat exchanger cooling system is sometimes used where a source of cool water is available. Sources of water may be city, sea, river, lake, or well water. In a heat exchanger system, the engine cooling water flows in a closed loop from the engine to the heat exchanger and back to the engine. Raw water from the city, sea, etc, flows in a separate circuit within the heat exchanger and removes heat from the engine cooling water. If a city water supply is being evaluated as a source of water from the heat exchanger, the possibility of interruption of city water during a prolonged emergency has to be considered. For health care facilities, this method of cooling is not recommended if one of the other methods is available.

Also, if the water from the heat exchanger is to be dumped into the sewage system, it should not violate local conservation or natural resource ordinances, or overload the sewage system. Some heat exchangers may require a pressure reducing valve to limit the pressure supplied by a city water system to an acceptable valve for the heat exchanger.

Remote radiators fall into two categories:

(1) Radiator located horizontally remote from the engine.

(2) Radiators located vertically remote (above) the engine.

The primary concern when a radiator is horizontally remote is that the water pipe resistance to flow not exceed the engine driven water pump capability. The engine manufacturer will normally list the total permissible pressure on the pump and the maximum allowable external friction head. External pipe should be free of obstructions, excessive bends, elbows, tees or couplings. It should be clean and free of rust, scale, weld slag, or corrosive material. It should not collapse while being formed or while in service. The internal diameter should be greater than the water pump inlet diameter. Figures 37 and 38 may be used for estimating pressure drop in pipe, fittings, reducers, etc. The external circuit should be coupled to the engine via a flexible connection which permits engine movement without restraint and thermal expansion of the line.

Valves and couplings should normally be provided between the engine and the remote cooling system. By closing the valves, the engine may be serviced without draining the entire cooling system. Care should be taken to prevent the valves from being left closed accidentally. If this occurs, the generator set will be rendered useless.

Many engine coolant systems are not readily compatible with an auxiliary booster pump. Consult the engine manufacturer before specifying an auxiliary booster pump. It is good practice in health care facilities to avoid designs, when possible, that depend on auxiliary power systems energized by the system that they support or by other external power systems subject to the same disturbance.

Installations where the radiator is below the engine level are rare and can cause problems. The primary problem is usually an air lock which prevents water circulation. A prime requirement in such installations is the proper location of air vents in areas where air pockets are likely to form in the cooling system.

Installations where the radiator is above the engine level are quite common. The maximum height of the radiator above the engine is limited by the static pressure which can be imposed on the cooling system seals and gaskets without leakage. The engine manufacturer should be consulted if a limiting head or pressure is not available. The friction head should still be within the engine manufacturer's limits and may be estimated from Figs 37 and Fig 38. Flexible couplings at the engine are required for connection to the remote cooling system.

If a higher radiator position is necessary, the engine should be separated from the radiator circuit. Figure 39 illustrates such a system although many variations are possible. Both circuits circulate from a common reservoir, commonly called a "Hot Well," "Hot Tank," or "Compound Cooling" system. With the basic Hot Well the engine merely pumps coolant to and from the tank. The tank acts as a blending tank, an expansion tank, and holds the radiator and line coolant when the radiator auxiliary coolant pump is shut down. When vertical radiators are used, it may be beneficial to put coolant in at the bottom of the radiator. This keeps the radiator filled during operation. The tank should be vented to the atmosphere in order to accommodate the large changes of coolant volume in the tank. A sight glass on the hot tank is recommended with markings for the "run" and "stopped" levels. High and Low marks on both levels are helpful. It is good practice to design cooling systems to allow for a 10% reduction in cooling capability owing to deterioration over the operating life.

5.2.7 Temperature. Provisions should be made to maintain the generator room at not less than 50 °F (10 °C) or the engine water jacket temperature at not less than 70 °F (21.1 °C).

Electric coolant heaters are the most common method of maintaining the engine coolant above 70 °F. In order to assure fast starts and good load acceptance, one engine manufacturer recommends that standby generator set engine coolant be maintained at a minimum of 120 °F (49 °C). Thermostatically controlled tank type jacket water heaters provide coolant circulation which heats the entire engine. These heaters must be turned off when the engine is running.

Electric oil immersion heaters may be used to maintain lubricating oil temperatures. Oil heaters are frequently controlled by the same thermostat as the jacket water temperature.

5.2.8 Starting. Battery electric systems and compressed air systems are used for starting standby generator sets. The selection of a starting system depends upon the type of engine, readily available energy source such as compressed air, and customer preference. Each system has certain advantages under specific conditions.

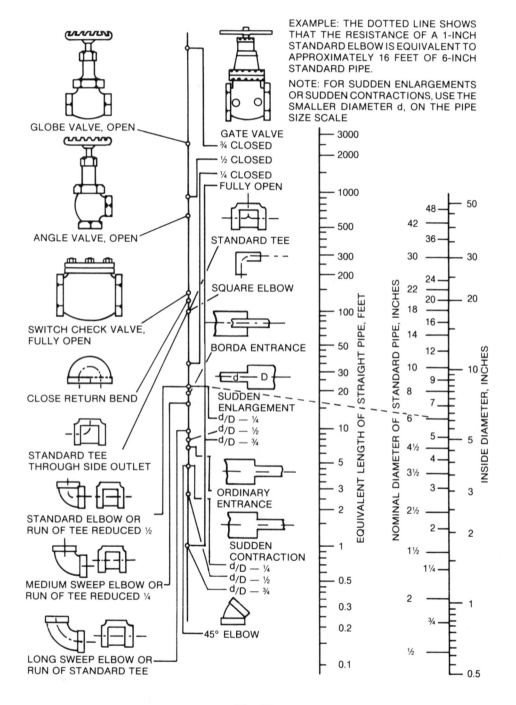

**Fig 37
Resistance of Valves and Fittings to Flow of Fluids**

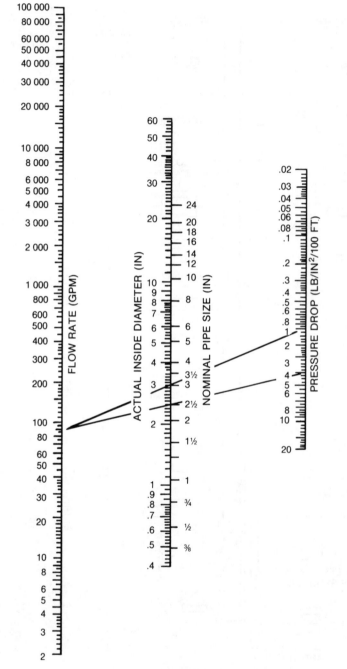

**Fig 38
Fluid Flow in Pipe**

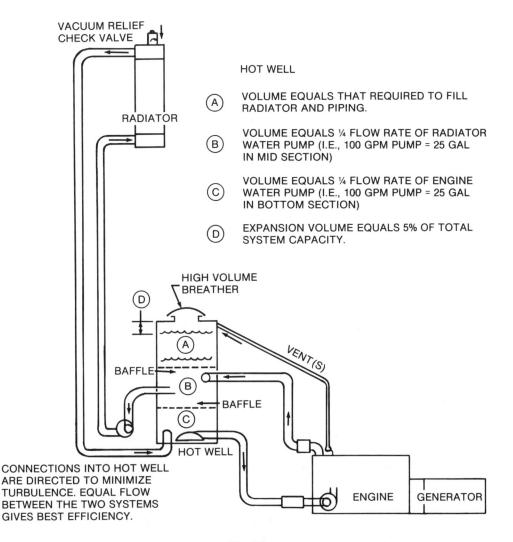

**Fig 39
Hot Well Cooling System**

Electric starting is the most common starting method and offers a compact, convenient, economical, and dependable method of starting engine driven standby generator sets. The engine portion of the system consists of a starting motor, batteries and some method of connecting and disconnecting the starting motor to the batteries. In standby power applications the batteries are normally maintained and recharged by a battery charger powered by the essential electrical system.

Many engine starters are "positive engage" type. In this type of starter motor, the starter pinion must be fully engaged with the engine ring gear before cranking commences. The system works quite well about 98% of the time. However, approximately 2% of the time a pinion tooth abuts directly with a ring gear tooth and the motor does not crank. To eliminate this problem, "cycle cranking" is preferred. In cycle cranking, a cranking period is followed by a reset period. This is followed by subsequent crank and rest periods. The starter pinion is turned slightly at the start of each rest period and the probability of successive tooth abutments approaches zero. The timing of the crank and rest cycles is usually combined in an automatic cranking panel. The automatic cranking panel should also include some means to terminate cranking when the engine starts and a method of disabling the engine safety shutdown controls (other than overspeed and overcrank) during starting.

ANSI/NFPA 99-1984 [3] requires that internal combustion engine starting batteries have sufficient capacity to provide 60 seconds of continuous cranking. The engine manufacturer will normally define the battery capacity required to meet this requirement. The definition will usually be in terms of CCA (Cold Cranking Amperes) as defined by SAE J537-82 [8]. This standard is essentially applicable to lead-acid batteries (and variations thereof) only. Nickel-cadmium batteries are widely used for engine cranking. EGSA ECB1-1977 [6] may be used to specify either lead-acid or nickel-cadmium battery performance.

When a plentiful supply of compressed air is available, air can be an economical method of starting a standby generator set. Two types of compressed air starting are used.

(1) *Air motor.* An air motor drives a ring gear from the air starter motor pinion. This is similar to the electric starter. It is usually used on 1200 and 1800 rpm engines.

(2) *Direct air injection.* Compressed air is injected into the individual cylinders by an air distributor system. This system is usually found on only the larger engines which operate at 900 rpm or below. It has the advantage that full engine torque is produced during cranking. This produces rapid acceleration.

To prevent problems, air starting systems require a sufficiently sized air tank and an auxiliary source of compressed air. An air tank with sufficient capacity to provide five 10-second cranking attempts, as required by ANSI/NFPA 99-1984 [3], will take up considerable space and could be a significant factor in determining which starting method should be used. Electric motor driven air compressors are the most convenient means of recharging air tanks. However, during a utility power failure, these compressors are unavailable. An auxiliary gasoline engine driven air compressor is one solution to this common problem and is recommended for air start installations in health care facilities.

When a facility does not have a reliable supply of compressed air readily available, the electric start method is more practical and economical.

5.2.9 Governor. A governor regulates the standby generator set engine speed which is directly proportional to frequency. Although gear reduction is used to couple gas turbines to ac generators, it has not been widely accepted on internal combustion engines. When an engine is directly coupled to an ac generator, the engine must run at 3600, 1800, 1200 or other lower synchronous speeds to produce 60 Hz. The governor regulates the amount of fuel delivered to the engine at various loads to keep the speed or frequency relatively constant.

The traditional governor utilizes rotating flyweights to sense speed and a spring (speeder spring) as a reference. More sophisticated flyweight governors use hydraulic pressure to turn a shaft which is connected to the engine throttle or rack. Many hydraulic governors can operate isochronously, that is, same speed at no load and full load and maintain the speed or frequency steady state stability within +0.25%.

All electric and electro-hydraulic governors are available which sense speed from pulses generated by a magnetic pickup mounted adjacent to an engine gear, usually the flywheel ring gear. Electric governors provide the same characteristics as hydraulic governors, but have the advantage of a quicker response time. They act faster. Electric governors are also available with numerous accessories which may be useful in specific applications. These include:

(1) Electric load sensing for isochronous load sharing among paralleled generator sets.

(2) Electric load sensing for "load anticipation" to further reduce response time.

(3) "Ramp acceleration" to provide a controlled acceleration rate and reduce frequency overshoot on start-up.

(4) Electronic speed adjustment to adjust engine speed for synchronizing generators.

(5) Reverse and forward power monitors that provide an output signal if power flows toward the generator or when a preset output power level has been reached, or both.

A reduction in the frequency response time of single unit generator sets with the "load anticipation" option is observable on a frequency strip chart recorder. However, this decrease in response time of a few tenths of a second is not readily discernible in a health care facility. "Load anticipation," on single unit generator sets, essentially doubles the governor cost and is ten times as difficult to connect correctly. Load sensing governors for single unit engine applications are rare.

Lights, motors, heating and most other power equipment will operate satisfactorily if the frequency remains between 60 and 62 Hz. This is approximately three percent frequency droop, that is, 61.8 Hz at no load, 60.0 Hz at rated load. For many computers to function properly, the frequency must be 60.0 ±0.5 Hz. If any of these computers are to be operated directly (not through a UPS or uninterrupted power supply) from a standby generator set, an isochronous governor is required.

5.2.10 Fuel Supply. In order to operate properly, an engine should have an adequate supply of fuel which meets the engine manufacturer's recommendations. All installations should incorporate a fuel filter to remove flakes, dirt, metallic chips, and water from whatever source, including condensation.

A day tank, sometimes called a "service tank" or "ready tank," is recommended for all standby generator set installations. A day tank provides an ample supply of clean fuel at a relatively constant head, regardless of the fuel level in the bulk storage tank. The day tank does not necessarily hold a day's supply of fuel. More commonly, a day tank is specified to hold at least the amount of fuel that would be burned in one hour at rated load. A day tank provides a readily available supply of fuel independent of bulk storage and acts as an emergency supply in the event of failure of the auxiliary fuel pump, connecting fuel lines, or float-control switch. For diesel engines, it also acts as a relief and bypass tank for diesel fuel that is circulated to the injectors. When the bulk storage fuel level is far enough above the day tank to give adequate gravity flow, a float valve or float switch and fuel shut-off solenoid should be used. In other installations a day tank fuel transfer pump should be used. A primary filter is usually recommended between the bulk storage tank and the day tank. In multiple engine installations, a single common day tank is sometimes used. Such arrangements should be equipped with appropriate fuel isolation valves for maintenance of individual systems.

The capacity of the bulk storage tank is essentially determined by the expected length of a disaster which might interrupt fuel delivery. Since this is a very subjective criteria, it is noted that bulk storage tanks usually have less than a 30-day and more than a 3-day fuel supply. A common recommendation is that 14 days of fuel storage capacity be installed. However, the user should carefully review his own particular problem and specific needs. Many diesel engines operate satisfactorily on boiler fuel oil. When oil fired boilers are used, a common bulk storage tank is often used for the furnace and the standby diesel generator set.

Water condensation and contamination is the primary problem with long term storage of fuel. There will also be some evaporation, particularly of the more volatile parts of gasoline. Sometimes there are comments that bacterial action may contaminate diesel fuel, but these claims are difficult to substantiate. Storage of diesel fuel up to one year is satisfactory. After this, samples should be taken at six month intervals to assure that fuel deterioration has not occurred. Check for water in the fuel storage tank should be made every two weeks. This is particularly important in above ground storage tanks.

5.2.11 Ratings. Internal combustion engines are rated in hp or kW, or both, output at a given speed, intake air temperature and barometric pressure or altitude. Although gas turbines use a gear reduction to produce a synchronous generator speed, gear reducers have not been widely accepted on gasoline or diesel engine driven generator sets. Most internal combustion engines must therefore operate at the synchronous speeds of 3600, 1800, 1200, 900, etc, rpm to produce 60 Hz. As the speed is decreased, the mass and cost increases in a generally linear relationship. However, 3600 rpm internal combustion engine generator sets are, in general, limited to 25 kW output or below.

Engines are rated in hp and kW output. The engine kW rating should not be confused with the generator kW rating. As a rule of thumb, 1½ hp is required from an engine to produce 1 electrical kW from an engine. Some of the engine power is required to drive the radiator cooling fan while the largest power loss is within the ac generator itself.

Non-turbocharged gasoline and diesel engines have an inherent limit on the power they can produce at a given speed. The limit is essentially established by the amount of air which can be pulled into a cylinder for combustion. If excess fuel is used, combustion is incomplete and the excess fuel goes out the exhaust as carbon (smoke or soot), carbon monoxide, and unburned hydrocarbons.

This limitation does not apply to turbocharged engines. As engine load increases, the turbocharger forces more air into each cylinder, which can now burn additional fuel to produce additional power and additional air into the cylinders. If the fuel or air is not limited by some means, this can become a self-sustaining continuity until stresses exceed the breaking point or something melts. Any turbocharged engine can be fueled to produce 10% additional power, but the useful life of the engine will probably be reduced. The engine manufacturer's published standby ratings of engines are normally the maximum ratings that the manufacturer believes, from experience and test, will give satisfactory service. Standby ratings are frequently published with no overload 'capability although additional capability can usually be demonstrated.

5.2.12 Sizing the Alternator. The alternator should be sized based on two types of loading. These are the maximum continuous load the alternator will carry and the motor load which the alternator will be required to start.

First, consider the maximum connected load. This load includes the lighting, heating, and running motor loads which the alternator will be required to carry at one time.

As an example, consider a small facility with a 100 kW lighting load, 50 kW of water heaters, a 25 hp blower motor on the heating and air conditioning system, a 50 hp air conditioning compressor motor and two 25 hp elevator motors.

Therefore, the total connected running load is as follows:

25 hp Code G blower motor

$$kW = \frac{68 \text{ running A} \cdot 230 \text{ \# V} \cdot 0.8 \text{ pf} \cdot \sqrt{3}}{1000} = 21.7 \text{ kW}$$

50 hp Code G air conditioning compressor motor

$$kW = \frac{130 \text{ A} \cdot 230 \text{ \# V} \cdot 0.8 \text{ pf} \cdot \sqrt{3}}{1000} = 41.4 \text{ kW}$$

25 hp Code G elevator motor

$$kW = \frac{68 \text{ A} \cdot 230 \text{ \# V} \cdot 0.8 \text{ pf} \cdot \sqrt{3}}{1000} = 21.7 \text{ kW}$$

25 hp Code G elevator motor

$$kW = \frac{68 \text{ running A} \cdot 230 \text{ \# V} \cdot 0.8 \text{ pf} \cdot \sqrt{3}}{1000} = 21.7 \text{ kW}$$

$$\text{Total Running Load} = 256.5 \text{ kW}$$

Now consider the total motor load the alternator will be required to start. It is virtually impossible for all four motors to start at the same time; however, since there is nothing to prevent it from happening, consider this to be the worst case condition. Since most motor starters will drop out at about 60% voltage, we should limit the voltage dip on motor starting to 35%.

Motor starting capability of alternators will vary depending on the alternator, type of exciter, voltage regulator and voltage regulator accessories used.

Most present-day alternators have a minimum across-the-line motor starting capability of .5 hp/kW with a 35% voltage dip. The total connected motor load in our example is 125 hp; therefore, the required alternator motor starting kW would be:

$$kW = 125 \text{ hp} \times \frac{kW}{.5 \text{ hp}} = 250 \text{ kW}$$

The continuous running load of 256.5 kW is slightly larger than the 250 kW motor starting requirement and would be the determining load. Since the demand for electric power is continually increasing with new appliances and lighting added from time to time, an allowance for future requirements should be made. A general industry practice is for the load to be not more than 80% of the alternator rating on a new installation. Applying this rule to this example, the kW requirement would then be an alternator of $\frac{256.5 \text{ kW}}{.8}$ = 320.6 kW. Since this is not an even rating, the next higher rating of 325 kW would be utilized.

5.2.13 Voltage Regulators. There are four basic types of voltage regulation systems available today. They include:

(1) The static exciter-regulator which not only regulates the alternator voltage but also supplies the excitation power to the alternator field.

(2) The brushless self-excited automatic voltage regulator.

(3) The brushless separately excited automatic voltage regulator.

(4) The self-excited self-regulated system which does not use a separate voltage regulator.

The first three systems provide typical voltage regulation of 0.25 to 2% and the fourth provides typically 4% regulation. All systems may be adequate for health care facilities provided the connected loads can withstand the voltage variations. Refer to Chapter 9 which deals with voltage variation susceptibility of hospital medical equipment and instrumentation.

(a) *Static Exciter-Regulator.* The static exciter-regulator is a solid state device which takes its supply from the main stator output voltage for both the input reference and the power input. The input power is rectified to direct current and is the controlled input through brushes and slip rings to the main field of the alternator. This system has a fast response to load changes and has the motor starting capability of a half horsepower per kilowatt with a 35% voltage dip (see Fig 40).

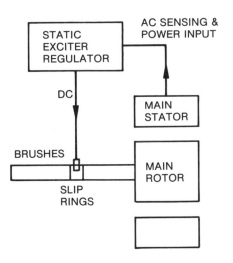

Fig 40
Static Exciter-Regulator System

The static exciter-regulator is not self-exciting and requires an external dc source to flash the field for initial voltage build-up of the alternator. This is usually accomplished by a dc circuit connected to the engine starting batteries which is automatically disconnected when the ac voltage builds up.

(b) *Brushless Self-Excited Automatic Voltage Regulator*. The brushless self-excited automatic voltage regulator also takes its supply from the main stator windings for both the reference input and the power input. The input power is controlled by the reference voltage and control portion of the regulator. It is rectified to dc and becomes the outpower to the exciter stator. This regulator is self-exciting from the residual voltage of the alternator. Typically, the contacts of a normally closed relay or a solid state relay are used to apply the alternator residual voltage directly to a full wave bridge and to the exciter field. As the ac voltage builds up, the relay picks up, disconnecting the build up circuit (see Fig 41).

(c) *Brushless Separately Excited Automatic Voltage Regulator*. The separately excited automatic voltage regulator receives input power from a separate source but receives reference voltage input from the alternator windings. Separate input power is usually provided by a permanent magnet generator mounted on the same shaft as the exciter and main rotors.

The permanent magnetic generator provides a nearly constant power source under all operating conditions and is not affected by external load. Excitation is greater than the full load requirements of the alternator and is usually high enough to sustain a short circuit current of three times rated current.

Whereas the static exciter-regulator, the self-excited voltage regulator, and some separately excited regulators sense a lower than normal output voltage and "turn on" to increase the excitation to the exciter field to bring the output voltage

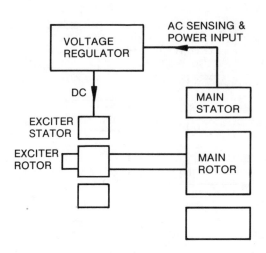

Fig 41
Self-Excited Regulated System

back up to normal, some separately excited voltage regulators work in reverse. Since the permanent magnet generator always provides more excitation than is required for normal voltage output, the voltage regulator must act to suppress the excitation. Therefore, when a lower than normal output voltage is sensed, the voltage regulator "turns off" to increase the excitation to the exciter field to bring the output voltage back up to normal (see Fig 42).

Fig 42
Separately Excited System

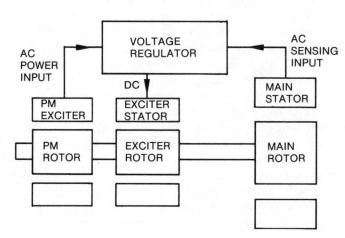

This system has a fast response to load changes and has the motor starting ability of ¾ hp/kW with a 35% voltage dip.

(d) *Self-Excited Self-Regulated System.* The self-excited Aself-regulated system does not use a separate voltage regulator. There are various methods to accomplish this, but in almost all systems voltage build-up occurs from residual voltage or residual voltage plus the addition of permanent magnets in the field circuit. The excitation required for no load voltage is supplied by a portion of the main stator winding voltage. The output voltage is maintained under load by using the load current to provide excitation to the exciter. Most exciter fields utilize direct current; however, one manufacturer uses alternating current in the exciter field (see Fig 43).

Since these systems utilize the load current for exciter power, they are very responsive to load changes and have a motor starting ability of 1 hp/kW with a 35% voltage dip.

5.2.14 Parallel Operation. To operate two or more generators in parallel, provisions should be made for the generators to share the reactive load current proportionally and prevent circulating currents. Proportional sharing of the real kW load current is controlled by the engine governor.

Fig 43
Self-Excited Self-Regulated System

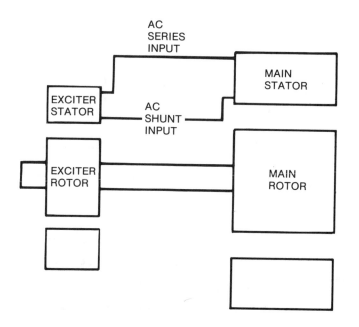

The static exciter-regulators, self-excited regulators and the separately excited regulators are all capable of parallel operation when equipped with parallel provisions.

There are two methods of controlling or sharing reactive load current when paralleling generators: (1) Voltage droop method, and (2) Cross-current compensation method.

(1) *Voltage Droop Method.* The parallel module for the voltage droop method consists of a low secondary current transformer installed in generator phase 2 when the regulator sensing is from line 1 to line 3. If three-phase sensing is used, a second CT installed in phase 1 is also required. Figure 44 shows a single-phase sensing arrangement. The current transformer develops a voltage signal across an adjustable resistor connected across the CT secondary which is proportional in amplitude and phase to the generator line current. This voltage is connected in series with the voltage applied to the voltage regulator sensing circuit. The result is that the voltage applied to the voltage regulator sensing circuit is the vector sum of the generator ac voltage and the voltage developed by the paralleling module. The voltage supplied by the paralleling module is small in comparison to the generator voltage.

When a resistive load (unity power factor) is applied to the generator, the voltage across the paralleling resistor leads the sensing voltage by 90 degrees and the vector sum of the two voltages is nearly the same as the original sensing voltage and no change occurs in the generator output voltage.

Fig 44
Interconnection—Single-Phase Sensing

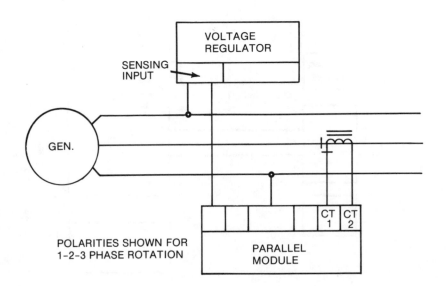

When a lagging power factor (inductive) load is applied to the generator, the voltage across the paralleling resistor becomes more in phase with the sensing voltage and the vector sum of two voltages results in a larger voltage being applied to the sensor circuit. Since the action of the regulator is to maintain a constant voltage, as in sensing terminals, the regulator reacts by decreasing the generator voltage.

When a leading power factor (capacitive) load is applied to the generator, the vector sums result in a smaller voltage at the regulator sensing terminals and the regulator reacts to increase the generator output voltage.

With two generators operating in parallel, if the field excitation on one generator should become excessive and cause circulating currents to flow between generators, the current appears as a lagging power factor (inductive) load to the generator with excessive field current and a leading power factor (capacitive) load to the other. The parallel compensation circuit will cause the voltage regulator to decrease the field excitation on the generator with the lagging power factor load so as to minimize the circulating currents between the generators.

This action and circuitry is called parallel or voltage droop compensation. It allows two or more paralleled generators to proportionally share inductive loads by causing a decrease or droop in the generator system voltage.

(2) *Cross-Current Compensation Method.* The parallel modules described for the voltage droop method of paralleling provide the necessary circuit isolation for the cross-current compensation method of paralleling. Cross-current compensation allows two or more paralleled generators to share inductive reactive loads with no decrease or droop in the generator system output voltage (see Fig 45). This is accomplished by the action and circuitry described in the voltage droop method and the addition of cross connecting leads between CT secondaries. The output of the first unit CT is connected to the input of the second unit CT, the output of the second unit CT is connected to the input of third unit CT, etc, until all CT's are connected in series.

The final step is to connect the output of the last CT to the input of the first unit CT. This forms a closed series loop which interconnects the CT's of all generators to be paralleled. The signals from the interconnected CT's cancel each other when the line currents are proportional and in phase (no circulating currents) and no drop in system voltage occurs.

Cross-current compensation can be used only if the *regulators are identical* and if the regulators on all the generators operating on a common bus are interconnected into a cross-current loop. Generators of different kW ratings may be operated with cross-current compensation if parallel CT's are selected that give approximately the same secondary current at each generator's rated load.

Voltage droop compensation does not require the above interconnection between generator regulators nor matching CT output for different size generators. For this reason, and the simplicity of the voltage droop method, it is the most popular method of paralleling generators.

Some self-excited, self-regulated generators are capable of parallel operation. The previously mentioned self-excited, self-regulated unit using ac voltage in the

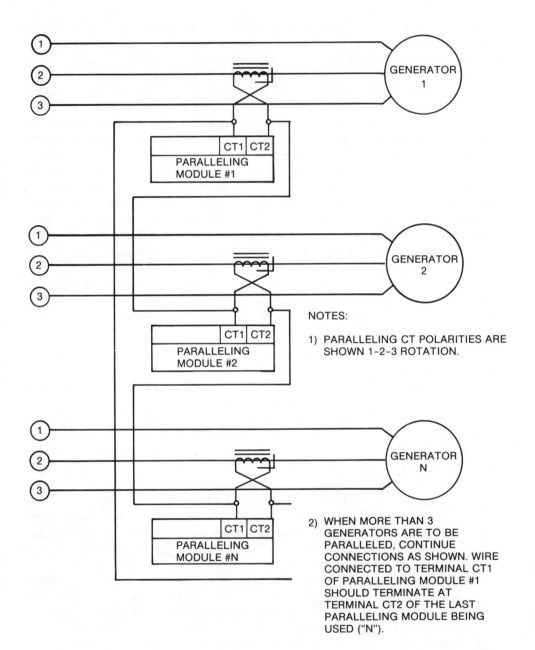

NOTES:

1) PARALLELING CT POLARITIES ARE SHOWN 1-2-3 ROTATION.

2) WHEN MORE THAN 3 GENERATORS ARE TO BE PARALLELED, CONTINUE CONNECTIONS AS SHOWN. WIRE CONNECTED TO TERMINAL CT1 OF PARALLELING MODULE #1 SHOULD TERMINATE AT TERMINAL CT2 OF THE LAST PARALLELING MODULE BEING USED ("N").

Fig 45
Cross-Current Compensation CT Interconnection

exciter field can be paralleled with like units and share reactive load. In addition to the normal requirements for paralleling (same voltage, same frequency, same phase rotation), the units must have drooping voltage with reactive load and their output voltages must be within 2%.

If the voltage on one of the paralleled units is higher than the other, it will try to take the reactive load. The higher reactive load will cause the generator voltage to droop, thus decreasing the voltage and balancing the reactive load between both generators.

5.2.15 Exciters. There are two basic exciters in use today. They are the static exciter and the rotating brushless exciter.

(1) *Static Exciter.* The static exciter is a solid state device which derives its input from the output voltage of the main stator. The ac input is rectified to dc, controlled by the voltage regulator and supplied through brushes and slip rings to the main field of the alternator. The static exciter must supply all the power to the main field. Typical power required by the main field on a 200 kW generator is 3 kW.

(2) *Rotating Brushless Exciter.* The rotating brushless exciter is actually a three-phase generator with a rotating armature on the same shaft with the main generator rotor. The voltage regulator supplies excitation current and voltage to the stationary field. The three-phase output from the rotating armature is rectified by a three-phase rotating bridge and the dc voltage is supplied to the main generator field.

The power input to the brushless exciter for a 200 kW generator is 0.3 kW.

5.2.16 Load Pickup. Motor starting is the most severe requirement for the generator in terms of voltage dip. As stated earlier, voltage dip should not exceed 35% in order to prevent motor starters from dropping out. A study should be made to determine that other connected loads will operate satisfactorily when this dip occurs. Refer to Chapter 9. The engine power required during motor starting is relatively small since the power factor is low, in the 0 to 0.4 range.

Full load pickup at rated power and 0.8 power factor will cause a voltage dip in the area of 15 to 20%. However, this is a more severe requirement for the engine. Since the real kW load will not cause a large voltage dip, the engine must pick up full load. This is usually not a problem for smaller naturally aspirated engine generator sets, but on larger sets with turbochargers the sudden loading can cause the engine to stall before the turbocharger can come up to speed.

To prevent this from happening, loads can be picked up in sequence. The first loads to be picked up consist of the emergency system transfer switch circuits. These loads must be on the line in ten seconds. After a delay, the equipment system transfer switches feeding the motor loads are sequenced to the generator. For more information, refer to Paragraph 5.3.1(3).

5.2.17 Exercising. No load operation of diesel engines eventually results in the formation of carbon within the engine. In order to avoid this condition as well as to check the complete standby power system, the complete generator set should be exercised with the facility load. According to ANSI/NFPA 99-1984 (Paragraph 8-2.1.2.5) [3], "Generator sets serving Emergency and Equipment systems shall be inspected weekly, and shall be exercised under load and operating temperature conditions for at least 30 minutes at intervals of not more than 30 days. The 30-minute exercise period is an absolute minimum, or the individual engine manufacturer's recommendations shall be followed."

5.3 Automatic and Nonautomatic Transfer Switches. Automatic transfer switches are used where alternate sources of power are required to automatically assure power continuity to designated electrical loads in health care facilities. An automatic transfer switch may be defined as an inherently double throw emergency device that automatically transfers electrical loads from a normal source to an emergency source whenever the normal source voltage fails or is substantially reduced. The switch automatically retransfers the load back to the normal source when it is restored.

Because of its unique position in the electrical system the transfer switch should be a highly reliable device with long life and minimum maintenance. Transfer switches applied in health care facilities should have electrical characteristics suitable for the operation of all functions and equipment they are to supply. The main characteristics to be considered here are:

(1) Types of load to be transferred.
(2) Voltage rating.
(3) Continuous current rating.
(4) Overload and fault current withstand ratings.
(5) Type of overcurrent protective device ahead of the transfer switch.
(6) Source monitoring.
(7) Time delays.
(8) Input/Output control signals.
(9) Main switching mechanism.
(10) Ground fault protection considerations.
(11) System operation.
(12) Nonautomatic transfer switches operation.
(13) Multiple transfer switches versus one large transfer switch per system.

Reliability and economics are the prevailing factors in deciding the best selection for the application.

5.3.1 Types of Loads

(1) *Load Classification.* The types of loads to be served in health care facilities are defined in Chapter 2.

Loads are classified by ANSI/UL 1008-1983 [4] as:

(a) Total System Loads.
(b) Motor Load.
(c) Electric Discharge Lamp Loads.
(d) Resistive Loads.
(e) Incandescent Lamp Loads.

UL requires marking of transfer switches to indicate the type of load they are capable of handling. The marking, "Total System Loads" indicates that the transfer switch can be used for any combination of the loads described above under (a) through (e). However, the incandescent load shall not exceed 30% of the total load unless the transfer switch is specifically marked as suitable to transfer a higher percentage of incandescent lamps. Most transfer switches are rated for transfer of Total System Loads, though some may be marked Resistance Only, Tungsten Only, etc, or a combination of these markings. The burden of the system designer is lessened when he chooses switches listed and rated for Total System Loads.

(2) *Motor Load Transfer Considerations.* Two special design considerations to be weighed by the system designer when motor loads are to be supplied from alternate power systems:

(a) How to avoid nuisance breaker tripping and possible damage to the motor and related equipment when the motor is switched between two energized power sources that are not synchronized.

(b) How to shed motor loads prior to transfer and delay reconnection to prevent overloading the power source to which the load is being transferred.

Depending on the makeup of the load, either one or both of the above may require consideration for any given dual power arrangement.

1) *Avoiding Damage to Motors.* Motors and related equipment can be damaged when switched between two live power sources. During routine testing of the system, or during retransfer from the alternate power source back to the normal power source, both power sources are at full voltage. Experience has shown that motors, especially large three-phase motors of 50 hp or more, when transferred from one energized power source to another energized power source, can be subjected to abnormal inrush currents. This in turn can lead to damage of motor windings, insulation, couplings, and, in some cases, the driven load. The motor overcurrent device may also trip out due to abnormal inrush current, and require resetting. The abnormal currents are caused by the motor's residual voltage being out of phase with the voltage source to which it is being transferred.

The situation is similar to paralleling two unsynchronized power systems. Various control methods that are being used to overcome this problem are:

    a) In-phase transfer.

    b) Motor load disconnect control circuit.

    c) Transfer switch with a timed center-off position.

    d) Overlap transfer to momentarily parallel the power sources.

2) *In-phase Transfer.* In-phase transfer schemes have been applied to health care facility equipment loads for many years. With thousands of installations such as shown in Fig 46, in-phase transfer is perhaps the most popular method of transferring low-slip motors driving high-inertia loads on secondary distribution systems.

A primary advantage of in-phase transfer is that it can permit the motor to continue to run with little disturbance to the electrical system and the process which is being controlled by the motor. Some motor loads should not be interrupted and shut down. Concern has been expressed about the slowdown of auxiliary motors which result in pressure surging of boilers or cavitation of pumps [15]. Where it may be desirable to avoid intentionally delayed interruptions so

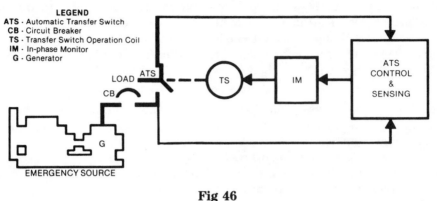

Fig 46
In-phase Motor Load Transfer

motor controllers will not have to be reset, the in-phase transfer approach is the most practical.

Another advantage of in-phase transfer is that a standard double throw switch can be used with the simple addition of an in-phase monitor. The monitor samples the relative phase angle that exists between the two sources between which the motor is transferred. When the two voltages are within the desired phase angle and approaching zero phase angle, the in-phase monitor signals the transfer switch to operate and reconnection takes place within acceptable limits. The faster the transfer switch operates, the wider the frequency difference can be between the two power sources without exceeding normal motor starting current at time of transfer [12].

Under certain conditions, the in-phase monitor should be omitted. Fast transfer has been recognized as a means for the transfer test of power station auxiliaries [10]. Fast operating transfer switches have been in use on secondary distribution systems for many years. When a motor is being transferred between two synchronized sources, such as two phase locked utility company lines from the same source, a transfer switch with fast operating time is usually sufficient for successful transfer since the motor does not have time to slow down significantly.

3) *Load disconnect control circuit.* Motor load disconnect control circuits, such as shown in Fig 47 and similar relay schemes, are also a common means of transferring motor loads [13]. This arrangement and the following arrangement (Timed Center-Off Position) should not be used if the motors cannot be deenergized momentarily during transfer. Momentary deenergization may result in unacceptable disturbances to the electrical system and the process being controlled by the motor.

As Fig 47 indicates, the motor load disconnect control circuit is a pilot contact on the transfer switch which opens to deenergize the contactor coil circuit of the motor controller. After transfer, the transfer switch pilot contact closes to permit the motor controller to reclose. For these applications, the controller should reset automatically.

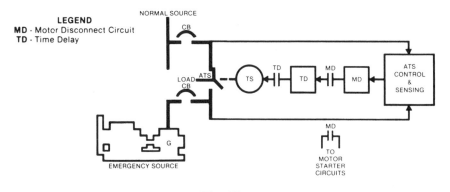

Fig 47
Motor Load Disconnect Circuit

The transfer switch motor load disconnect control circuit positively isolates each motor through its own controller thus preventing possible interaction with other system loads.

A proper motor control disconnect circuit should be arranged to open the pilot contact for approximately three seconds before transfer to the alternate power source is initiated. This pretransfer delay should be nontemperable as time must be allowed for the motor controller to open and extinguish all arcing before the transfer switch operates. Depending on the motor's time constant, or whether timed reclosing is provided in the motor controller circuit, it may also be necessary to add a second delay in the motor load disconnect control circuit. If the motor controller circuit does not have timed reclosing and the motor's time constant exceeds three seconds, an additional delay should be included in the motor load disconnect control circuit. A three-second delay is usually satisfactory. An exception might be large high inertia motors, which may have time constants of four to five seconds. In such cases, it may take six or more seconds for the residual voltage to decay to an acceptable value for reclosing.

If several motors are being transferred and it is desirable not to reconnect them simultaneously so as to prevent excessive inrush currents if they start simultaneously, the secondary delay can be a sequencer with several timed and sequenced pilot contacts (one contact for connection to each motor controller circuit).

As these arrangements require interconnection of control wires between the transfer switch and the motor controller, some consideration should be given to the design and layout of the system to minimize control line runs. To overcome this problem, the transfer switch is frequently located adjacent to or within the motor control center.

4) *Timed Center-Off Position.* Transfer switches with a timed center-off (neutral position) have been used as a means of switching motor loads. Figure 48 shows a typical arrangement. This arrangement achieves results similar to the motor load disconnect control circuit described earlier.

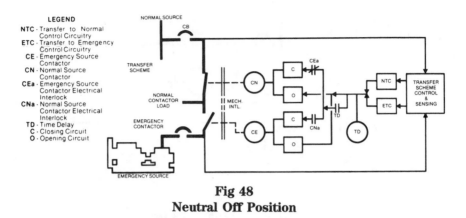

Fig 48
Neutral Off Position

One advantage, provided that timed sequence reclosing is not required, is that interconnections between the transfer switch and motor controller are not required.

    5) Closed Transition Transfer. Closed transition transfer with momentary paralleling of the two power sources appears to be an ideal solution at first glance (see Fig 49). An uninterrupted load transfer should provide the least amount of system and process disturbances [14]. However, overlap can only be achieved when both power sources are present and properly synchronized by voltage, frequency and phase angle. In the case of a failing source, overlap transfer may be extremely difficult, if not impossible, to achieve. Overlap transfer can only be used during test transfers and retransfer back from the generator to the utility when both sources are at full voltage.

    While the overlap arrangement is technically feasible, it is not always practical because of the reluctance of the utility companies to permit paralleling of extraneous power sources to their lines. However, there are indications that this reluctance may be tempered in the future because of the energy crisis.

Fig 49
Closed Transition Transfer

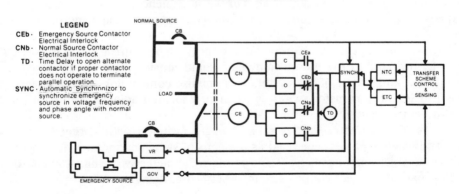

(3) *Sequential Loading of the Generator.* What methods are available to prevent overloading of the alternate source operator? Such generator sets often have limited capability to supply the total inrush and starting currents of the connected load. For economical purposes, generator sets are often sized to provide full load current plus a limited motor starting capability [11]. In such cases, it becomes essential to delay reconnection of loads when transferring from the normal power source to the on-site generator.

Article 517 of the NEC requires that the equipment system load (primarily motor load) transfer switches in hospitals be equipped with time delay relays that will delay transfer of the connected load to the generator set. The purpose is to assure that the more important emergency system loads are connected first and established within 10 seconds of failure. The transfer switches feeding the motors are then sequentially transferred to the generator set.

Another reason for load shedding is the need to "power down" certain loads, such as those utilizing silicon controlled rectifiers (SCR's) to avoid damage to, or failure of, such components during transfer. Following are various solutions in use today to help solve these problems by adding circuit features to transfer switches.

(a) *Transfer switches with individual time delay circuits on transfer to emergency.* This arrangement is in frequent use today. If there are several transfer switches in an installation, the time delay can be adjusted slightly different on each transfer switch so that the transfer switches close sequentially onto the generator. Consideration should be given to individual motor inrush requirements, the remaining available starting kVA of the generator, and the importance of the respective loads when determining the sequence of transfer.

(b) *Transfer switches with signal circuits for definite disconnection of a single load prior to transfer and reconnection after transfer.* This arrangement was described previously under "Load Disconnect Control Circuit." With the additional delay described in the text, the control circuit not only assures that the motor is disconnected before transfer, but also prevents the motor load from being reconnected until several seconds after the transfer switch has transferred and reconnected any other loads which are fed by the same transfer switch.

(c) *Transfer switches as in (b) but with multi-signal circuits to sequence several loads onto the generator.* A further refinement of the system described above utilizes several signal circuits when several motors are to be fed by the same transfer switch and it is desired to reconnect them sequentially rather than all at once. Two to nine circuits are commonly provided. The time delay between reconnection steps is adjustable from 2–60 seconds to allow the starting current to reduce to a safe value before the next motor is signalled to be reconnected. Once the delay is set, it is the same for each step.

(4) *Hospital Isolation Transformer Load Considerations.* Isolation transformers are frequently used in anesthetizing locations and in special environments of health care facilities. See Chapter 6.

The transformers are generally located on the load side of the transfer switch supplying the critical branch.

The electrical and mechanical construction of some of these transformers is such that very high inrush currents frequently occur when the transformer is energized. The inrush currents are sometimes high enough to cause nuisance trip out of the overcurrent protective device. These transformers use grain oriented square loop steels. The magnetic flux stays in the last position it was in when the input voltage was removed.

There are various solutions to overcome nuisance tripping depending on the manufacturer of the transformers. Sometimes, series reactance, impedance starting, and special overcurrent devices are considered as solutions. A solution beyond the transfer switch is necessary because other interruptions, such as momentary outage on the high lines, can cause a similar problem.

5.3.2 Voltage Ratings. An automatic transfer switch is unique in the electrical distribution system in that it is located where two unsynchronized power sources are commonly connected to it. This means that the voltages impressed on the insulation may actually be as high as 960 V on a 480 Vac system. A properly designed transfer switch should provide sufficient spacings and insulation to meet these increased voltage stresses.

For this reason, the electrical spacing on a transfer switch should not be less than those shown in ANSI/UL 1008-1983 (Table 15.1) [4] regardless of what type of component may be used as part of the transfer switch.

The voltage ratings for this discussion will be limited to Health Care Facility Essential Electrical System applications where transfer switches are rated 600 V or less.

The ac voltage ratings of automatic transfer switches are normally 120, 208, 240, 480 or 600 V, single or polyphase. Standard frequencies are 50–60 Hz. Automatic transfer switches can also be supplied for other voltages and frequencies when required.

5.3.3 Continuous Current Rating. A continuous current (load) is defined by the NEC as one which is expected to continue at its maximum value for three hours or more (ANSI/NFPA 70-1984 [2]). Transfer switches differ from other emergency equipment in that they must continuously carry the current to critical loads, whereas an engine generator set generally supplies power only during emergency periods. Current flows continuously through the transfer switch whether the switch is in the normal or the emergency position. Automatic transfer switches are available in continuous ratings ranging from 30 through 4000A.

Most transfer switches are capable of carrying 100% of rated current at an ambient temperature of 40 °C. However, some transfer switches, such as those incorporating integral overcurrent protective devices, may be limited to a continuous load current not to exceed 80% of the switch rating.

When selecting an automatic transfer switch, it is only necessary to determine the maximum continuous load current which the transfer switch must carry. Momentary inrushes, such as occur when lighting or motor loads are energized, can be ignored provided the switch is ANSI/UL 1008-1983 [4] "Total Systems Load" rated. Select an automatic transfer switch that is at least equal to, or greater than, the calculated continuous current.

For new projects, the system designer may specify a transfer switch that will be able to carry future anticipated loads. In such cases, it is advisable to select a transfer switch with a continuous current rating equal to the total anticipated load.

The transfer switch continuous current rating is found by totaling the amperes required for all loads. Electric heater and tungsten (incandescent) lamp load currents are determined from the total wattage. Fluorescent, mercury vapor and sodium vapor lamp load currents must be based on the current of each ballast or autotransformer draws, not on the total watts of the lamp. Motor loads are determined by motor full load running currents. Motor inrush and locked rotor currents need not be considered in sizing a transfer switch UL listed for total system loads.

5.3.4 Overload and Fault Current Withstand Ratings. Transfer switches are often subjected to currents of short duration exceeding the continuous duty ratings. The ability of the transfer switch to handle higher currents is measured by its overload and withstand current ratings. A discussion on overload ratings and fault current withstand ratings can be found in Chapter 3.

5.3.5 Protective Device Ahead of Transfer Switch. The type and size of overcurrent device ahead of the transfer switch play a significant role in transfer switch application. Refer to Chapter 3 for a discussion on coordinating the protective device and the transfer switch.

5.3.6 Source Monitoring. Most often the normal source is from an electric utility company whose power is transmitted many miles to the point of utilization. The control panel continuously monitors the voltage of all phases. (Because utility frequency is, for all practical purposes, constant, only the voltage need be monitored.) For single-phase power systems, the line-to-line voltage is monitored. For three-phase power systems, all three line-to-line voltages should be monitored to provide full phase protection.

In addition to feeder failure, monitoring protects against operation at reduced voltage, such as brownouts, which can damage loads. Since the voltage sensitivity of loads varies, the pickup (acceptable) voltage setting, and drop out (unacceptable) voltage setting of the monitors should be adjustable. Typical range of adjustment for the pickup is 85% to 100% of nominal while the pickup setting is 75% to 98% of the pickup selected. Usual settings for most loads are 95% of nominal for pickup and 85% of nominal for drop out (90% of pickup).

As long as normal voltage is available at or above the preset limit, the transfer switch should remain connected to the normal source. Likewise, if voltage is lost to only one of several transfer switches, then only that transfer switch should transfer to emergency. The remaining switches should stay on normal.

Sensing of the alternate source voltage need only be single-phase since most applications involve an on-site generator with a relatively short line run to the automatic transfer switch. In addition to monitoring voltage, the alternate source's frequency should also be monitored. Unlike the utility power, the engine generator frequency can vary during startup. Frequency monitoring will avoid overloading the engine generator while it is starting and can thus avoid stalling the engine. Combined frequency and voltage monitoring will protect against transferring loads to an engine generator set with an unacceptable output.

5.3.7 Time Delays. Time delays are provided to program the operation of the automatic transfer switch to avoid unnecessary starting and resultant transfer to the alternate supply. A time delay, up to six seconds, will override momentary interruptions and reductions in normal source voltage but allow starting and transfer if the reduction or outage is sustained. The time delay is generally set at one second, but may be set higher if reclosers on the high lines take longer to operate or if momentary power dips frequently exceed one second. If long delay settings are used, care must be taken to insure that sufficient time remains to meet 10-second power restoration requirements.

Once the load is transferred to the alternate source, another timer delays retransfer to the normal source until that source has time to stabilize. This timer is controlled by the preferred source voltage monitors and is adjustable from 0 to 30 minutes. It is normally set at 30 minutes. Another important function of this retransfer timer is to allow an engine generator to operate under a load for a preselected minimum time to insure continued good performance of the set and its starting system. This delay should be automatically nullified if the alternate source fails and the normal source is available as determined by the voltage monitors.

Engine generator manufacturers often recommend a cooldown period for their sets which will allow the set to run unloaded after the load is retransferred to the normal source. A third time delay, usually five minutes, is provided for this purpose. Running an unloaded engine for more than five minutes is neither necessary nor recommended since it can cause deterioration in engine performance.

It is sometimes desirable to purposely sequence transfer of the loads to the alternate source where more than one automatic transfer switch is connected to the same engine generator such as on the equipment branch of the essential electrical system. Refer to Paragraph 5.3.1(3). Utilization of such a sequencing scheme can reduce starting kVA capacity requirements of the generator. A fourth timer, adjustable from 0 to 5 minutes, will delay transfer to emergency for this and other similar requirements.

5.3.8 Input/Output Control Signals. When the transfer switch control panel detects a sustained failure of the normal source, a set of contacts, one normally open and one normally closed, operates to signal starting of the alternate source. These contacts should be rated to handle the low dc voltages and currents encountered on most engine starting systems.

Additional dry contacts, normally open and normally closed, should be provided on the transfer switch unit for remote indication of transfer switch positions and other control functions.

5.3.9 Main Switching Mechanism. The main switching mechanism of a transfer switch should have the following characteristics:

(1) *Electrical operation.* It is usually desirable to electrically operate the transfer switch using control power from the source to which the load is to be transferred. This arrangement assures an adequate source of power for switch operation.

(2) *Mechanically held.* Electrically held transfer switches are limited in size, will drop out and disconnect the load if the main coil fails, and have very low fault current withstandability. Conversely, mechanically held mechanisms are not limited in size, will not drop out and can withstand higher fault currents.

(3) *Mechanically interlocked—double throw.* The switch mechanism should be of the mechanically interlocked double throw type permitting only two possible positions—closed on normal or closed on emergency. If the interlocking permitted both sets of contacts to close at the same time, a system-to-system short circuit can occur.

5.3.10 Ground Fault Protection Considerations. Ground fault protection of electrical systems that have more than one power source (that is, a load fed by either a utility or engine generator set) requires special consideration when the neutral conductor of the engine generator set is required to be grounded at the generator location, thus creating multiple neutral-to-ground connections. The system must be properly designed to avoid improper sensing of ground fault currents and nuisance tripping of overcurrent devices. Transfer switches are often furnished with neutral transfer contacts to provide the necessary isolation between neutrals.

Ground fault protection as applied to emergency power systems is covered in depth in Chapter 3.

5.3.11 System Operation. The emergency system and the equipment system should be so arranged that, in the event of failure of the normal power source, an alternate power source is automatically connected within 10 seconds to the emergency system loads and to the switching devices (time delay or nonautomatic) supplying the equipment system loads.

The automatic transfer switch is arranged to achieve this operation. An automatic transfer switch consists of two major components: (1) an electrically operated, double throw transfer switch and (2) a control panel (see Fig 50).

The essential electrical system is normally served by the utility power source except when the utility power source is interrupted or drops below a predetermined voltage level as sensed by the voltage monitor VM. Settings of the sensors should be determined by careful study of the voltage requirements of the load.

Chapter 3 describes the overall essential electrical system. Failure of the normal source will automatically start the alternate source generator after a short delay (TD1). When the alternate power source has attained a voltage and frequency that satisfies minimum operating requirements of the essential electrical system as sensed by the combination voltage/frequency monitors V/FM, the load is connected automatically to the alternate power source through the transfer controls TC and main transfer switch operator TO.

Upon connection of the alternate power source, the loads comprising the emergency system are automatically reenergized. The load comprising the equipment system is connected automatically after a time delay (TD2) and in such a manner as not to overload the generator.

When the normal power source is restored, and after a time delay (TD3), the automatic transfer switch disconnects the alternate source of power and connects the loads to the normal power source.

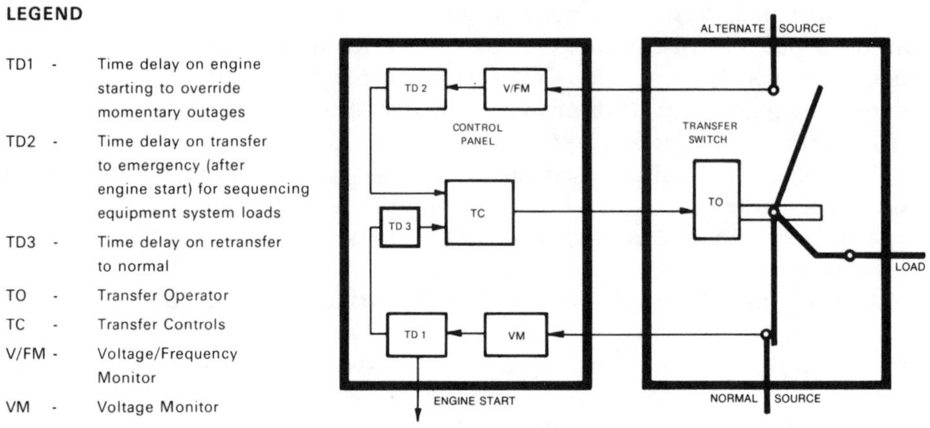
LEGEND
TD1 - Time delay on engine starting to override momentary outages
TD2 - Time delay on transfer to emergency (after engine start) for sequencing equipment system loads
TD3 - Time delay on retransfer to normal
TO - Transfer Operator
TC - Transfer Controls
V/FM - Voltage/Frequency Monitor
VM - Voltage Monitor
ALTERNATE SOURCE
TD 2
V/FM
CONTROL
PANEL
TRANSFER
SWITCH
TO
TC
TD 3
LOAD
TD 1
VM
ENGINE START
NORMAL SOURCE

Fig 50
Automatic Transfer Switch (Consists of the Control Panel, Left, and the Switch Unit, Right)

If the emergency power source should fail and the normal power source has been restored, retransfer to the normal source of power is immediate, bypassing the retransfer delay timer.

5.3.12 Nonautomatic Transfer Switches. Nonautomatic transfer switches are sometimes considered for certain code defined portions of the equipment load and various nonessential loads when permitted. For these installations it is necessary that operating personnel be present to effect an operation and that the load not be of an emergency nature requiring immediate automatic restoration of power. For these reasons it is recommended that all loads be transferred automatically, whenever possible. When possible overloading of the generator is a concern, it may be more practicable to manually transfer nonessential loads.

Devices used as nonautomatic transfer switches should have the same electrical characteristics, rating and features as an automatic transfer switch except that the control panel is omitted. Operation is achieved either through an externally operable quick make-quick break manual operating handle or by electrical remote push-button control.

Electrically operated nonautomatic transfer switches should derive control power from the source to which the load is being transferred to assure an adequate power supply to the main electrical operator. Control relays are often used at the transfer switch to avoid voltage drops owing to long control line runs.

5.3.13 Multiple Transfer Switches vs. One Large Transfer Switch. In small hospitals and nursing homes, ANSI/NFPA 77-1984 [2] permits one large transfer switch rather than multiple branch transfer switches.

Which approach is better? The system designer should consider the following:

(1) One single large automatic transfer switch close to the incoming service controlling the entire emergency load, in lieu of individual automatic transfer switches in each branch of the emergency system, may reduce the overall reliability and design flexibility of the system. Maximum protection is better achieved by locating the transfer switches downstream as close to the loads as possible. At this location, the automatic transfer switch will not only monitor the external utility power supply but also the internal conductors feeding the transfer switch.

(2) A second consideration deals with maximizing physical isolation of the separate branches and feeders in the essential electrical system by using separate transfer switches in each feeder. Separate transfer switches, in each of the essential load feeders, increase total system reliability because separation of the conductors is maintained all the way back to the utility and generator main distribution switchboards. If one large transfer switch were used, it might require a long main power conductor run. If something happened to this one conductor or the single automatic transfer switch, the complete essential electrical system would be shut down; whereas, with the multiple automatic transfer switch approach, only one branch of the system would be affected.

(3) A third design consideration is the need to sequentially transfer the loads in blocks so as not to overload the generator. Multiple automatic transfer switches with adjustable delay on transfer to the generator are generally used for this purpose. If one large transfer switch were used, it might require oversizing the generator or development of a load-shedding, load connect system.

(4) Economy is a further consideration. While several small transfer switches equal the ampacity of one large switch and might cost about the same, the additional cost of separate feeders and installation is a factor favoring the use of one large switch.

When branch circuits on the load side of the transfer switch are required to be extra reliable because they are life-sustaining, area protection devices [9] might be a consideration. These devices can sense failures at the load side of the individual panelboard overcurrent devices or directly at the point of utilization. Such devices can signal for remedial action when overcurrent device opening (inadvertent, mechanical failure or circuit actuated), circuit wiring failure, equipment failure or unintentional equipment disconnection occur.

5.4 Engine Generator Controls

5.4.1 General. The engine generator control panel contains the devices that monitor and control the status and operation of the engine operator system. Interfacing with control components on the engine and the transfer switch is generally required. The control panel should be located near the engine generator set. The assembly and conductors should be protected from the effects of vibration.

ANSI/NFPA 99-1984 [3] requires that the generator sets be equipped with certain visual prealarm and alarm devices, automatic safety shutdown, and an audible alarm device to indicate activation. It further requires a remote annunciator to indicate alarm conditions outside of the generating room at a regular work station (undefined). Where the regular work station periodically is unattended, an audible and visual derangement signal should be provided at a continuously monitored (24 hours a day) location. Generally the annunciator is located in the boiler plant, fire station, telephone switchboard or nurses station.

5.4.2 Safety Controls. It is usually preferable to shut down a standby generator set and correct a problem rather than continue to operate the unit and possibly destroy it in the process. For this reason, safety shutdown controls are required on standby generator sets.

(1) The controls are arranged to shut the engine down for:

   (a) Overspeed

   (b) Low lubricating oil pressure

   (c) Excessive engine temperature

   (d) Reverse power (in paralleling applications)

In addition, pre-shutdown anticipatory alarms for low lubricating oil pressure and excessive engine temperature are also provided in health care facilities. When warned of an impending shutdown, an attendant may take corrective action to prevent shutdown for low lube oil pressure and excessive engine temperature. If a governor loses control, engine speed may increase from rated speed to overspeed in less than one second and no corrective action is possible. Therefore, a pre-shutdown alarm is not practical for overspeed.

(2) Additional indicator lights or alarms, or both, are specified for:

   (a) Overcrank (fail to start)

   (b) Battery charger malfunction

   (c) Low fuel level

   (d) Low water temperature, that is, coolant heaters not operating

   (e) Standby generator set operating

   (f) Low coolant level

Indicator lights to show malfunction of many other items may be desirable in specific installations. These may include excessive engine room temperature, remote radiator fan failure, etc.

Some U.S. Government Health Care Facility specifications require exhaust pyrometers with individual cylinder port thermocouples. The probable damage from a broken thermocouple entering a turbocharger would appear to overshadow any benefit derived from the observation of individual cylinder exhaust temperatures in a standby generator set.

5.4.3 Automatic Starting. The alternate source generator(s) in health care facilities are normally automatically started and stopped as a function of a control contact on the automatic transfer switch. Refer to Paragraphs 5.3.8 and 5.3.11. The control contact closes to initiate engine start and run, and opens to initiate engine stopping.

The engine generator control panel (see Fig 51) includes an automatic engine start control which operates upon signal of the control contact on for the transfer switch to control the various devices on the engine for engine start and run. For example, on a diesel engine, a fuel solenoid valve may be energized to permit fuel to flow into the fuel injectors. At the same time, the cranking motor relay circuit is energized to initiate cranking. The automatic engine starting con-

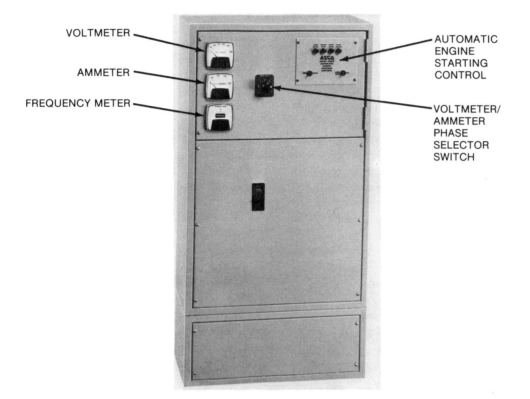

Fig 51
Typical Engine Generator Control Panel

trol includes an overcrank time delay which will sound an alarm and lock out any further cranking if the engine fails to start after a programmed period. A common cranking sequence is four cycles of ten seconds crank and ten seconds rest.

When the engine fires, the cranking circuit is automatically disconnected via any one or more methods such as speed governor switch, oil pressure switch, ac generator voltage buildup and battery charging generator voltage buildup. The selection of the proper crank disconnect method is best made at the recommendation of the engine manufacturer.

The automatic engine starting controls also monitor the various engine protective devices described above to sound alarms, give visual indication and shut the engine down when failures occur. The failure lockout circuit requires resetting before the engine can be restarted.

5.4.4 Engine Generator Control Panel Features

(1) In addition to the automatic engine starting control, the engine generator control panel also includes:

(a) Voltmeter

(b) Ammeter

(c) Frequency meter

(d) Voltmeter/ammeter phase selector switch

(e) Current transformers

(f) Overcurrent protective device

(g) Vibration isolators when engine mounted

(h) Remote annunciator interface

(2) Various other accessories are furnished depending on the application. These might include:

(a) Elapsed time meter

(b) Panel illumination lamp with on-off switch

(c) Governor motor raise-lower switch

(d) Voltage adjust rheostat

(e) Voltage regulator

(f) kW meter

5.4.5 Remote Annunciator

(1) Health care facilities require a remote annunciator panel (see Fig 52) to provide visual and audible indication of:

(a) Low fuel level

(b) Low water temperature

(c) Low oil pressure

(d) High water temperature

(e) Overspeed

(f) Overcrank

(2) Visual indication only is required for the following:

(a) Battery charger malfunction

(b) Generator is supplying the load

In addition to the above, a derangement contact should be supplied to close for signalling to a regularly attended work station that an alarm condition has occurred.

5.5 Battery Chargers for Cranking Batteries

5.5.1 General Description. There are a great variety of battery chargers available. The type selected for a generator set installation will depend upon the electrical equipment used on the engine. Most chargers fall into two categories:

(1) *Full battery recovery.* The full recovery type charger is required on standby generator set installation when a charging generator is not used to restore the battery charge. It is usually a high-low rate charge which can be either manual or automatic in operation. The high rate will recharge the battery, and the low rate will maintain the batteries in prime starting condition.

(2) *Maintenance trickle charge.* The trickle type charger is sometimes used when a charging generator is supplied on the engine. With a trickle charging rate

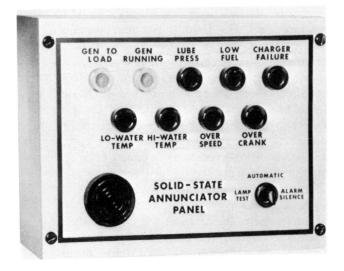

Fig 52
Typical Remote Annunciator Panel

of 2 A, it maintains the battery condition at whatever level the charging generator leaves the battery at. It is not designed to recharge a discharged battery and for this reason it may be more reliable to provide a high-low full battery recovery charger even if a charging generator is furnished on the engine.

A battery charger for engine cranking batteries is similar if not identical to a dual rate battery charger for standard float application. The primary difference between the chargers is sizing. In engine cranking applications, the battery load is usually several hundred A (possibly a few thousand A) for only a few seconds. The batteries may need to be relatively large to provide the high breakaway and rolling currents for the starter motor. On the other hand, the charger is usually small in comparison to the battery ampere hour (Ah) capacity because only a small amount of battery capacity is removed with each crank cycle.

Example: 1000 A for 10 seconds equals:

$$(1000\,\text{A})\ \frac{(10\ \text{s})}{(3600\ \text{s/hr})} = 2.77\ \text{Ah removed}$$

In lead acid batteries, the individual cell voltages will begin to drift apart and will need to be brought back to the full charge by increasing the charger voltage approximately 10% for 25–30 hours every 30 days. This is referred to as "equalizing" the battery. Nickel cadmium batteries have much less self-discharge over longer periods of time under similar conditions.

Whether it is lead acid or nickel cadmium, both types of batteries need a high rate of charge to achieve a fully charged state.

Many nickel cadmium battery users have been allowed to believe that because their type of battery does not require periodic "equalizing charges" such as required for lead acid, that they did not need a dual rate battery charger. They have, as a result, used only a single rate float charger. This type of charger will adequately maintain a fully charged nickel cadmium battery until it is discharged by an external load. However, once the battery is discharged, it will not recharge to more than 85% at float voltage regardless of the current capacity of the charger. It is also true that with each successive discharge, the nickel cadmium battery in such a charging circuit will continue to lose capacity. This phenomenon has from time to time been referred to as "memory effect." However, it is simply a result of inadequate recharging of the battery. It can be corrected with a sequence of several high charge and deliberate discharge cycles.

5.5.2 Definitions of Terms

(1) *Ambient Temperature.* The ambient temperature is the temperature of the medium, usually air, surrounding the battery charger.

(2) *Battery Charger.* As defined in this standard, a battery charger is static equipment which is capable of restoring and maintaining the charge in a storage battery.

(3) *Charge.* Charge is the conversion of electrical energy into chemical energy within the battery.

(4) *Charging Rate.* The charging rate of a battery charger is the current expressed in amperes at which the battery is charged.

(5) *Constant Potential Charge.* A constant potential charge is a charge in which the voltage at the output terminals of the charger is held to a constant value.

(6) *Current Limit.* Current limit is the maximum output of the battery charger delivered to a discharged battery and load, usually stated as a percentage of output rating and with nominal input voltage supplied to the charger.

(7) *Float Voltage.* The float voltage is the voltage maintained across the battery by the charger in order to keep the battery at its best operational condition with minimum water loss. Float voltage is expressed in volts/cell (V/C).

(8) *Equalize Voltage.* The equalize voltage is a voltage approximately 10% higher than the float voltage. This higher voltage is used for periodic equalizing of lead acid and nickel cadmium batteries. Equalize voltage is expressed in volts/cell.

(9) *Nominal Value.* The nominal value is an arbitrary reference value selected to establish equipment ratings.

(10) *Overcurrent Protection.* Protection of the battery charger against excessive current, incuding short circuit current.

(11) *Short Circuit Current.* The short circuit current of a battery charger is the current magnitude at the output terminals, when the terminals are short circuited and with nominal input voltage supplied to the charger.

5.5.3 Charger Ratings

(1) The continuous duty output current rating must be adequate to supply the engine cranking battery charging current plus all auxiliary load requirements.

(2) The charger output voltage rating is dictated by the type of battery and the number of cells being charged.

(3) Float voltage ranges per cell at 77 °F (25 °C) are:

Lead Plante @ 1.210 Sp. Grv. (Specific Gravity) Electrolyte 2.15–2.19 V

Lead-Antimony @ 1.210 Sp. Grv. Electrolyte 2.15–2.19 V

Lead-Antimony @ 1.265 Sp. Grv. Electrolyte 2.29–2.33 V

Nickel-Cadmium 1.35–1.45 V

(4) Equalize voltage ranges per cell at 77 °F (25 °C) are:

Lead Plante @ 1.210 Sp. Grv. Electrolyte 2.25–2.35 V

Lead-Antimony @ 1.210 Sp. Grv. Electrolyte 2.25–2.35 V

Lead-Antimony @ 1.265 Sp. Grv. Electrolyte 2.4–2.5 V

Nickel-Cadmium @ 1.50–1.60 V

(5) The ac input ranges for 60 Hz are:

Normal Voltage	Minimum	Maximum
120	106	127
208	184	220
240	212	254
277	245	293
480	424	508
575	508	600

(6) The rated alternating current supply frequencies are 50 or 60 Hz.

(7) Rated ambient temperature range is 32–122 °F (0–50 °C).

5.5.4 Charger Sizing. The worst case load on the charger is when the battery is discharged and the charger must recharge the battery plus power the load. There are many considerations such as the number of cells, voltage window of the load, input voltage, input frequency, single-phase, three-phase, output regulation, ripple, recharge time, etc, all of which can affect the charger selection.

In general, because engine cranking batteries are seldom discharged very deeply, it is common practice to size the charger by the following equation:

$$I \text{ (chg)} = \frac{0.6 \text{ (Ah)}}{HR} + I \text{ (load)} \qquad \text{(Eq 3)}$$

where

I (chg) = Current capacity of charger

Ah = Ah capacity of battery

HR = Hours to recharge

I (load) = Continuous dc load on the system

(1) It should be understood that battery recharge time actually relates to two different parameters of the charger:

(a) The current capacity of the charger.

(b) The voltage setting of the charger.

Refer to Fig 53. T_1 is almost completely determined by the current capacity but the charger's current capacity has almost no effect on T_2.

T_2 is almost completely determined by the output voltage setting of the charger, although this setting has virtually no effect on T_1.

The charger will be in its current limit mode during the first part of T_1 and, as the battery voltage begins to increase, the charger will come out of current limit. A typical curve is illustrated by Curve A. T_1 can be cut in half simply by doubling the current capacity of the charger.

(2) The only way to shorten T_2 is to shift up to a higher charging curve, such as shown in Curve B, by applying more volts/cell to the battery. This is done by adjusting the "recharge" mode ("equalize" for lead acid systems) of the charger output up to a higher voltage. Caution: This may not be as simple as it first appears. There are various potential problems which must be considered:

(a) Lead acid batteries are more sensitive to high charging voltages than nickel cadmium. The extra heat buildup in the plates may cause plate warpage.

(b) The voltage window of the applied load may not accommodate the increase in charger voltage.

Fig 53
Battery Recharge Time

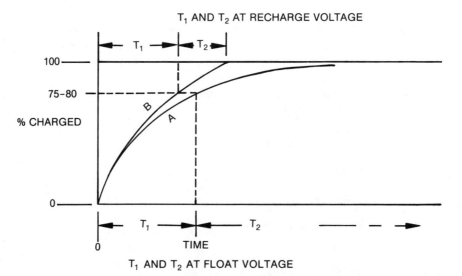

T_1 = The time required to recharge a fully discharged battery to 75–80% charged.

T_2 = The time required to bring the battery from 75–80% charged to 100% charged.

The charger can be adjusted up to 1.65–1.7 volts/cell for pocket plate nickel cadmium cells without any damage to the battery, but all loads have some maximum voltage above which serious damage will result. One of two standard methods is commonly used to effect desired recharge times without damage to the load.

Method 1 (Oversizing).
Since T_1 is a function of current capacity of the charger, but only restores the battery to 75–80% of full charge, the battery can be oversized by 25% and a larger charger used. Even though the battery will not be fully recharged during time period T_1, it will be recharged sufficiently to carry another duty cycle for the specified time period. (Note: When specifying the charger, it may be desirable to require "a charger which will restore the battery sufficiently to carry another duty cycle as specified for the battery" instead of "fully recharged" in a given period of time.)

Method 2 (Dropping Diode).
Although damage to the battery is possible for lead acid batteries being rapidly recharged, the nickel cadmium pocket plate battery can accept current as quickly as it can release it. There is no danger to the battery as long as the electrolyte level is kept above the surface of the plates (see Fig 54).

5.5.5 Advantages and Disadvantages of Lead Acid and Nickel Cadmium Cells. Although the lead acid battery and its nickel cadmium counterpart can be used interchangeably in most applications, there are certain advantages and disadvantages to each type.

The primary advantage to the lead acid battery is its lower initial cost.

Fig 54
Dropping Diode Circuit (CEMF)

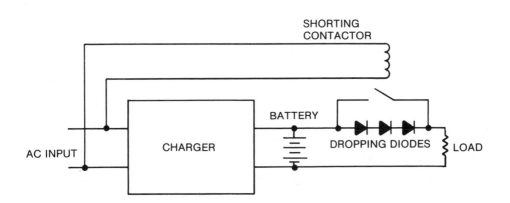

The primary advantage to the nickel cadmium battery is that it is a lower maintenance, longer life, more physically rugged battery. For engine cranking applications, a properly sized and maintained nickel cadmium battery will have an expected useful life of 18-20 years, compared with 2-4 years for the engine cranking lead acid battery.

It should also be acknowledged that the possibility of a battery failing prematurely and without warning is greatly reduced with a nickel cadmium battery because of the improved quality of materials and workmanship in the more expensive product.

5.5.6 Memory Effect on Nickel Cadmium Batteries. There is a phenomenon in all electrochemical couples which are being inadequately recharged that causes the cell to appear to lose capacity with each recharge cycle.

All batteries have an optimum voltage which is ideal for continuous "float" charging. This voltage results in maximum battery life and minimum water usage. For lead acid batteries at 1.230 specific gravity acid, this voltage is 2.15-2.17 V/cell. For nickel cadmium batteries, the voltage is 1.4-1.42 V/cell.

In lead acid cells and nickel cadmium sinter plate cells, even if the battery is not discharged the individual cell voltages will begin to drift apart. Approximately every 60 to 90 days, the lower voltage cells will need to be brought back to full charge by increasing the charger voltage approximately 10-15% (2.33-2.36 V/cell for lead acid cells and 1.60-1.65 V/cell for sinter plate nickel cadmium cells).

Pocket plate nickel cadmium batteries have much less self-discharge and as a result if a pocket plate nickel cadmium battery is not discharged with an external load, it will remain fully charged for many years at 1.4 V/cell. It is, therefore, a true statement that pocket plate nickel cadmium cells do not need to be "equalized." However, lest we create real problems in the battery room, it must be understood that we are not saying you do not need the dual rate recharging mode of the "Float/Equalize" battery charger.

Whether it is lead acid or nickel cadmium, both batteries need the approximate 10-15% higher voltage to restore the discharged battery to a fully charged state. Many pocket plate nickel cadmium battery users have been allowed to believe that because their type of cell does not require periodic "equalizing charges" they did not need a dual rate battery charger. They have as a result used only a single rate float charger. This type of a charger will adequately maintain a fully charged pocket plate nickel cadmium cell until it is discharged by an external load. However, once the cell is discharged, it will not recharge to more than about 85% at a voltage of 1.4 V/cell regardless of the current capacity of the charger. It is also true that with each successive discharge the nickel cadmium cell in such a charging circuit will continue to lose capacity. This phenomenon has from time to time been referred to as "Memory Effect." It is really simply a result of inadequately recharging any battery. Memory effect is also experienced in lead acid batteries. However, usually, before the loss of capacity is noted in the lead acid battery it is destroyed by sulfation of the positive plates as a result of undercharging.

5.5.7 Typical Performance Features

(1) The battery charger should be a solid state, constant potential device whose output potential is regulated by sensing the battery voltage.

(2) The charger should deliver full rated capacity to a discharged battery with a line variation as shown in 5.5.3(5).

(3) The output float voltage should be maintained within ±1% of the nominal setting.

(4) The output equalize voltage should be maintained within ±2% of the nominal setting.

(5) A device should be provided to change the output voltage from float to equalize when conditions warrant.

(6) Controls should be provided to adjust the voltage over the range specified in 5.5.3(3) and 5.5.3(4).

(7) The back drain from the battery should not exceed 50 mA with the loss of ac input.

(8) The battery charger should be self-protected and the output current shall be limited to a safe value under cranking loads.

(9) Surge suppressors should be provided to protect the rectifier from line and load transients. The input and output circuits shall be protected with fuses, circuit breakers, or both.

(10) An ammeter should be provided to indicate the output current. The meter shall have minimum accuracy of 5%.

(11) The charger design and manufacture should satisfy the performance and safety codes of NEMA PE5-1983 [7] and EGSA BCES1-1980 [5].

5.5.8 Optional Accessory Features

(1) A voltmeter should be considered to indicate the dc output voltage. The meter should have a minimum accuracy of 5%.

(2) An alarm device can be furnished to actuate up on the loss of proper charger output.

(3) High dc voltage alarm devices are available to actuate when the charger output voltage exceeds the preset alarm level. This level can be adjustable from equalize voltage to 2.6 V/cell lead acid or 1.7 V/cell nickel cadmium. The device should maintain its alarm set-point adjustment within ±1%.

(4) A low dc voltage alarm device can be provided to actuate when the charger output voltage falls below the present alarm voltage level. This level should be adjustable from float voltage to 1.75 V/cell lead acid or 1.0 V/cell nickel cadmium.

(5) AC power failure alarm devices are available to actuate on loss of ac input.

(6) An equalize timer can be provided to cover a range of 0–24 hours or 0–72 hours. When manually activated, this timer will place the battery charger in the equalize mode. At the end of the specified time period, the timer will automatically return the charger to the float mode.

(7) An automatic equalize timer can be furnished to be activated by ac power failure or low dc battery voltage and will place the battery charger in the equalize mode. At the end of the specified time period, the timer will return the charger to the float mode.

5.5.9 Installation and Maintenance Data

(1) Wire between the battery charger and the battery should be sized to min-

imize voltage drop.

(2) Adequate clearance should be provided to allow convection cooling of the charger.

(3) All auxiliary loads should be connected to the battery bus, not to battery terminals or charger terminals.

(4) The charger shall be installed in accordance with the ANSI/NFPA 70-1984 [2].

(5) Periodic inspections, dust and dirt removal, and connection tightening should be scheduled.

5.6 Synchronizing and Paralleling Control Systems for Multigenerator Set Installations. To supply large loads, two or more engine generator sets are often operated in parallel on a common bus as an emergency power supply. Successful operation of mutliple engine generator sets in parallel requires a control system that can provide all the functions needed to operate the generator automatically, plus automatically handle synchronizing, load sharing, isochronous operation, and load control operations.

The system designer is faced with a number of considerations. Some of the more important are:

(1) Parallel operation or one engine generator set
(2) Load considerations
(3) Engine generator set considerations
(4) Types of paralleling
(5) Dividing the load
(6) Establishing load priorities
(7) Load shedding
(8) Load switching means
(9) Typical system operation
(10) Sensing
(11) Control logic
(12) Instrumentation
(13) The generator power breaker

5.6.1 When to Parallel. Emergency power systems having one engine generator are often preferred and are generally more economical. However, there are many situations today that can be handled better by paralleling two or more engine generator sets. Parallel operation is usually justified for one or more of the following reasons.

(1) *For economy.* One reason for paralleling two or more sets is for economy. For example, the distribution system may be such that it is not practical to split one large load into several sections to be handled by individual generator sets.

Another example of economy is the cost of multiple small sets versus the cost of one large set, such as 500 kW, 1800 rpm sets instead of the 2500 kW, 600 rpm set.

A third example is where the load is expected to grow substantially, but because of economics, the initial investment must be minimized. The designer has the option of making provisions only for add-on in the generator paralleling switchgear for future generator sets and distribution or of actually providing all of the gear for future sets in the initial installation.

Another example is where an existing system is to be expanded. (It is more economical to run one large bus instead of several independent feeders.)

(2) *For reliability.* An important reason for paralleling two or more engine generator sets is for reliability. For example, part of the emergency load may be so essential that it is desirable to have more than one generator set that can handle the load. Here, when there is a power failure on the normal line, all sets are signaled to start at the same time. The probability that at least one set will start is higher than an installation with only one set. The first one ready to handle the emergency load does so. Then the other sets pick up the remaining loads as generators become ready.

Another example is where all sets are running, but one fails. In this case, some or all of the less important load, such as equipment system load, is dropped so that the remaining sets will handle the emergency load.

(3) *To minimize downtime.* When preventive maintenance or overhaul is being done on an engine, it may be necessary to provide back-up power. To do so, an additional, ready-to-go engine generator set is available when needed.

5.6.2 Engine Generator Set Governor Considerations. The engine generator sets should be furnished with electronic governors and voltage regulators to make them suitable for unattended automatic paralleling and load sharing. The electronic governor provides isochronous operation (constant speed regardless of load), and automatic proportionate load division which enables automatic paralleling of dissimilar size sets. The electronic governor will permit paralleling at any time without necessitating adjustment or requiring droop. Similarly, voltage regulators should be able to achieve automatic reactive load division to provide constant voltage systems.

5.6.3 Random Paralleling. Random paralleling, or more accurately, random access to the bus employs a synchronizing device for each engine generator set in the system. The reliability of the paralleling control system is high because of a redundance of parallel logic paths.

Random access permits simultaneous synchronizing of each set to the bus and therefore achieves parallel operation of sets in the shortest possible time. This is important in health care facilities because the emergency branch must be "on line" in 10 seconds.

In a random access system, the first set to achieve nominal voltage and frequency is connected to the bus to make emergency power available within 10 seconds to the emergency branch transfer switches and their respective loads and provide a basis of comparison for synchronizing the remaining sets. As the remaining sets come up to voltage and frequency, they are synchronized and paralleled to the bus at which time the equipment branch transfer switches transfer in delayed sequence to connect the equipment loads.

5.6.4 Dividing the Load. When paralleling two or more engine generator sets, it is necessary to consider the capacity of each set relative to the total load. The system should be arranged to inhibit the connection of additional loads to the alternate source power bus until sufficient generating capacity is on the bus. To do this, the essential electrical system load should be divided into parcels, or blocks, which can be safely connected to the alternate source bus without overloading the engine generator sets. The size of the load blocks is a function of the individual engine generator set capacity.

For example, if the load is 1800 kW and the engine generator sets are to be 500 kW each, then the load may be divided into three blocks of 500 kW each, with a fourth block at 300 kW. Such a system would require four 500 kW engine generator sets. However, if it were decided to use two 900 kW engine generator sets, the same load would be divided into two blocks of 900 kW each.

Sometimes it is necessary to examine the load in terms of how it can be suitably divided and still satisfy the needs of the various essential loads. In this case, the size of the load blocks determines the size and number of generator sets needed.

5.6.5 Establishing Load Priorities. Once the load block size is determined, then the sequence in which these loads are added to the bus should be decided upon. Each load block is assigned a priority rating. This rating specifies how many engine generator sets must be on the bus before a particular load may be transferred. For example, the first priority would be the emergency system loads, the second priority the "delayed automatic" equipment loads, and the third priority the manually switched (nonautomatic) equipment loads.

5.6.6 Load Shedding. As with adding loads to the bus, the ability to shed loads is also determined by the size and number of engine generator sets. Load shedding is necessary when the connected load exceeds the capacity of the on-line engine generator sets. This situation can occur on malfunction of an engine generator or on a drop in bus frequency. The initiation of load shedding and resulting reduction in connected load will allow the surviving engine generators to service the highest priority (emergency system) loads without interruption in, or degradation of, the power delivered.

5.6.7 Load Switching Means. There are several ways to switch loads on and off the generator bus. Inasmuch as the system is a dual source power system, there is already a built-in switching means in the system, which is the automatic transfer switch. It is generally a simple modification to cause the automatic transfer switch to be controlled in both directions for load connect and load dump operation.

When more than one class (priority) of load is fed from a given automatic transfer switch, a remote control switch can control the lower priority load on the load side of the automatic transfer switch. Another method would permit the load connect to be controlled by the automatic transfer switch, with the load dumping achieved by shunt tripping circuit breakers. However, care should be taken in the application of the shunt trip approach if molded case breakers are used, because shunt tripped breakers must be manually reset. It may be desirable to have automatic resetting means. Also, consideration should be given to the anticipated number of operations to which the device will be subjected.

There are as many approaches to load switching as there are applications for emergency power. The preferred approach for any application is determined by the requirements of the application with due consideration to reliability, flexibility and economics.

5.6.8 Typical System Operation. A typical multiengine automatic paralleling system depicting some of the load switching schemes previously mentioned is shown in Fig 55. The following sequence of operation refers to the line diagram in Fig 56. The system is comprised of four engine generators as the emergency source.

The operation is for a random access paralleling system, and the loads are connected to the bus in random order, as they become available.

The loads, however, are always connected to the emergency bus in ascending order of priority beginning with priority one. For load shedding, the loads are disconnected in descending order of priority beginning with the last priority of load to be connected.

Fig 55
Typical Automatic Paralleling System for Four Engine Generator Sets,
Including Nine Automatic Transfer Switches

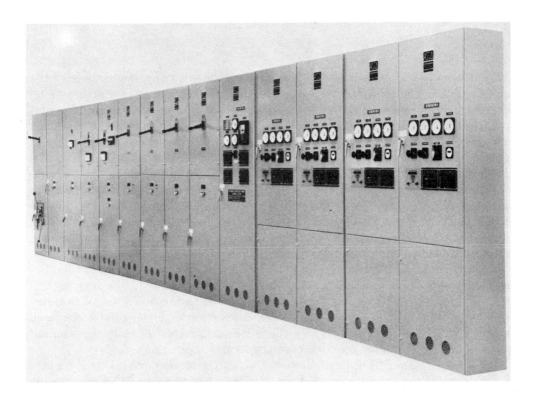

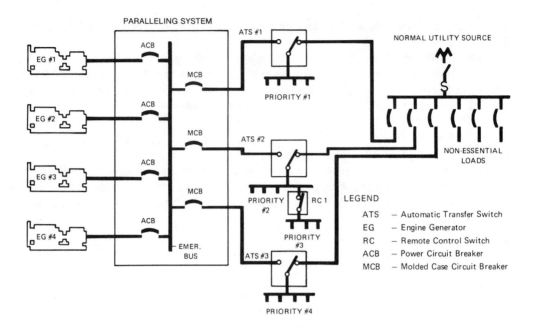

PARALLELING SYSTEM

NORMAL UTILITY SOURCE

NON-ESSENTIAL LOADS

LEGEND

ATS	— Automatic Transfer Switch
EG	— Engine Generator
RC	— Remote Control Switch
ACB	— Power Circuit Breaker
MCB	— Molded Case Circuit Breaker

Fig 56
Typical Multiengine Automatic Paralleling System

Upon a loss of normal source voltage as determined by any one or more of the automatic transfer switches shown in Fig 56, a signal initiates starting of all engine generator sets. The first set to come up to 90% of nominal voltage and frequency is connected to the alternate source bus. Critical and life safety loads are then transferred via ATS #1 and #2 to the bus upon sensing availability of power on the bus. As the remaining engine generator sets achieve 90% of the nominal voltage and frequency, their respective synchronizing monitors will control the voltage and frequency of these oncoming units to produce synchronism with the bus. Once the oncoming unit is matched in voltage, frequency, and the phase angle with the bus, its synchronizer will initiate paralleling. Upon connection to the bus, the governor will cause the engine generator set to share the connected load with the other on-line sets.

Each time an additional set is added to the emergency bus the next load is transferred in a numbered sequence via additional transfer switches, such as ATS #3, until all sets and essential loads are connected to the bus. Control circuitry should prevent the automatic transfer or connection of loads to the bus until there is sufficient capacity to carry these loads. Provision is made for manual override of the load addition circuits for supervised operation.

Upon restoration of the normal source of supply as determined by the automatic transfer switches, the engines are run for a period of up to 15 minutes for cooling down and then shutdown. All controls automatically reset in readiness for the next automatic operation.

The system is designed so that reduced operation is automatically initiated upon the failure of any plant through load dumping. This mode overrides any previous manual controls to prevent overloading the emergency bus. Upon sensing a failure mode on an engine, the controls automatically initiate disconnect, shutdown and lockout of the failed engine, and reduction of connected load to within the capacity of the remaining plants. Controls should require manual reset under these conditions.

Protection of the engine and generator against motorization is provided. A reverse power monitor, upon sensing a motorizing condition on any plant, will initiate load shedding, disconnect the failing plant, and shut it down.

5.6.9 Sensing. The paralleling system is subject to various transients in voltage and frequency which are the result of changes in loading on the system. The sensing devices must ignore these normal transients while responding to harmful ones. Basically, four types of monitors are used in paralleling systems: voltage, frequency, synchronizing, and power.

(1) *Voltage Monitors.* There are various methods of sensing the magnitude of an ac sine wave. For example, there are peak, peak above average, and rms detection. Each method has its own distinct characteristics. The rms method is preferred.

The advantage of rms detection is that the trip settings of the monitor are directly related to the ability of the power line to supply the load. Therefore, the trip points of the monitor will coincide exactly with the values determined from rms metering regardless of power line distortion. Other monitoring techniques may provide erroneous trip points when compared to rms metering on high distortion power lines.

Because generator power capacity is small in comparison to the utility, load changes may generate large voltage transients. Consequently, the monitor must differentiate between transient and long-term conditions. Thus a means of distinguishing this difference should be included in the monitor. A preferred method is to include an adjustable time delay within the monitor to override momentary system transients. The time delay should start the instant the power line voltage goes below the preset monitor limits; it should reset to zero when the voltage is restored within those limits. This, in effect, provides zero differential around the monitor trip settings.

(2) *Frequency Monitors.* As in voltage detection, there are also many techniques for sensing frequency. Therefore, careful consideration should be given to selecting the proper type of frequency monitor to meet the needs of the power system and the load. The most important considerations in selecting a frequency monitor are the effects of wave form distortion, line voltage regulation, line transients, and ambient temperature on the monitor trip settings.

Wave form distortion is more often caused by nonlinear loads than by the power source or the distribution system. The distortion becomes more pronounced when the load causing the distortion approaches the size of the power source.

Distortion often occurs when the load is fed by or through semiconductors such as diodes, triodes, or SCR's. (These devices would commonly be found in uninterruptible power supplies, solid state motor controls, etc.) For example, where triacs or SCR's are "gated on" well within the voltage cycle, as in phase control, high currents can flow over only a portion of the cycle, resulting in nonlinear loading and wave form distortion. Figure 57 is a graphic representation of the effects of distortion on a fundamental sine wave.

Sudden load changes may, in addition to voltage transients, cause momentary frequency shifts. The frequency monitor selected to protect the power line should have the capability of discriminating between momentary and sustained frequency variations. The typical methods of protecting against momentary or sustained outages are to provide trip point differentials and time delays. The advantage of a trip differential is to provide acceptance of a power line frequency which may be perfectly adequate under sustained load conditions. Time delay on trip is normally used to prevent false monitor response due to large frequency transients.

To obtain the best possible operation, both types of protection should be incorporated into the same monitor.

Fig 57
Distorted Wave Shapes

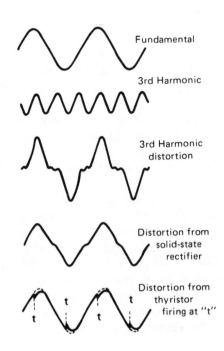

(3) *Reverse Power*. When power sources operate in parallel on a common bus, the voltage and frequency of each source is common. Neither voltage nor frequency monitors nor any combination of them can distinguish a malfunctioning engine generator set from an acceptable one. The only way to determine proper operation on the bus is to measure the power output of each engine generator set. When a set is delivering power to the bus, it is operating properly. When a set is drawing power from the bus, it is motorizing, and there exists the possibility of a malfunction. The reverse current flows are known as circulating currents. It is normal to have power flow to the set from the bus for short periods when the bus is lightly loaded. 5–10% or less of set capacity is normal. At this load level, all that keeps the sets in synchronism is the exchange of synchronizing currents causing this reverse power. Therefore, the monitor which measures for this condition should be set at a high enough value to ignore this harmless condition. However, it must be set at a low enough value to detect a malfunction. How much is enough? That depends on the engine. Some engines will draw only 1–2% of their full load rating when motorizing. Others will draw 8–10%. This determines the range of adjustability of the trip setting (that is, between 0–10%). In the absence of manufacturer's data, field tests may have to be run to determine proper settings.

There are many kinds of reverse power relays available. They fall into two general classifications: electromechanical and electronic. The electromechanical type utilizes induction disc sensing and is reasonably inexpensive. However, it needs frequent calibration checks due to its sensitivity to temperature, dust, age, moisture, etc.

The electronic type is a solid state reverse power monitor that provides repetitive accuracies without the need for constant calibration.

Whichever type is used, it should have an integral time delay to ignore transient conditions caused by light loading and switching large blocks of load.

Single-phase sensing is adequate since the generator, when acting as a motor, is a balanced load.

(4) *Synchronizing.* Sources are considered synchronized when their sine waves are equal. That is, the sources to be paralleled must be equal in (1) phase angle, (2) frequency, (3) voltage, and (4) rotation. All four of these conditions should be satisfied when paralleling engine generator sets.

Figure 58 shows five voltage sources. No two of them are synchronous.

Paralleling such sources can cause substantial damage to the engine, the generator, and/or the system. Synchronizing is, therefore, the most critical operation in the system. Due to tolerances in equipment, there should be some allowance for differences in parameters. However, when these differences become too great, the result is out-of-synchronism paralleling.

To produce minimum disturbances, the differences should be minimized. It is not unreasonable to expect the following maximum allowable differences.

Voltage	±5%
Frequency	±0.25 Hz
Phase Angle	±10°

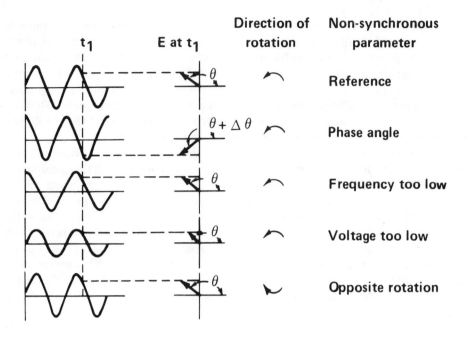

Fig 58
AC Sine Waves Representing Differences in
Phase Angle, Frequency, Voltage, and Rotation

The synchronizer should sense the existing difference in voltage, frequency, and phase angle, and then take corrective action if necessary to reduce the differences to the acceptable limits stated above.

Motorized potentiometers are often used to adjust the speed of the oncoming generator to reduce the frequency difference. However, greater reliability can be achieved where electronic governors are used to control the engine generator set. These governors are basically analog devices. Thus, the direct input of an analog signal proportional to the frequency difference will produce the necessary adjustment. This eliminates the need for a motorized potentiometer assembly which can be a potential source of malfunction.

5.6.10 Control Logic Power Sources. In the design of a control system for paralleling engine generator sets, the choice of power source is limited to the generator output, the engine starting batteries, or switchgear batteries.

(1) *DC Control Power.* In an emergency power application, the generators are normally not running. Consequently, upon an outage of the normal source, the only available power source is from batteries.

There are good reasons for using the same batteries for control power as are used for engine starting. For example, utilization of all engine batteries provides redundant power sources for the control logic. The minimal control power drain does not normally require any additional considerations in the sizing of the batteries. The control circuit burden is typically less than 1% of the engine battery Ah rating. In addition, this drain is only imposed while the system is in operation. When in the standby mode, the system does not normally draw control power. Choosing the engine starting battery as a control power source instead of a separate switchgear battery eliminates the need for maintenance and charging equipment for an additional set of batteries.

When engine starting batteries are used they provide redundancy in control power availability. An uninterruptible control power source selector device can provide for drawing control power from any combination of batteries with respect to an individual battery's ability to supply power. The device must provide positive isolation as well as prevent a fault in one bank from discharging the other batteries.

(2) *DC Control Logic.* The dc control logic provides for starting, stopping, and monitoring of the engines. When malfunctions occur, dc control logic removes the engine from service and initiates appropriate action to protect the remaining sets. In addition, the control logic for multiple engine systems must be adequate for operation at the voltage levels it is subject to.

The dc control logic should accept the generator-on-line signals in whatever order they occur to cause loads to be connected in a predetermined order of priority. The logic should also accept generator availability signals as determined by respective generator voltage and frequency monitors to permit the first unit available to be connected to the bus.

Each system should be furnished with an audible alarm to annunciate a malfunction, and a visual alarm to identify the source of malfunction. When a silencing circuit is used in conjunction with the audible type alarm, it should be reset automatically either upon correction and clearing of the malfunction, or upon the occurrence of another malfunction.

(3) *AC Control Power.* AC can be used in the control system only when the functions are such that they occur while a generator is operational and where load transients will not affect the operation. For example, it is desirable to use the generator as a power source for closing the generator main power breaker. Closing this power breaker at ac potentials requires substantially less current than at dc battery potentials. Opening current for this power breaker should be drawn from the battery source so that a generator set can be removed from the line upon loss of ac generator output. As shunt tripping requires substantially less current than closing, battery capacity is generally adequate for tripping purposes.

5.6.11 Instrumentation. Instrumentation helps to facilitate periodic inspection, preventative maintenance, and calibration essential to proper system operation and longevity.

Since the devices in the system are highly accurate, the instruments which measure the performance of these devices should also be accurate. Switchboard type 1% accuracy instruments are preferred as the application is comparable to service entrance type applications. Further, since the manufacture of a switchboard instrument requires closer tolerances than a panelboard instrument, longer life can be expected from the 1% instrument.

The minimum complement of instruments should include an ammeter for each generator with a means of switching to measure current in each line; a voltmeter with switching means to measure each line-to-line voltage; a frequency meter, preferably having a 55–65 Hz scale with division for $\frac{1}{10}$ Hz to measure engine speed; and a wattmeter to indicate engine performance.

The ammeter furnishes data on generator loading and voltage regulator performance and adjustment. The voltmeter permits adjustment of the voltage regulator for proper operating voltage. The frequency meter permits adjustment of the governor for proper operating frequency. The wattmeter permits adjustment of the governor for proper load division between engine generator sets operating in parallel. The wattmeter also permits engine adjustments based on loading.

5.6.12 Generator Power Breaker. The generator power breaker serves two functions. First, it provides protection to the generator against overload and short circuits. Second, it operates as a switch to make on inrush loads and break continuous current as well as stalled motor currents. In either case, the breaker must be capable of repetitive operations.

Air circuit breakers, and the newer insulated case (not molded case) circuit breakers, are the most commonly used devices for the generator breaker. The insulated case breakers are being used more frequently because their switching endurance life is about four times that of an air breaker. The insulated case breaker also incorporates solid state elements which provide a degree of flexibility to match virtually any overcurrent coordination protective scheme.

Fig 54 illustrates how the generator power circuit breaker fits into a typical system. For more specific information on health care facility essential electrical systems including protection, coordination, and selectivity, refer to Chapter 3. However, it's important here to reiterate the need for selectivity in essential system overcurrent protective devices. The purpose of the generator breaker is not to disconnect faulted circuits from the generator. This function is handled by downstream devices which are selectively coordinated with the generator breaker.

The generator power breaker should be of the five cycle closing type, include dc shunt trip, alarm contacts and interlock contacts for interfacing with the system. Sensing and trip units for proper coordination of trip curves within the distribution system are required with the breaker for overcurrent and short circuit protection.

The code requires the overcurrent protective device to be located at the generator, which is the source of supply for the emergency conductors. For installations where the generator switchgear is not located immediately adjacent to the generator, separate switching devices for paralleling should be furnished in the generator switchgear cubicles.

5.7 Utility Peak Demand Reduction Controls. The control of utility peak demand within a health care facility is somewhat different from the usual peak demand control systems employed in most other types of facilities. There are generally no loads that may be shed at the time which coincides with the peak demand without having significant effect on operations. Many other types of facilities are able to control peak demand by use of a load demand controller which deenergizes such items as electric space heating, electric water heating, air conditioning chillers and auxiliaries, blowers, fans and other comfort loads.

5.7.1 Special Requirements for Health Care Facility Loads. In a health care facility, none of the loads described above is suitable for dumping on an indiscriminate basis. The loss of almost any such service for an extended period could seriously compromise patient care. For this reason, ANSI/NFPA 99-1984 [3] has provided an exception to its Paragraph 8-2.3.2 as follows:

"3-3.2 *Exclusive Use for Essential Electrical Systems.* The generating equipment used shall be either reserved exclusively for such service or normally used for other purposes. If normally used for other purposes, two or more sets shall be installed, such that the demand and all other performance requirements of the Essential Electrical System shall be met with the largest single generator set out of service.

"Exception: A single generator set shall be permitted to operate the Essential Electrical System for (1) peak demand control, (2) internal voltage control, or (3) load relief for the external utility, provided any such use will not decrease the mean period between service overhauls to less than three years."

The purpose of this exception, which first appeared in the 1977 edition, is to allow the use of the standby plant for the purposes described in the exception. See Paragraph 5.7.5.

5.7.2 Nature of Electrical Load Billing. Health care facilities are generally served by a commercial utility. Billing by the utility is normally based on the following:

(1) Total consumption of the facility in kWh.

(2) Peak demand charge computed on the highest average power consumption recorded during the billing period. Demand charges are determined by the utility by measuring the power consumption during a given interval (usually 15 minutes). This procedure is repeated for each succeeding interval during the billing period (usually one month) with the demand charge being based on the highest recorded value. The demand hand indicates the highest interval (for example, 15 minutes) and is manually reset to zero each time the meter is read. The consumer is frequently billed for a percentage of the maximum demand charge (often 90%) for the next 12 months, or a percentage of the contracted capacity (often 75%), whichever is larger. In addition, other miscellaneous charges such as fuel adjustment charges, low power factor penalties, etc, may be assessed.

5.7.3 Advantages of Load Demand Control. In a health care facility, load demand control is not generally an energy conserving feature. Loads are not normally suitable for indiscriminate shedding on a programmed basis. However, it may be seen from the nature of utility billing described above, that control of demand will save dollars for the user. If the demand is closely controlled, the user will be able to avoid high demand charges, which will be used for billing not only for the month in question, but also for the subsequent 12 months. In addition, contracted capacity charges can be reduced because smaller demands will be made upon the utility's capacity.

5.7.4 Load Demand Controllers. There are many different types of load demand controllers. The simplest type is a time clock or a group of time clocks which will cause various loads to be shed on a programmed basis. Such a system is not generally suitable for health care facilities. A more sophisticated system utilizes a microprocessor which receives information from a standard kWh meter with a pulse initiator. This information is stored and accumulated during the demand interval (for example, 15 minutes) and the average kW computed. The monitor receives these signals continuously, and updates its prediction of peak demand. The unit thus becomes a predictor of when a predetermined peak demand will be reached, and also when the load will fall to acceptable levels. Loads will be transferred to the generating system when the demand approaches this predetermined level, and shed as the load is reduced back to the acceptable level. Therefore, the demand can be reduced without compromising the routine of the health care facility by using the in-house generating system.

5.7.5 Load Demand Control. Two methods of load demand control are available. The methods are operation in parallel with the utility, and operation independent of the utility. The selection of the system to use is based on the policies of the utility company. If the utility company will permit parallel operation with its service, parallel operation is usually the preferred method. However, many utility companies either prohibit this practice, or place such restrictions on its use as to make it impractical. When this is the case, operation independent of the utility is mandatory. Obviously, the first step in system selection is to ascertain the practices of the utility involved.

(1) *Operation in Parallel with the Utility—Manual.* When the load demand controller senses that the preset peak demand is being approached, the controls will start the generating set and operate an audible and visual signal to alert the operator of the condition. The operator will then manually synchronize the output of the generator with the utility source and assume its rated portion of the load through the systems controls. When the load has fallen to within acceptable limits, a second set of signals will direct the operator to manually transfer all of the load back to the utility source, and after the prescribed unloaded running time, shut down the machine. If during the operation of the system in the load demand control mode, there should be a failure of utility power, the system will revert to an emergency power system, serving the essential electrical system through the systems automatic (and manual) transfer switches.

(2) *Operation in Parallel with the Utility—Automatic.* When the load demand controller senses that the preset peak demand is being approached, the controls will start the generating set, automatically synchronize its output with the utility and cause its rated portion of the load to be assumed by the plant. When the load has fallen to within acceptable limits, the load will be automatically retransferred to the utility, and after the prescribed unloaded running time, the controls

will shut down the machine. Appropriate audible and visual signals should be provided to indicate the various conditions of the system. If during the operation of the system in the load demand control mode there should be a failure of utility power, the system will revert to an emergency power system, serving the essential electrical system through the systems automatic (and manual) transfer switches.

(3) *Operation Independent of the Utility.* Unlike the systems employing operation in parallel with the utility, which requires no interruption of power for its operation, operation independent of the utility requires an interruption of power to the various loads. For this reason it is suggested that loads served from the essential electrical system not be selected as those to be served by the system when it operates in the load demand control mode. Rather, such loads as noncritical electric cooking equipment; air conditioning chillers, fans and pumps; electric heat and loads of a similar nature be selected. This can be accomplished by providing a separate panel or panels designated to serve these loads and providing a system of mechanical key interlocks to allow such loads to be served either from the utility or from the generator. The system would operate as follows.

(a) When the load demand controller senses that the preset peak demand is being approached, the controls will start the generating set, and operate an audible and visual signal to alert the operator of the condition. The operator should take the following steps to transfer the loads to the output of the generator:

1) Trip the overcurrent device(s) serving the load demand control panel(s) from the utility source.

2) Remove the key from the key interlock device for the overcurrent device above, place it in the key interlock device for the overcurrent device(s) serving the load demand control panel(s) from the generator, and operate the key.

3) Close the overcurrent device(s), placing the loads on the output of the generator. When the load demand controller senses that the load has decreased to within predetermined limits, a second set of signals will be initiated, notifying the operator to manually retransfer the loads by reversing the procedure described above.

(b) If during the operation of the system in load demand control mode there should be a failure of utility power, the system will revert to an emergency power system, serving the essential electrical system through the systems automatic (and manual) transfer switches.

(c) The above system can also be arranged for complete automatic operation.

5.7.6 Determination of Mean Period Between Service Overhauls. In order to determine compliance with Paragraph 8-2.3.2, exception, of ANSI/NFPA 99-1984 [3], the engineer should establish that the mean period between service overhauls will not be decreased to less than three years. In order to determine this, he must know the expected hours of operation of the engine as an emergency power unit, the expected hours of operation in the peak demand reduction mode, and the manufacturer's anticipated mean operating hours between major service overhauls. Published data from manufacturers is difficult to obtain. A good rule of thumb, based on a high quality of maintenance, is shown in Table 8.

Table 8
Mean Period Between Service Overhauls

Engine Speed	Minor Overhaul* Operating Hours	Major Overhaul Operating Hours
1800 rpm	6000 and 12 000	18 000
1200 rpm	8000 and 16 000	24 000

* A minor overhaul is defined as replacement of valves, inserts, valve
guides, injection capsules, rings, and gaskets.

5.8 Elevator Emergency Power Selector Systems. The need for limited continuous elevator service in hospitals, nursing homes and related health care facilities is obvious. For this reason every applicable code and standard requires that such limited electrical service be maintained. For hospitals, both ANSI/NFPA 99-1984 [3] and ANSI/NFPA 70-1984 [2] require that elevators be on the equipment system of the essential electrical system, and both, in identical verbiage, require:

"Elevator service that will reach every patient floor, ground floor, and floors on which are located surgical suites and obstetrical delivery suites. This shall include connections for cab lighting and control and signal systems.

"In instances where interruption of power would result in elevators stopping between floors, provide throwover facilities to allow the temporary operation of any elevator for the release of patients or other persons who may be confined between floors."

This does not require that all elevators in multi-bank installations be served from the essential electrical system, but does require that each elevator be capable of being connected to the system one at a time on a selective basis.

General practice dictates that one elevator, on a selected basis, be connected to the essential system, with provisions to disconnect this elevator from the system and to connect any other.

The obvious advantage of such a system is to keep the use of the alternate source generator within reasonable limits without unduly compromising passenger safety or movement of patients during an interruption of normal power.

In the design of such systems, several problems should be addressed. These are problems associated with regenerative power and problems associated with providing proper controls to establish sequencing of the elevators when they are receiving power from the generators. Special problems are introduced into the emergency and normal power systems by elevators utilizing silicon controlled rectifiers in lieu of motor generator sets. Elevator manufacturers proposing the use of such equipment should be consulted during design in order to avoid complications.

5.8.1 Problems Associated with Regenerative Power. The nature of the electrical load imposed by elevators on either the normal or emergency power supply is very similar to that imposed by any other piece of alternating current motor-driven equipment of equivalent horsepower, except in one very important respect which is of major consideration to the electrical engineer. Under certain load conditions, an elevator actually generates electrical energy which is fed back into the power supply. For example, a fully loaded elevator moving in the down direction is actually producing energy which ultimately takes the form of electric power which is also supplied to the elevator. This same situation also occurs to a lesser degree when an empty elevator is traveling up. This phenomenon produces two problems which must be dealt with in the design of the emergency power system. The first of these problems applies only where a relatively small emergency generating plant is utilized, in which case the regenerative power from the elevator can actually cause overspeeding of the emergency generating plant and possible speed governor tripping. This problem is solved by making certain that the total emergency power load which is connected to the emergency generator is at least twice the size of the elevator load. If the load is distributed in this manner, the regenerated power from the elevator system is easily absorbed by the other devices which comprise the emergency power load. For example, if the total electric load imposed by the elevators which are required to operate on emergency power, is 150 kW, then the total emergency power load including these elevators should not be less than 300 kW.

The second of these two regenerative problems becomes more evident during the actual transfer from normal to emergency power, or from emergency to normal. If this transfer is permitted to take place at a time when the elevator system is regenerating voltage which is out of phase with the power source to which it is being reconnected, power transients can be introduced into the supply source which may trip the circuit breakers controlling the power supply. The solution to this problem requires that the transfer function take place only when the sources are in phase or the elevators are at rest. Intentional time intervals to permit the elevators to come to rest before transferring to the alternate power source is one solution. Operation is normally initiated via control contacts on the transfer switch.

A transfer switch with an "in-phase monitor" is another solution. These devices are capable of monitoring the phase angles of both power supplies, and signalling for transfer when the normal power and emergency power are in phase (see Fig 46). The transfer is then made automatically and the timed intervals as described above are not required when this device is furnished. It is not necessary to have the elevators at rest prior to restoring the service from emergency to normal power or when switching to emergency power during a routine test of the emergency power plant while normal power is available.

A second consideration would be the use of a timed center-off position transfer switch. This device would normally function with an off time of 25 cycles to possibly 60 cycles. It may also be furnished with time delays beyond these values if desired. Utilizing such a device would allow normal starting current surges for motor applications.

5.8.2 Sequence of Elevator Operation on Emergency Power. On normal power supply failure, all elevators will be brought to a stop by the automatic application of a brake which brings the car to a rest and holds it in that position. This almost invariably results in "trapping" elevator passengers in the stalled car between floors. After the establishment of emergency power and the expiration of the above interval, one elevator in each group of elevators descends automatically to a lower floor where it parks with its doors open in an inoperative condition. Each elevator in each group then goes through this same sequence one at a time until all elevators have returned to the lower floor. At this time, one preselected elevator in each group resumes normal automatic operation. The elevator control system prevents any more than one elevator in each group from operating at any given time in order to avoid overloading the emergency power supply source. All elevators will continue to be illuminated.

When the system is ready to return to normal power service, each elevator in emergency condition will stop at the next available floor where it will park inoperative with its doors open. At this time, the system can be transferred back to normal power operation and all elevators can resume normal service to the building. The above operation requires that a signal be provided to the elevator control equipment indicating that the system is ready to transfer back to normal power. This signal must be given prior to the time at which the transfer back to normal power is to occur.

If an elevator has been removed from automatic service for inspection, independent service, fire service, etc, it does not receive an automatic return signal.

If an elevator failure occurs during the sequential lowering operation which takes place on the establishment of emergency power, that car is automatically removed from service, and the next car in order assumes the lowering sequence. If an elevator is in normal service operating on emergency power and it becomes inoperative, that car is automatically removed from service, and another elevator commences operation from the emergency power supply.

(1) *Examples of Available Options.* The following are some of the options available as emergency features.

(a) *Automatic Car Selection, Express to Lobby.* In the event of normal power power failure, the elevators can be arranged to automatically return on emergency power to a preprogrammed floor, one car at a time. Operational features such as independent service shall be overridden allowing the elevator return. After all cars have been returned to this floor, a preselected elevator shall remain on emergency power. Emergency power shall be supplied through the normal machine room feeders. A pair of wires carrying emergency power is supplied to the controller designated by the elevator contractor in each machine room to supply a signal indicating power failure and activation of emergency operation. All other controls and provisions for operation of each elevator on the emergency power supply is generally provided and installed by the elevator contractor.

(b) *Manual Car Selection, Express to Lobby.* In the event of normal power failure, the elevators shall be controlled by a manual selector switch located in the lobby control panel. When actuated, this manual selector switch selects which elevator will receive emergency power. After receiving emergency power, the elevator will automatically express directly to the floor where the selector switch is located. After all elevators have been returned in this manner, a single elevator may be selected to continuously operate. Operational features such as independent service are overridden, allowing the elevator return. Emergency power is supplied through the normal machine room feeders. A pair of wires carrying emergency power should be supplied to the controller designated by the elevator contractor in each machine room to supply a signal indicating power failure and activation of emergency operation. All other control and provision for operation of each elevator on the emergency power supply is generally provided and installed by the elevator contractor.

(c) *Automatic Car Selection, Stop at Nearest Floor.* In the event of a normal power failure, the elevators can be arranged to automatically start on emergency power, travel to the nearest floor and shut down. This is done one car at a time. Operational features such as independent service must be overridden allowing this operation. After all cars have been stopped at a floor, a preselected elevator remains on emergency power. Emergency power is supplied through the normal machine room feeders. A pair of wires carrying emergency power should be supplied to the controller designated by the elevator contractor in each machine room to supply a signal indicating power failure and activation of emergency operation. All other controls and provision for operation of each elevator on the emergency power supply is generally provided and installed by the elevator contractor.

(2) *Integral Controls.* All controls for the elevators, including all of the equipment required for the automatic power selection, should be provided as an integral part of the elevator system. Modern equipment normally includes these features.

(3) *Independent Controls for Emergency Power Transfer.* In some cases, primarily in existing facilities, it may be impractical to incorporate the controls and devices required for emergency power transfer into the elevator manufacturer's equipment. Systems are available which provide group mounted automatic transfer switches, control logic devices and sensing, and a remote selector panel. The operation of the system is essentially as described for the integral systems. The system should be carefully coordinated with the elevator manufacturer to insure proper operation. One advantage of the independent system is that it can be designed such that the equipment system automatic transfer switch can be smaller than with integral systems (see Fig 59).

5.8.3 Summary. In the design of emergency power requirements for elevator systems, the following items should always be considered:

(1) Determination of number and location of elevators which will be required to operate on emergency power.

(2) Determination of whether regenerated power will be a problem, and if so, determination of steps required to absorb it.

(3) Determination of required control connections between the emergency power system and the elevator control system for selected transfer scheme.

5.9 Bypass/Isolation Switches for Automatic Transfer Switches. In many health care facilities, it is very difficult to perform regular testing or detailed inspections on the emergency system because some or all of the loads connected to the system

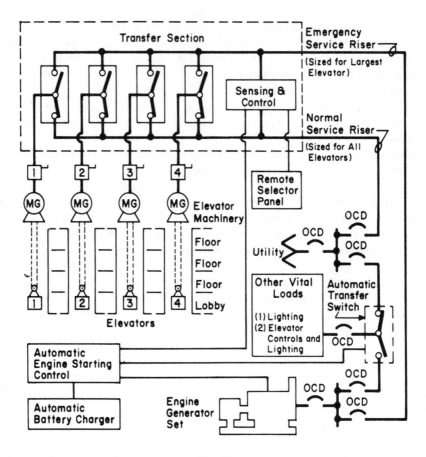

Fig 59
Elevator Emergency Power Transfer System

are vital to human life. Deenergizing these loads for any length of time is difficult. This results in a lack of maintenance. In such installations, a means can be provided to bypass the critical loads directly to a reliable source of power without downtime of the loads. The transfer switch can then be isolated for safe inspection and maintenance.

ANSI/NFPA 99-1984 (Appendix A-8-2.1.2(a)) [3] states that health care facilities should consider "properly designed and installed bypass arrangements to permit testing and maintenance of system components that could not be otherwise maintained without disruption of important hospital functions." Two-way bypass/isolation switches are available to meet this need. A typical two-way bypass/isolation switch combined with an automatic transfer switch is shown in Fig 60.

These switches can perform three functions:

(1) Shunt the service around the transfer switch without interrupting power to the load. One manufacturer interrupts the load for a few cycles during opera-

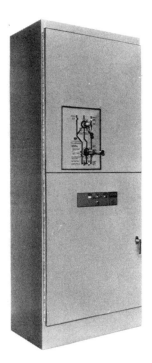

Fig 60
Typical Automatic Transfer and Two-Way Bypass/Isolation Switch

tion. In Fig 61 the bypass (upper) handle is in the bypass-to-normal (PB-NORM) position. The load gets power directly from the normal source through the right-hand BP contact. The isolation (lower) handle is shown in the closed position.

(2) Allow the transfer switch to be tested without interruption of power to the load. In Fig 62 the isolation (lower) handle is in the test position, so the transfer switch can be tested without disrupting the load.

(3) Electrically isolate the transfer switch from both sources of power and load conductors to permit inspection and maintenance of all transfer switch components. In Fig 63 the isolation handle is moved to the open position, and the load is fed directly from the normal; the automatic transfer switch (ATS) is completely isolated and can be removed without interrupting the load.

The functions outlined above are accomplished by operating two handles in an easy-to-follow sequence. The equipment can be furnished as a complete automatic transfer and bypass/isolation switch for new installations or as a replacement for existing equipment. Some arrangements can be supplied with a drawout mechanism so the transfer switch can be easily removed for maintenance.

In addition to the two-way switches, one-way switches are also available which bypass to only one preselected source. Experience has shown that the somewhat higher price for a two-way switch is fully justified when considering its over-

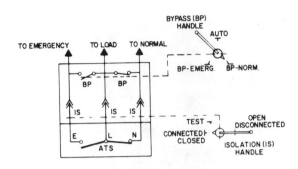

Fig 61
Bypass-Isolation Switch in Bypass-to-Normal Position

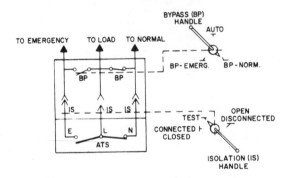

Fig 62
Bypass-Isolation Switch in Test Position

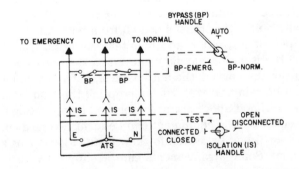

Fig 63
Bypass-Isolation Switch with Transfer Switch Removed

whelming advantages over one-way switches. For example, a two-way bypass/ isolation switch allows either power source to be selected to feed the load during bypass. The operator can choose the source that is the more dependable at that time. Furthermore, when the transfer switch is in the test or open position as shown in Figs 62 and 63, a two-way bypass/isolation switch can be used to transfer the load to the alternate source if the source to which it has been bypassed fails. One-way devices cannot provide these features.

Essential loads that warrant bypass switches to permit periodic maintenance of transfer switches should be provided with the capability to transfer in two directions. Such an arrangement assures the backup capability to transfer critical loads to an available normal or emergency power source even if the automatic switch is inoperable.

As a minimum, two-way bypass/isolation switches should be furnished for the transfer switches on the emergency system in a health care facility.

5.10 Uninterruptible Power Supplies. Uninterruptible power supplies (UPS's) are highly efficient power converting devices that provide a regulated ac voltage at their output terminals regardless of the quality of the source at their input terminals.

In the event of a total power loss at the UPS input, output power is generally provided by means of a bank of batteries. An inherent, additional benefit of the UPS is its ability to filter spikes and power aberrations from the ac source between the input and output terminals. These power problems could result from natural causes, buffer line disturbances on the utility power, or they could be caused by disturbances, such as load switching, within the facility itself.

Uninterruptible power is generally not specified by code requirements for hospitals or health care facilities. However, UPS systems are increasingly being incorporated into such electrical designs. Typical applications include backup support for sensitive laboratory and diagnostic equipment, life-support equipment in intensive care units, data processing systems, and for illumination in life-support areas.

UPS's are generally static devices, although there are hybrid systems available that combine static and mechanical components.

A UPS consists of a rectifier to convert the input ac power to dc, a bank of batteries, an inverter to reconstitute the ac sine waves, and a static switch. Refer to Fig 64 for a typical one-line diagram.

The static switch is part of a transfer system which provides a means to transfer the critical load back to utility power without interruption in the event of a system overload, an inverter malfunction, or for planned maintenance.

The battery most often used in UPS installations is the lead-calcium cell. It is ideally suited for UPS applications because of its discharge characteristics, its low hydrogen evolution, and consequently its low water usage.

The normal UPS configuration is called "reverse transfer." This term is used because the output of the UPS supplies power to the critical load during normal operation. The system transfers to the utility only in one of the alternate modes of operation, as previously noted.

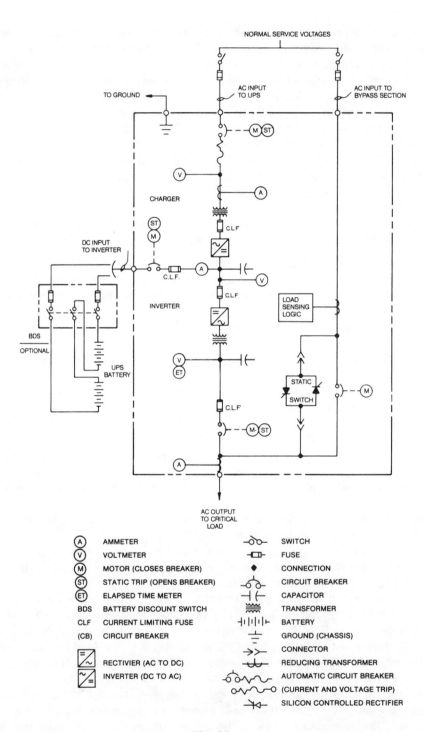

Fig 64
Typical UPS One Line

The rectifier derives its power from the utility and feeds dc power to the input of the inverter. In the event of loss of utility power, the inverter receives its power from the battery source. When the input voltage returns to the predetermined level, the rectifier begins supplying power to the inverter and also begins recharging the discharged battery bank.

Reverse transfer UPS can supply single-phase or three-phase outputs. Single-phase output units can have either a single-phase or a three-phase input. Typical single-phase units are sized to supply a load ranging from .5 kW to 50 kW, and three-phase units from 15 kW to 600 kW. A number of UPS manufacturers have the capability of paralleling units for additional capacity. They can also offer a forward transfer unit in the 0.5 kW to 10 kW range that prepackages the UPS and batteries in a common enclosure.

The design of a UPS system involves both electrical and environmental considerations. The first step is to calculate the UPS module size (rectifier, inverter, static switch combination). Determining factors are the present load, power factor, diversity of application, and future load additions and deletions. An alternate approach would be to size the UPS module to handle the anticipated load and the battery bank for the present load. Expansion can be achieved by paralleling an additional battery bank in the future. A common reserve time for the battery bank is 15 minutes.

The power connections to a UPS involve the battery bank, the input to the rectifier, the bypass circuit, and the output. The output and bypass feeders should be sized to handle the output capability of the UPS module. The rectifier is sized to handle the output of the inverter plus recharging a discharged bank of batteries. The input feeder must be sized larger than the load to handle the additional current. The battery feeder is determined by the maximum dc discharge current. As the battery begins discharging, the dc current rises as the voltage falls. Maximum dc current occurs at the point of low dc voltage shutoff. A rule of thumb is to allow a maximum 2 V drop in the cable (calculated at maximum dc current).

A separate disconnecting/overcurrent device should be provided for both the input and the bypass feeders. Additionally, an overcurrent/disconnection device should be incorporated in the total scheme and located near the battery bank for required protection. In larger UPS modules, care should be taken to limit the dc voltage to 250 V. A convenient method of achieving this would be to split the battery bank into two equal segments and connect the two across the center pole of a 3-pole battery disconnect switch as shown in the one-line diagram.

Isolation of the UPS module can be incorporated into the design through a maintenance bypass scheme. This is accomplished by first placing the UPS in a bypass mode, then closing a maintenance bypass device, and lastly opening a nonautomatic breaker or unfused device at the output of the UPS. The UPS is then completely isolated both from the critical load and from the building electrical system. This transition is accomplished without an interruption in the power supply to the critical load.

Most UPS manufacturers supply a remote annunciator panel to monitor the status of the UPS system. This is a desirable feature and should be located in the same area as code-required annunciator panels.

A final electrical consideration in the UPS design is the coordination between sizing of the protective devices at the output of the UPS inverter (usually a circuit breaker) and those downstream. Consideration should also be given to the same coordination for the situation when the UPS is in either its bypass or maintenance bypass modes.

There are three environmental considerations in the installation of a UPS: (1) the heat output of the UPS, (2) maximum ambient operating temperature and relative humidity of both the UPS module and the batteries, and (3) the hydrogen emission of the batteries.

The heat output of the UPS is a measure of the module efficiency. This heat must be removed to prevent exceeding the maximum operating temperature of both the UPS module and the batteries. Generally, the maximum operating temperature of the UPS module is considerably higher than a temperature that would adversely affect the batteries.

Provisions should be made for sufficient diffusion and ventilation of hydrogen emitted from the batteries to prevent the accumulation of an explosive mixture. This means keeping the hydrogen from reaching a level of 1% by volume of the room. If the battery room is air-conditioned, the exhaust air should not be returned to the building's air distribution system. The battery room should have its own exhaust system connected to the outdoors.

Ideally, the batteries should be located in their own room. If this is not possible, a substantial screen should partition off the batteries to limit access only to qualified persons. There are a variety of rack configurations available. The UPS manufacturer should be consulted to determine proper space and location limitations. In earthquake-prone areas, seismic battery racks should be specified. Lastly, an eyewash area should be located in the vicinity of the battery bank.

UPS's are state-of-the-art systems for which technical improvements are constantly being made. An example of this is the use of microprocessor diagnostics that enable the rapid identification of equipment problems based on critical point monitoring. This feature is of particular benefit to the health care industry where uptime of the UPS is important to its proper operation.

5.11 Maintenance. ANSI/NFPA 99-1984 [3], which is generally considered a minimum by authorities having jurisdiction, requires certain testing and maintenance procedures. Appendix C, included in ANSI/NFPA 99-1984 [3] for information purposes only, provides a maintenance guide to assist in the establishment of a maintenance program.

The equipment manufacturers have publications prescribing their recommended minimum requirements. Failure, either during initial start-up of the installation or later during an emergency situation, cannot be readily diagnosed by the designer or the owner when it is found that the manufacturer's recommendations for installation, testing, and maintenance have not been followed.

Unless space is critical, the designer should lay out the generator based on the manufacturer's largest dimension recommendations. Working space for doors, oil drainer, and minor maintenance should be considered.

For new facilities, where testing and maintenance programs have not been previously established prior to start-up, a manual should be prepared that includes:

General description of operation
Manufacturer's technical manuals
Test log
Maintenance log
Piping diagrams
Wiring diagrams
Spare parts list
Special tools
Source of emergency assistance
Maintenance schedule

Testing may be either automatic or nonautomatic. In either case personnel are required. Maintenance personnel may grow lax when automatic exercisers are used as they are likely to skip witnessing of the test. Many hospitals prefer manual testing since there is always the risk of a nonscheduled surgery being performed at the time an automatic timer may call for a load interruption test.

For installations with limited personnel capability, a maintenance and testing contract may be desirable.

When the emergency generator set is down for maintenance or repair, the essential loads may be vulnerable in the event a utility power failure should occur. The emergency system designer may want to give some consideration to the design of the system so that a portable generator can be readily connected during these periods. Nonautomatic push-button operated transfer switches, such as described in 5.3.12, may help to readily facilitate the connection of a portable generator into the system.

5.12 References

[1] ANSI/IEEE Std 446-1980, IEEE Recommended Practice for Emergency and Standby Power Systems for Industrial and Commercial Applications.

[2] ANSI/NFPA 70-1984, National Electrical Code.

[3] ANSI/NFPA 99-1984, Standard for Health Care Facilities.

[4] ANSI/UL 1008-1983, Safety Standard for Transfer Switches.

[5] EGSA/BCES1-1980, Battery Chargers for Engine Starting and Control Batteries Constant Potential Static Type. Electrical Generating Systems Association performance standard.[22]

[6] EGSA ECB1-1977, Engine Cranking Batteries. Electrical Generating Systems Association performance standard.

---

[22] EGSA documents can be obtained from EGSA, PO Box 9257, Coral Springs, FL 33065.

[7] NEMA PE5-1983, Constant Potential-Type Electric Utility (Semiconductor Static Converter) Battery Chargers.

[8] SAE J537-82, Storage Batteries.[23]

[9] Area Protection Assures Emergency Power When Failures Occur Down-Stream. *AscoFacts*, vol 2, no 6. Automatic Switch Company, Florham Park, NJ.

[10] AVERHILL, E.A. Fast Transfer Test of Power Station Auxiliaries. *IEEE Transactions on Power Apparatus and Systems*, vol PAS-95, no 3, May/June 1977.

[11] FISCHER, M.J. Designing Electrical Systems for Hospitals. Vol 5 of *Techniques of Electrical Construction and Design*. New York: McGraw-Hill, 1979.

[12] GILL, J.D. Transfer of Motor Loads Between Out-of-Phase Sources. Conference Record, Industry Applications Society, IEEE-IAS 1978 Annual Meeting.

[13] KELLY, A.R. Relay Response to Motor Residual Voltage During Automatic Transfers. *AIEE Transactions*, vol 74, Part II, Applications and Industry, Paper 55-427, September 1955.

[14] LEWIS, D.G. and MARSH, W.D. Transfer of Steam-Electric Generating-Station Auxiliary Busses. *AIEE Transactions*, vol 74, Part III, Power Apparatus and Systems, Paper 55-96, June 1955.

[15] SQUIRES, R.B. Analytical Studies of Large Induction Motor Behavior During Bus Transfer. Gibbs & Hill, Inc. A paper presented at the conference for Protective Relay Engineers, Texas A&M University, College Station, Texas, April 27, 1973.

---

[23] This document can be obtained from Customer Service Department, SAE, 400 Commonwealth Drive, Warrendale, PA 15096.

6. Electrical Safety and Grounding

6.1 General Discussion

6.1.1 Purpose. The purpose of this chapter is to discuss the basic engineering involved to obtain electrical safety in health care facilities through proper design of the electrical distribution system. This chapter will provide the background as to why electricity can be a hazard, and will give a perspective to the hazards so that a rational design may be made. Factors involved in making design decisions among the various options available will be discussed.

6.1.2 Overview. The incorrect application of electricity can cause both minor and serious problems. There were serious problems and accidents in the period from 1940 and 1970, which required major additions to the codes and standards. While some of the measures taken at that time may be considered too stringent today and require some modification because of cost containment restraints, the ratio of electrical safety to the increase of complexity of instrumentation has greatly increased even as the level of complexity has been rising. The designer must remain vigilant to electrical hazards and take appropriate safety steps. It is also important that unnecessary safety measures not be specified if they are not justified.

The general level of safety requirements for electrical devices and installations has increased over the past years. Examples of this are changes in the NFPA National Electrical Code and the Underwriters Laboratories standards. It should be pointed out that the National Electrical Code or any other NFPA standard can only be enforced if it is adopted as being applicable by an authority having jurisdiction. Any governmental body or administrative agency may or may not incorporate the NFPA codes into its own health, building or construction codes. Familiarity with local standards is mandatory for any designer.

This chapter will concentrate on the special requirements of a health care facility over and above those normally required for a commercial facility. Principal differences are in layout, care of installation, quality of components and special devices required.

Since all of the details contained in referenced documents cannot be duplicated in this chapter, it is highly recommended that these be obtained, studied, and their applicability to a particular facility determined.

The patients in a hospital are either ill or incapacitated and rely on others for care, and as such, are often physically incapable of taking self-protective action. These patients may be brought in contact with electrical equipment routinely, and this may take place in a wet environment or in the presence of flammable vapors, such as alcohol or ether, plus supplemental oxygen. The patient may also be subjected to invasive procedures of various types.

The design must take into consideration the electrical safety of not only the patient, but also of the nurse, doctor and any other health care provider working in the environment. Hazards can exist not only in the familiar ampere ranges, but also at the milliamp and microamp levels.

Among basic safety features required are overcurrent protection, adequate dependable power, (especially for life support equipment), reliable grounding, and coordinated protection to guard against shock or burns from leakage and fault currents.

6.2 Physiological Parameters. An understanding of some of the physiological parameters involved should give the designer of hospital care facilities a better understanding of the factors involved in the development of a safe environment for the patient.

6.2.1 Cell Excitability. The individual nerve and muscle cells have a small inside-to-outside potential of the order of 90 mV because of chemical differences. Excitation of the cell for transmission of a nerve impulse or muscle contraction can be produced by chemical or electrical imbalance from the normal resting state. The levels involved are nonlinear in amplitude and time, so that creation of perceived shock and contraction is not simple. To a certain extent, this explains the variances in expressing levels of shock in ranges rather than specific values. There are many variables of nonlinearities present.

6.2.2 Nerve Reaction to Electrical Stimuli. Nerve reaction to electrical stimuli is to send to the brain a message of exposure to an unsafe condition. A current density at a nerve location sufficient to stimulate one or more nerve cells is required. The same current density in different areas of the body may create different sensations.

6.2.3 Muscle Reaction to Electrical Stimuli. A current introduced into the heart through the diffused connection provided by a liquid filled catheter may cause no cardiac reaction, while the same current could produce a cardiac reaction if introduced through a very small metal electrode. At low levels, the nonlinearities become a factor, so that the difference between a constant current source and a constant voltage source becomes important.

Improper stimulation of the cardiac muscle can create disorganized contractions called fibrillation, with little or no pumping of blood. Severe contraction of hand muscles can create grasping of an energized conductive object without the ability to let go. Heavy currents across the chest can cause contraction of muscles controlling breathing and possibly cause suffocation.

6.2.4 Tissue Reaction to Heat. The principle of current flowing through resistance generating heat can also cause harmful burning in a tissue. This phenomenon is also used for cutting tissue and coagulation of bleeding sites.

6.2.5 Body/Tissue Resistance. Body tissue has, in general, a specific resistance that is useful in calculating expected currents. During defibrillation where massive currents are produced through large electrodes, good electrical contact with the skin is necessary.

The skin, in general, provides a high impedance barrier to most sources from which leakage currents could flow. Well prepared contacts for EKG's, etc, provide about 1000 Ω between electrodes. Dry, calloused skin may have an impedance approaching one million ohms.

6.3 Shock Levels. The susceptibility of humans to electrical current has often been demonstrated in powerline accidents. Burns, ventricular fibrillation, respiratory paralysis, hemorrhage and neural dysfunctions are frequent results of contact by a human body between a power source and ground. These effects can also be caused in daily work hazards through misuse of electrical appliances and wiring.

The following values relate to alternating current applied to the unbroken skin:

6.3.1 Perception. The lowest levels of current that are perceptible to a person start at about 100 μA through a very sharp point, resulting in a high current density. A large contact area, such as a bed handrail, may require 1 mA for perception.

6.3.2 Contraction. Arm muscle contraction and pain may develop with 1–5 mA, and is assured at 10 mA.

6.3.3 No-Let-Go. Uncontrolled contraction (no-let-go), can start at levels of 6 mA and higher. Up to 30 mA, these reactions increase in intensity, and although such currents are usually non-fatal, temporary respiratory paralysis can occur. Above 30 mA, the chances of a fatality from a variety of causes, including ventricular fibrillation, increase.

For the general patient, the above levels may be lower. The patient may be weak, helpless to free himself, suffering from a damaged or stressed heart, an infant, in a wet environment, or experiencing an increased electrical sensitivity as a result of drug therapy.

There is another class of patient for whom the level of dangerous current is appreciably lower. For these patients, direct electrical pathways to the patient's heart may exist through pacing wires or fluid-filled catheters. Current in the range of 20 μA to 300 μA at 60 Hz is sufficient to cause ventricular fibrillation under such circumstances.

6.3.4 Cardiac Fibrillation. Cardiac fibrillation is a phenomena in which the muscles of the heart contract in a disorganized manner so that little blood is pumped. Cardiac fibrillation is a complex phenomenon related to concentration, location, duration of current and timing in the cardiac cycle. Part of the complication of determining a threshold level is that the mere physical placement of an electrode within the heart may cause fibrillation with no current. Under controlled conditions when fibrillation is intentionally produced by direct stimulation, currents of 80 μA and higher are usually required from constant current sources.

Other clinical parameters which may cause the heart to become susceptible to induced fibrillation in the presence of low levels of 60 Hz are: alternating current and electrolyte imbalance, myocardial ischemia, hypothermia, hypoxia, and the use of drugs such as digitalis, alcohol or vasodilators. Good engineering design today sets 10 μA at 60 Hz as the maximum allowable leakage current available from any device having leads that may enter the heart.

6.4 Areas of Potentially Increasing Hazards. The following list is arranged in a general order of increasing electrical hazards. No such arrangement is absolute as practices, usage and maintenance vary. In addition, for most areas the true increase from type-to-type is so slight, this order can easily be changed.

6.4.1 Waiting Rooms, Offices. Good standard commercial specifications can be followed in these areas.

6.4.2 Corridors. Corridors have historically been high abuse areas as far as electrical receptacles are concerned. Therefore, receptacles should be selected to withstand heavy physical abuse. Oftentimes, corridor receptacles are used for supplying power to cleaning machines, which are taken into a patient room. Requirements would therefore also include green wire ground and metal conduit. Hospital grade receptacles or equivalent are recommended.

6.4.3 Psychiatric Patient Room. Psychiatric Patient Room is to be treated as a general care patient room. For the number of circuits and outlets see ANSI/NFPA 70-1984 [2]* and ANSI/NFPA 99-1984 [3]. While not common, it is possible to have a psychiatric ICU or CCU room, in which case it would be treated as a critical patient care area as outlined in the aforementioned documents. Green wire ground and metal conduit, as well as tamper proof receptacles, are mandatory. Hospital grade receptacles or the equivalent are recommended.

6.4.4 General Medical Care. Number of circuits and receptacles should conform to ANSI/NFPA 70-1984 [2] and ANSI/NFPA 99-1984 (Chapter 8) [3]. Green wire ground and metal conduit are mandatory. It is recommended that all receptacles be hospital grade or equivalent.

6.4.5 Critical Care Patient Room. Number of circuits and receptacles should conform to ANSI/NFPA 70-1984 [2] and ANSI/NFPA 99-1984 [3]. Green wire ground and metal conduit are mandatory. Emergency power provisions are also mandatory by these standards. It is recommended that all receptacles be hospital grade or equivalent. While isolated power is not mandatory, it is often used in these areas and invasive procedures are common. When isolated power is used, the same specifications must be followed as when it is used in an anesthetizing location. These specifications can be found in ANSI/NFPA 70-1984 [2] or ANSI/NFPA 99-1984 (Chapter 3) [3].

6.4.6 Recovery Rooms. This is a very difficult area to categorize since areas under this heading can widely vary in use and application. Most often it is an intensive nursing area where the patient is held and observed until he recovers from anesthesia. The area should be equipped with green wire ground, emergency power service, and metal conduit. It is recommended that all receptacles be hospital grade or equivalent. If the hospital does plan to use the recovery room for

---

*The numbers in brackets correspond to those in the references at the end of this chapter.

patients requiring life support and invasive monitoring, it should be treated as a critical patient care area. Most hospitals, however, take critical patients directly to the intensive care or coronary care units rather than hold these patients in the recovery room.

The codes do not address the recovery room with regard to the number of receptacles and circuits required for patients. Consultations with local code authorities and with hospital personnel using this area are recommended before determining these service requirements.

6.4.7 Wet Locations. The use of ground fault circuit interrupters is appropriate and required for areas such as those used for hydrotherapy. Where power interrruption cannot be tolerated, the use of isolated power is required by NEC.

A controversy exists as to whether patient dialysis units should be considered wet locations. It depends upon the design of the unit, the type of equipment and the intended operation. Operating or procedures rooms that often have spilled liquids, lots of metallic grounded objects and grounded drains need ground fault circuit interrupters or isolated power if interruption of power is not acceptable. Where inhalation anesthesia is used, isolated power is required by NEC Code at the time of this writing.

6.4.8 Laboratories. The special precautions for this area relate to the type of receptacle to be used. These should be the best grade available. Where these are mounted in a continuous raceway, it is very important to use a good grade of receptacle. Extra care is needed in specifying bonding between receptacle and raceway and various raceway sections in any single location or room. Green wire ground is highly recommended and may be required by local codes.

6.4.9 Outpatient Care Units with Invasive Procedures. Follow the same specifications as those for an equivalent area for inpatient units.

6.4.10 Heart Catheterization Rooms. Follow grounding procedures as outlined in ANSI/NFPA 70-1984 [2] and ANSI/NFPA 99-1984 [3]. Determine whether this is a multi-function room with hospital administration, and if it is used as a general anesthesia area follow anesthetizing location specifications as given in ANSI/NFPA 70-1984 [2] and ANSI/NFPA 99-1984 [3]. Careful and precise grounding is mandatory in this area as well as hospital grade receptacles. It is recommended that at least one grounding jack be provided since some devices used for dye injection require a redundant ground.

6.4.11 Operating Rooms in Which Only Local Anesthetic Agents Are Used. There are times when this area would not have to receive complete treatment as an inhalation anesthetizing location. However, documentation of the intent of use should be obtained from the hospital administration and careful review with local code authorities should be made. In many cases the facts will indicate full treatment as an anesthetizing location.

6.4.12 Inhalation Anesthetizing Locations. Follow specifications as they appear in ANSI/NFPA 70-1984 [2] and ANSI/NFPA 99-1984 (Chapter 3) [3]. Isolated power, green wire grounding, and hospital grade receptacles are all mandatory. Recent code changes, as covered in ANSI/NFPA 99-1984 (Paragraph 3-2.3.1.1) [3], may not require some inhalation anesthetizing locations to have isolated power.

6.4.13 Inhalation Anesthetizing Locations Which Become Wet Locations. This covers almost all operating rooms, with the exception of some highly specialized areas (such as those exclusively used for ophthalmology). Follow the specifications for "Wet Locations" as shown in ANSI/NFPA 70-1984 [2] in addition to the specifications for "Anesthetizing Locations" in ANSI/NFPA 70-1984 [2] and ANSI/NFPA 99-1984 (Chapter 3) [3]. Isolated power, green wire grounding, hospital grade receptacles, and metallic conduit are all mandatory. Emergency power requirements should be provided as specified in ANSI/NFPA 99-1984 (Chapter 8) [3].

6.4.14 Inhalation Anesthetizing Locations in Which Invasive Thoracic Procedures Are Performed. Same as 6.4.12 on p. 209.

6.4.15 Inhalation Anesthetizing Locations in Which Flammable Anesthetizing Agents Are Used. Same specifications as 6.4.12 except follow additional requirements as outlined for "Hazardous Areas" in ANSI/NFPA 70-1984 [2] and ANSI/NFPA 99-1984 (Chapter 3) [3].

6.5 Fire and Explosion Hazards

6.5.1 Flammable Anesthetizing Agents. Many of the requirements for electrical safety were developed to minimize the fire and explosion hazards when ether and other flammable agents were used. The use of flammable anesthetics in the operating room and the potential problem of explosion required that special electrical safeguards be developed. Since flammable gases can be ignited by static electric discharge, comprehensive methods minimizing the build-up of static charge were developed and used. These included high impedance conductive floors, conductive footware, clothing for minimum generation of static charge, high impedance conductivity of elastomeric tubing used within the anesthesia airway path, and grounding of patient electrical devices and exposed metal. Isolated power systems were installed and monitored to indicate when the first line-to-ground fault current would exceed a μA level, where the arc from the current could ignite the gas.

Unfortunately, the concentrations of ether used for anesthetizing purposes are those that are the most explosive. Most explosions have either occurred within the anesthetizing machine or within the patient. Static discharge, as well as sparks from electrically powered devices, introduced in the explosive atmosphere can cause fires and explosions. Since most flammable anesthetizing agents are heavier than air, the area in an anesthetizing area up to the 5 foot level must be treated as a Class I, Group D location as covered by the National Electrical Code.

The use of flammable anesthetizing agents is continually decreasing, and as a result, the designer must establish the client's intentions in this regard.

While many of the new operating rooms are being designed for exclusive use of nonflammable inhalation anesthetizing agents, the current National Electrical Code and ANSI/NFPA 99-1984 (Chapter 3) [3] both require the use of isolated power in all operating rooms. The use of isolated power measurably reduces the risk of electrical shock and completely eliminates the risk of explosion due to flammable inhalation anesthetizing agents.

6.5.2 Flammable Cleaning and Preparation Agents. Several agents, such as alcohol which is used as a cleaning and antiseptic agent, are volatile and may be ignited, if not properly used, by the spark from electrosurgery devices.

The current resulting from the high impedance leakage path produced by splashing or spilling liquids either on the equipment or into the electrical receptacles may cause an alarm of the isolated power system. Carefully followed grounding procedures help to reduce the hazard from this type of situation. It should be noted that these same spills in the absence of an isolated system would probably cause a power interruption or, at a minimum, cause higher current to flow.

6.5.3 Oxygen Enriched Atmosphere. The same fire hazards from electrical short circuits that cause fires in electrical devices in other environments can cause fires in health care facilities. These may be aggravated by the fact that the air may be more often enriched with oxygen in the hospital than in other types of environments.

6.5.4 Conductive Flooring. Conductive flooring is used to control static electricity in anesthetizing locations where flammable anesthetic agents are administered. In older operating rooms the floors are often constructed of special terrazzo that incorporates carbon to form conductive pathways throughout the floor. The floor usually includes a metallic grid so that no point on the floor is more than a few inches from a grounded conductive element.

Some conductive floors are made of conductive ceramic tiles. This method results in a floor that is very stable with regard to the resistance but is apt to have tiles break loose when heavy equipment is rolled over it. The reason for this seems to be that when adhesives are made conductive they lose those characteristics that contribute to their durability as an adhesive.

Another type of conductive floor is sheet vinyl which is manufactured with a cushioned backing. It maintains the proper conductivity very well but is prone to be damaged by wheeled operating room tables and portable X-ray equipment, and it is easily cut when sharp surgical instruments are dropped on it.

A very common conductive floor is made of squares of hard conductive vinyl. These are placed over a grid of copper tape which is to insure that there is an uninterrupted path of conductivity between any two points on the floor.

The NFPA standard test method calls for a minimum and a maximum resistance between 5 pound circular electrodes, 2½ inches in diameter and covered with metal foil.

Under current NFPA rules, it is not necessary to have conductive floors in nonflammable anesthetizing locations. Where conductive floors exist, it is required that they be tested at lease once per year. There is no upper limit of resistance for conductive floors in these nonflammable anesthetizing locations and the lower limit is 10 000 ohms to insure that the conductive floor does not increase the hazards of electrical shock by offering too low an impedance to ground.

6.6 Environmental Conditions Relating to Electrical Safety

6.6.1 Source of Leakage Currents. Leakage current comes primarily from capacitive coupling between energized conductors and grounded objects, and secondarily from high resistance paths through or along the surface of insulating materials.

When two conductors in close proximity are energized from the secondary of a distribution transformer, a small current flows between them due to the dielectric properties of the conductor insulation. When these conductors are run in grounded metallic conduit, there will also be leakage between the "hot" wire of a grounded system and the conduit. In an isolated system neither power conductor is grounded, so there will be leakage from both power conductors to ground (that is, to the conduit or grounding conductor). The path is from one conductor to the conduit and on to the other conductor. Current does not flow in the conduit since there is no direct return path to the current source from ground. See Tables 9 and 10.

Table 9
Table of Leakages Contributed by Wiring

Materials Used	Result
TW Wire Metal Conduit wire pulling compound with ground conductor	3 μA per ft of wire
XLP Wire Metal Conduit *No* wire pulling compound with ground conductor	1 μA per ft of wire

Table 10
Table of Leakages Contributed by Equipment

Device	*Leakage Range in μA
OR Table Light (single light without track)	75–175
OR Table Light (track mounted)	300–400
Portable OR Light	10–100
X-ray Viewer (single)	50–150
Electro-Surgery Machine	100–300
Vacuum Pump	50–125
Physiological Monitor (single channel)	30–200
Physiological Monitor (eight channel)	275–350
Heart-Lung Machine	350–450
Defibrillator	50–125
Portable X-ray (120 V capacitor charge)	30– 50
Cardiac Fibrillator	15– 50
Respirator	100–150
Cardiac Synchronizer	75–125
Hyperthermia Unit (single patient unit)	125–175

NOTE: Excessive power cord lengths will add measurably to the total leakage of the equipment; i.e., a 60 ft power cord can add from 60–130 μA of leakage to an electro-surgery machine.

*Ranges given are from tests of equipment found in the field and in good working condition. Older equipment exhibited higher leakage currents.

6.6.2 Limits Set by Standards. Table 11 shows leakage current and voltage limits set by present standards ANSI/NFPA 99-1984 (Chapter 9) [3], ANSI/NFPA 70-1984 [2], and ANSI/AAMI SCL 12-78 [1]. These safety values are based upon physiological parameters. In general, particularly for the voltage, the actual values measured at time of acceptance should be much lower than these. Values approaching these indicate that something is wrong with the design or the installation.

6.6.3 Protective Measures for Leakage Current. The grounding system is the primary safeguard for bypassing the leakage and fault currents to prevent shock from these sources. The green grounding wire is the required ground and by itself may provide an effective grounding impedance of the order of 0.1 to 0.3 Ω at the end of a branch circuit. Metal conduit lowers the effective grounding impedance by providing another parallel path.

It should be emphasized that when an ungrounded electrical system is used, it does not diminish the need for an effective, low resistance grounding system. While the ungrounded distribution system limits the amount of fault current that flows in the fault, it does not eliminate the fault current completely. The grounding conductor is an effective shunt for this current in parallel with the patient and personnel.

The ungrounded system response to line-to-line fault is exactly the same as that of a conventionally grounded system, in that it will activate the overcurrent protective devices and interrupt power to the area. Most faults which occur within appliances are, however, line-to-ground type faults as opposed to line-to-line faults.

An ungrounded electrical system is more expensive than a grounded system to install, since an isolation transformer and line isolation monitor (LIM) must be

Table 11
Maximum Safe Current Leakage Limits

	ANSI/NFPA 99-1984 [3]	ANSI/AAMI SCL 12-78 [1]
Domestic Devices (Appliances, Lamps, etc)	500 μA	500 μA
Patient Contact (ECG Machine)	100 μA	100 μA
Patient Connected (ECG Electrode)	100 μA	50 μA
Intercardiac Leads (Catheter electrodes inside heart)	20 μA	10 μA

Maximum Safe Voltage Differential

	ANSI/NFPA 99-1984 [3] New Construction	ANSI/NFPA 99-1984 [3] Existing Construction	ANSI/NFPA 70-1984 [2] New & Existing Construction
General Areas	20 mV	500 mV	500 mV
Critical Care Areas	20 mV	40 mV	40 mV

provided. The package convenience of an isolated system in a single enclosure allows its installation in less time than installing individual components. Periodic tests should be performed on this equipment as well as the isolated power system, and records kept of the results of these tests. Ten minutes per month should be allowed for each ungrounded system within the hospital. For a conventionally grounded system, maintenance to insure the integrity of the ground, and to insure that the equipment is satisfactory, is at least as demanding. The cost of an isolated power system and the line isolation monitor must be evaluated against the benefits, the code requirements and the insurance premium, if it is not present. The isolated system is still recognized as the safest possible system by ANSI/NFPA 70-1984 (Article 517) [2] and ANSI/NFPA 99-1984 [3] even though it is an optional requirement in the CCU and ICU areas.

Usually modern construction adds one or more parallel, redundant grounding paths to the green grounding wire in terms of metal conduit, metal piping and metal structural members. These paths provide an effective grounding impedance at the receptacle in the order of 2 to 20 milliohms (mΩ). In addition to providing a low impedance, these elements provide a multi-path grid for fault currents so that voltages that do develop within the patient vicinity, even during a severe fault, seldom cause hazardous conditions. Hazardous conditions generally develop when device grounding wires or the connection to the distribution grounding system, or both, fail. Ground fault circuit interrupters (GFCI's) and isolated distribution systems minimize these hazards. GFCI's should only be applied where interruption of power is tolerable.

6.6.4 Design Factors Affecting Leakage Current. Specific inductive capacity (SIC) is a term which is used by wire manufacturers to evaluate the dielectric properties of the insulation characteristics of a particular wire. Dielectric constant is a term used to define the properties of insulating materials. The two terms, although closely related, are not exactly the same.

The National Electrical Code recommends that the secondary conductors of an isolated power system have an insulation with a dielectric constant of 3.5 or less. It should be recognized also that most manufacturers will state the SIC number which is usually higher than the dielectric constant of the insulation material. Care should be taken to define a particular wire for these low leakage applications.

It is important to recognize that for the consideration of leakage currents, the insulation quality and thickness limit the capacitive coupling between the conductors and ground. Capacitive coupling is determined by the dielectric constant of the insulation, the conductor length, and the spacing between the conductor and ground. Wire insulation with the lowest dielectric constant may have other properties which are unacceptable. Polyethylene has a lower dielectric constant than cross-link polyethylene but is also has a lower temperature rating.

6.6.5 Neutral to Ground Short Circuits. This is a phenomenon which does not cause problems directly with equipment operation. Such a fault is a common source of ground currents which can produce a serious secondary interference with measurements such as ECG and EEG. Most simple circuit testers do not test for this fault.

Another source that needs review is the grounding method used by X-ray and other heavy duty equipment with regard to the neutral. Sometimes these units use the ground as a neutral return.

6.6.6 Line-to-Line Faults. These should be protected by appropriate overcurrent devices coordinated in such a manner that a minimum portion of the system is affected. This requires careful coordination of the various devices in series. Careful design, installation and maintenance practices are required to minimize nuisance tripping when using GFCI's.

Branch circuits need to be planned with regard to occupant usage; the probabilities of a line-to-line fault in one room unintentionally interrupting the power supply to the life support system in another room, perhaps not even adjacent to the room with the fault, need to be minimized.

6.6.7 Line-to-Ground Faults. These can cause service interruption problems, the same as line-to-line faults. In addition, they introduce a current on the grounding system which can create further problems. Good electrical plugs, receptacles, device construction and adequate maintenance procedures will minimize these faults.

6.6.8 Transformer Vault Location and Electrical Disturbances. Since stray magnetic fields can cause problems with EEG or ECG laboratory measurements, precautions should be taken to assure that electrical installations which might create stray magnetic fields are not located adjacent to these measurement areas.

Switching devices may create electrical disturbances affecting electronic diagnostic devices such as cardiac monitors. A diagnostic device which is rendered incapable of providing the medical team with timely information or correct data is as great a hazard to the patient as a fire or an electrical shock. Radiation from the radio transmission on an adjacent building or transients from an elevator motor can also create problems which must be considered by the design engineer.

6.6.9 Wet Locations. An electrical shock is always possible when a line power device is operated in the presence of grounded conductive material and a person can bridge the gap between the two.

Large metal decks and floors covered with water present such a possible hazardous condition. A water-covered floor is potentially more hazardous than a dry metal deck since water can penetrate shoes and make better connection to the body than is possible from a dry metal deck. In addition there is always the possibility of having water splashed into electrical devices, creating contact with electrical sources.

The location of electrical devices near tubs or pools of water where a patient may be treated or where patients swim presents the possibility of shock.

Most operating rooms are considered wet locations since conductive liquids are frequently spilled.

A bed with an incontinent patient could possibly be considered a wet location. There have been reports of serious shocks when electrical beds had cord controls operated at line voltage. Using sealed, low voltage or pneumatic controls reduces the possibilities of these shocks.

Several precautionary steps need to be taken or considered whenever it is routine to have concentrations of conductive liquids on the floor while patients are present.

The first and most important step is to have equipment made for this type of environment properly installed, used and maintained with care. Steps should be taken to provide splash guards. Metal enclosures containing line powered equipment should be permanently grounded. Line powered equipment should be located as far from the wetted area as is practical. Particular care should be given to the placing of cord connected equipment where the cord might fall into a tub, basin or pool in which individuals will be working or treated. Electrocutions in home bathrooms have most often occurred when electrical appliances were placed near the tub and then were touched or fell into the tub.

Where portable cord connected line operated equipment will be used such as in a hydrotherapy room, GFCI's can be used to provide protection when accidents do occur. In the operating room the isolated power system shall be used, because power interruption cannot be tolerated.

At this writing the National Electrical Code requires GFCI's to be installed in new bathrooms in homes but not in hospital bathrooms. Accidents could occur with line-powered tooth brushes, shavers or hair dryers. An alternate to GFCI's would be to eliminate line powered receptacles.

6.7 Basic Safety Measures

6.7.1 Insulation. Energized conductors shall be insulated from each other, from ground, from patients and hospital personnel. This insulation is created both by the insulating material used and by space separation. Primary insulation protection of cardiac catheters can be provided by properly insulating the exposed end or by making the environment surrounding the catheter as safe as possible.

6.7.2 Grounding. Grounding provides a nonhazardous return path for leakage currents that exist and minimizes the hazard produced when a fault condition develops.

(1) *System Grounding.* Grounding in a critical patient care area and in an anesthetizing location is an important ingredient in safeguarding against shock and electrocution. Proper grounding provides a means for dissipating static charges and shunting fault currents and normal leakage currents away from patients and attendants.

A good grounding system requires a reference grounding point, usually the grounding bus in the distribution panel, previously referred to in some documents as an equipotential ground. All conductive surfaces in the patient vicinity that are likely to be energized are bonded to the reference grounding point with an effective conductance at least equal to #10 AWG copper wire. Two typical surfaces are the oxygen outlet and the plumbing fixture. All receptacle grounding terminals are grounded to the reference grounding point by means of the minimum #10 AWG insulated copper conductor. The conductor is insulated for corrosion protection and to prevent arcing points between the conduit and the conductor in case of a fault.

Grounding provides a low impedance path to safely conduct fault currents or leakage currents back to the source. It also is a means of bonding all conductive surfaces together such that the potential differences between such surfaces are minimal. Good grounding is more essential in health care facilities than other occupancies because of the vulnerability of the patients. Patients, especially those that are under an anesthesia, medication, or who are very ill cannot react to, or otherwise protect themselves from electrical shock as can a normal healthy individual and these patients are frequently connected to electrical equipment. In addition, potentials that are normally not hazardous to a clothed, healthy person might be dangerous in a health care facility. The nature of a patient's illness may lower his natural body resistance due to incontinence, perspiration or open wounds. The process of diagnosing a patient can make that patient more vulnerable to electrical shock. The grounding system in a health care facility is designed to minimize the voltage potentials that can be created on ground conductor surfaces due to circulating ground currents.

The National Electrical Code (1971, 1975 and 1978 editions) specified and dictated the use of a grounding system with maximum resistances for each branch of such a system. While these requirements have been considerably reduced in the 1981 and 1984 National Electrical Codes (ANSI/NFPA 70-1984 [2]) and ANSI/NFPA 99-1984 [3], the grounding requirements still remain more demanding than those shown in Article 250 for other occupancies. While the term "equipotential grounding" is no longer used in the codes and standards, the electrical engineer designing a hospital facility should be cautioned not to confuse the elimination of the code requirements with the elimination of all special grounding requirements in certain areas. Careful study of the code should be made to determine exactly what special grounding provisions must be provided in each project While the code allows building steel to be used as a grounding conductor if it can be proven it is equivalent to a #10 AWG copper conductor, the designer may not feel that this would be a viable alternative except where the building exists and resistance can be measured prior to any work being done. The expedient of specifying a copper conductor in a new building may be the safer path and, in the long run, the least expensive path to follow.

(2) *Power Cord Grounding.* The green grounding conductor provided in an equipment power cord prevents static potentials from building up to dangerous values on non-current carrying parts such as housings, cases and boxes of electrical appliances. If these parts are not properly grounded, a static charge could accumulate to some degree and may reach such a value that it will automatically discharge in the form of an electrostatic spark. Such a static discharge could be a hazard to the patient and the attendant, if it ignited some flammable gas or material or provided a shock.

The grounding conductor also provides a path for leakage current and fault current which could be conducted to an electrical appliance case. The magnitude of this leakage current is dependent on the characteristics of the appliance and the insulation associated with it. The leakage current could result in potential differences between pieces of equipment and could flow through vital organs of a patient, if a patient current path was established. One of these conditions is encountered in cardiac catheterization procedures where small amounts of current can cause ventricular fibrillation. An example would be a patient in an electrically operated bed with the patient having monitoring leads that are not isolated. The grounding path could be through the patient via the attendant and the cardiac leads. Since the resistance of the power cord ground conductor is significantly less than the path through the patient, almost all of the current will flow to the grounding conductor.

The resistance of the grounding conductor is of utmost importance. A #10 AWG only represents 0.001 Ω/ft. In anesthetizing areas design practice limits the potential differences between conductor surfaces that could come in contact with the patient to 40 mV.

(3) *Grounding Jacks.* In previous issues of the National Electrical Code, provisions for the connection of conductive non-electrical devices were dictated. These provisions had to be met by supplying each critical patient care area with a specified type of ground jack. Each operating room was required to have a minimum of six ground jacks. While this is no longer a code requirement, many engineers recommend that at least a single ground jack be provided in each critical care patient area. This ground jack will provide easy connection to the grounding system for the purpose of redundant grounding of any particular piece of exceptionally hazardous equipment and will further allow connecting to the ground system for testing purposes. While the cost of a single ground jack, or even several ground jacks in a room is very low and almost negligible, the benefits provided by having the connection to the ground system conveniently accessible are innumerable. If ground jacks are specified in the project, it is desirable to specify several ground cords that can be used with these ground jacks. See Fig 65.

Fig 65
Grounding Plugs and Twist Lock Receptacles

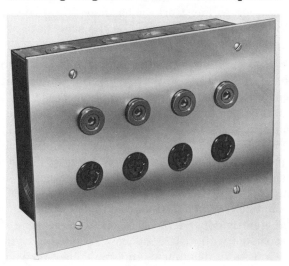

6.7.3 Overcurrent Protection. Little difference exists between that overcurrent protection which must be provided within hospital environments and that which must be provided for other commercial buildings. Where isolated power is used, the secondary circuits fed from the isolation transformer should be provided with 2-pole circuit breakers. Care should be taken to obtain the highest quality and most reliable equipment available.

6.7.4 Adequacy of Power. With electrical devices supporting life there is a strong need to supply a continuous adequate amount of power, where and when needed. There is a very reasonable expectation that the power requirements will increase with time, and this should be a design consideration.

6.7.5 Continuity of Power. See Chapter 5.

6.7.6 Isolated Power. The ungrounded electrical distribution system has been used in certain areas of the hospital for many years. It has been used in anesthetizing locations since 1948.

The term "isolated system" is normally used for an ungrounded electrical distribution system including (or comprised of) all of the necessary equipment as specified in ANSI/NFPA 99-1984 [3] and in ANSI/NFPA 70-1984 (Article 517) [2]. This system includes the shielded isolation transformer, line isolation monitor (LIM; see 6.7.9), circuit breakers, and the necessary power receptacles and associated grounding equipment. It is the responsibility of the electrical design engineer to specify each of the components required to establish the total system.

There was always a possibility of selecting imcompatible components and the labor for installing individual components was always quite high. Additionally, the integrity of the total system was difficult to ascertain.

In the early 1960's, the isolated system package or panel, as it was then called, began to appear. Initial units contained the isolation transformer, circuit breakers and the ground detector. Later, the line isolation monitor replaced the ground detector. In 1971, packages appeared which also contained power receptacles, ground buses and grounding jacks. Most present installations make use of these packaged components. UL standards have been established for these packaged units (UL 1047-1976 [5]) and they are available as labeled devices. The use of these packages assures the design engineer of compatible components and of the lowest possible installation cost.

While the National Electrical Code, JCAH and certain NFPA standards have reduced the number of places where isolated power is required, the use of an isolated system is mandated by ANSI/NFPA 70-1984 [2] and ANSI/NFPA 99-1984 [3] in all anesthetizing locations. Recent code changes as covered in ANSI/NFPA 99-1984 (Paragraph 3-2.3.1.1) [3] may not require some inhalation anesthetizing locations to have isolated power.

Prior to 1981, 2 mA of potential current flow was permitted before the alarm sounded. The permissible level today is 5 mA.

The isolated power system is also useful where wet conditions exist, and life support equipment must continue to operate in the presence of one fault to ground, such as in an open heart surgery operating room. There are other locations in the hospital such as intensive care or coronary care areas where isolated systems are considered optional but should be given consideration. There are some states which mandate the use of isolated systems in ICU/CCU areas. It is the responsibility of the electrical design engineer to point out to the hospital where isolated systems might benefit them. See Figs 66, 67, and 68. Clock timers are often included as part of a surgical facility panel (see Fig 69).

The benefits derived from the ungrounded electrical distribution system are:

(1) It limits the amount of current which can flow to ground through any single line-to-ground fault which may occur in the system. For all practical purposes, this eliminates the danger of massive electrical shocks (macroshock) to patients or personnel as a result of this type of fault. It also practically eliminates the possibility of high energy arcing as a result of this type of fault and thus provides protection against the accidental ignition of explosive or combustible materials being used in the area. This feature of the ungrounded electrical distribution system permits typical and practically sized grounding conductors to effectively protect even those patients who might be affected by very small amounts of elec-

Fig 66
Isolation Panel for the Operating Room

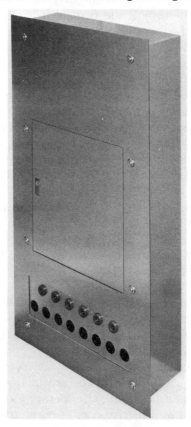

trical current. Internally isolated patient monitoring equipment also adds a large factor of safety.

(2) In a grounded distribution system, a line-to-ground fault on the system will operate the overcurrent protective device and interrupt power to the device or the area.

In most cases, this is a highly desirable feature. However, in any hospital area where life support devices are used, this loss of power may create a life support hazard. The ungrounded electrical distribution system responds quite differently to a line-to-ground fault. With this system the fault does not pose an immediate danger to the patient or to personnel and power is not interrupted. Only a visual and audible warning is issued. In many cases, the device in which the fault has occurred will continue to operate and can be safely used until replacement equipment is available. Without interrupting power, the LIM of the isolated power system warns of potential failure of equipment connected to the system, as long as the equipment has ground continuity. When the alarm sounds, the system is still safer than if a conventional grounded system were used in the first place. Any current that would flow would be less than if one of the conductors were solidly grounded, as is the case with the conventional grounded 120 V electrical system. The LIM used with the isolated system is the only device connected to the system that continuously monitors (and alarms when necessary) the integrity of the wiring of the room and the equipment connected to the system.

Fig 67
Isolation Panel for the Operating Room

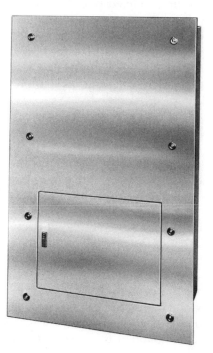

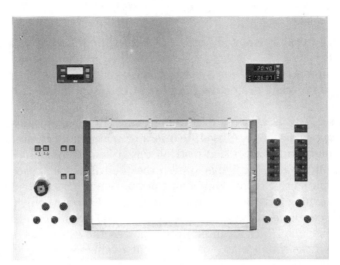

**Fig 68
Surgical Facility Panel**

The alternative is frequent laboratory testing of the equipment but there is no assurance that the equipment has not become degraded or defective between test periods. The integrity of the equipment and the integrity of the grounding conductor are especially important for life support systems.

Periodic LIM readings can provide a continuous record of the system and its operation. The LIM is a one-time only cost addition as compared to the continuing cost of periodically checking the system and equipment. With continous monitoring, the hospital engineering staff is kept on the alert to keep the equipment in excellent operating condition so that the LIM does not go into an alarm condition. The isolated power system gives the surgeon, or other users of the electrical equipment, macroshock protection, the same as if they were using double insulated or battery operated tools.

It should be emphasized that an ungrounded electrical distribution system provides an early warning that an appliance has a line to ground fault. The faults occurring within the appliances can be result of slowly degrading insulation or components. When the potential leakage caused by these conditions increases beyond the limits set for the ungrounded system, an alarm will sound and trigger preventive maintenance action. This feature is of great value even to institutions which have sophisticated preventive maintenance programs for their appliances and equipment. Even though an appliance is checked on a monthly basis, there is no guarantee that degradation of the unit will not become excessive the day after it has received its monthly check.

Radiologists and Pathologists sometimes use isolated power for CT Scanners and Multi-Channel Analyzers to protect devices from transients. As patient care areas become populated with computer chips, this may be the trend. The attenuation of the shielded isolation transformer produces as much as 52 dB reduction (300 to 1 voltage ratio) in the common mode noise transient.

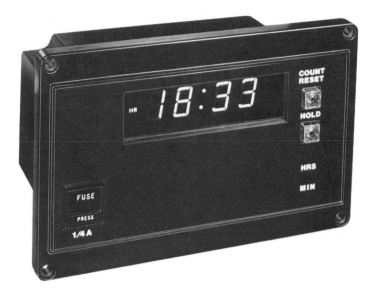

Fig 69
Clock Timer

6.7.7 Three-Phase Isolated System. In recent years there have been increasing demands for three-phase power within an anesthetizing location. Since the code requires that all power provided to the operating room must be isolated, three-phase ungrounded isolation systems have been developed and are listed under UL 1047-1976 [5]. It is generally not advisable to try to derive both the three-phase power requirements and the single-phase power requirements from a single isolation system. It is best to provide a separate three-phase isolation system for that equipment which requires it. Typical devices requiring three-phase power in the operating room are laminar air flow devices, photo coagulating equipment (laser), and special positioning, electrical surgical tables.

While much of this equipment is also available in single phase design, some of the devices available only in three-phase design have features not available in the single-phase machine and which the medical team requires. Once a situation of this type is established, it is the responsibility of the design engineer to properly specify and design a three-phase isolation circuit which will give the hospital trouble-free service.

The general rules and conditions for the effective three-phase isolation installation are identical to those for the single-phase isolation system previously described.

6.7.8 Limitations. The isolated distribution system has some limitations: (a) If the ground continuity of the system is lost, the predicted (potential) leakage current is not monitored on the LIM and this could give a false sense of security. (b) While chances of microshock are reduced, the level of alarm is too high to prevent microshock; the present level of 5 mA, as well as the previous level of 2 mA, still could produce microshock of a catherterized patient under the right circumstances. (c) High leakage conditions can result in alarms which may be disturbing during normal operating procedures.

While the line isolation monitor will not uncover all of the possible defects of instrumentation connected to the line isolation monitor (such as broken ground wires), it will sound an alarm when leakage currents above the National Electrical Code permitted values are encountered. While some hospital personnel may consider this alarm a nuisance, the line isolation monitor is a means of predicting the amount of leakage current that could be harmful.

To eliminate some of the so-called "nuisance alarm," the National Electrical Code was changed to permit a 5 mA alarm level rather than the previous 2 mA level. An attempt is being made to make the line isolation monitor (and, in fact, isolated power) optional in the operating room rather than mandatory. It should be noted that the 5 mA current is more likely to adversely affect members of the surgical team whereas 2 mA is less likely to create problems for individuals. The 5 mA line isolation monitor does, however, permit more equipment to be connected to the system without causing a "nuisance alarm." The shielded isolation transformer helps prevent electrical disturbances from passing into and out of the OR and CCU units. These electrical disturbances can affect monitoring and sensitive instrumentation.

6.7.9 Line Isolation Monitor. The LIM is an impedance measuring device used with isolated power systems which will sound an audible alarm, and give a visual warning when the impedance of the system has degraded to the point where current flow from any of the power conductors to ground would be in excess of the limits established by the standards (see Fig 70).

Fig 70
5 mA Line Isolation Monitor

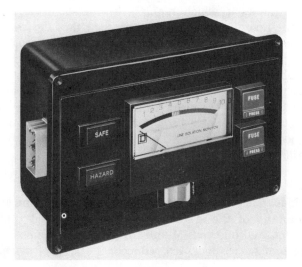

All LIMs shall provide a meter which will continuously predict how much current will flow through a ground fault if it should occur. It should be carefully pointed out to the hospital staff that the meter does not indicate current which is flowing but predicts the current which will flow if a fault to ground occurs.

All LIMs shall provide a means of silencing the audible alarm in the area of use so it does not distract the attention of the medical staff from the procedure being performed at that particular time. The standards do allow that any medical procedure being performed at the time the alarm sounds can be brought to its completion before service must be performed to remove the fault on the ungrounded system as indicated by the LIM. New procedures should not be started until the engineering or maintenance department of the hospital facility has located and corrected the problem and properly documented such action.

The monitor hazard current is defined as: "the measure of the degradation of the isolated system caused by connecting the LIM to the system." When a 2 mA trip level LIM is connected to a perfectly ungrounded system, if the amount of current that will flow after connection from either line-to-ground is 25 μA, then it is said that the monitor hazard current is 25 μA. A 5 mA trip level LIM would have a monitor hazard current of approximately 50 μA.

LIMs are provided with a means for testing their function. This is accomplished by a test switch that, when energized, will place a simulated fault on the LIM sufficient to cause it to alarm when operated at minus 15% or plus 10% of nominal rated voltage. This test verifies the proper function of the LIM and its associated alarms but does not verify the functioning of the total ungrounded electrical system. After installation, the system can be thoroughly tested by applying test faults at the outlets. A minimum of one similar annual test should be performed thereafter. The LIM function should be tested monthly as covered by ANSI/NFPA 99-1984 [3]. When in the test mode, the ground connection to the LIM is disconnected automatically so as not to cause "second fault" on the system and possibly endanger patients or personnel in the area where the test is being performed. All tests should be performed only when the system is not otherwise in use.

The LIM function test is not a means of checking the calibration of the LIM. Since most LIMs are basically complex network analyzers involving solutions of very complex network equations, it is desirable to have all calibrations performed at the factory where adequate and proper test equipment is available.

6.7.10 LIM Isolation Monitor Interpretation. In an operating room a LIM reading of 2 mA means that the impedance of one line-to-ground has deteriorated to 60 000 Ω on a 120 V system and the decision probably will be made to continue the surgical procedure. After the surgical procedure has been completed, the plugged-in equipment should then be examined and the fault corrected at the earliest opportunity.

If the indicator on the meter shows full scale deflection indicating a severe hazard condition, it indicates that one of the lines has shorted to ground or it could be caused by a combination of high leakage currents of several instruments. The isolated system is approaching a grounded system. This could create a serious hazard of electric shock to both the patient and the personnel in the event that a second fault occurs. The first fault should be located and corrected at least before starting another surgical operation. The full, let-through current of the circuit breaker could flow if any contact is made with a live (unshorted) conductor.

Because of the above reasons, the LIM meter should be in a "plainly visible place" in the operating theater. Means must be provided for conveniently silencing the audible alarm.

A similar analogy applies to the 5 mA LIM, with the exception that when the meter reads 5 mA, the impedance of one line-to-ground has deteriorated to 24 000 Ω on the 120 V system.

6.8 Design and Testing of Systems for Safety

6.8.1 Identifying Particular User Needs. It is very important to have a very clear understanding of the expected use of various areas in a health care facility. Various electrical codes, standards and regulations have different requirements for the various areas in a health care facility as contrasted to other types of occupancies. Many hospitals frequently have continuing changes in requirements, because of staff changes and because of advances in technology. Since cost is a very important consideration and since available funds are usually in short supply, it is very difficult to provide maximum flexibility in every area.

The first step would be to review with the administrator, or the owner of the facility, the expected initial use, and any anticipated modification in the future. Consideration should be given to changes in safety requirements as well as possible changes in applicable codes and standards.

6.8.2 Adjusting Special Design Features for Each Area. The second step is to apply the necessary special design features to those areas identified in Paragraph 6.8.1 as needing such treatment.

6.8.3 Distribution Systems. The choice of voltage of the distribution system can affect the safety in terms of continuity of service. Code changes for requiring ground fault protection on the main service, and reports of nuisance tripping of ground fault protection, indicates that extra careful selection, design, installation, testing, and training for maintenance are essential. Voltages and feeder loads should be carefully selected and analyzed to minimize the possibilty of nuisance outages.

6.8.4 Distribution Raceway Systems. There are a number of options available which have several economic and safety implications. One consideration is the use of either plastic or rigid metal raceways. The raceways provide two major functions; physical protection of the power conductors and redundant grounding. The physical protection becomes of greatest importance in facilities where renovation and changes are frequent.

The redundancy in grounding provided by metal conduit is twofold. The conduit provides a redundant path to the green grounding wire. In addition, the physical mounting of the conduit to other conduit, metal studs, other piping and structural steel members provides a network of redundant grounding paths. These design and inadvertent connections contribute to an effective low grounding impedance for current flow during fault conditions. Using electrical metallic tubing, frequently produces effective grounding impedances in the order of 1 to 10 milliohms. These values are low relative to that provided by a #10 wire having 1 milliohm per foot resistance.

This natural redundant grounding gains part of its safety advantage by causing fault currents to follow several paths and reducing possible hazardous conditions.

6.8.5 Distribution System-Grounded and Isolated Power. The grounded distribution system is the one usually found in most commercial installations throughout the United States. The grounded feature aids in tripping overcurrent protection devices during line-to-ground fault conditions. When line-to-ground faults include an individual as part of the circuit, serious shock hazards are possible. Line-to-ground faults also can cause arcing which is a hazard where any flammable gases are present.

The isolated distribution system is covered in Section 6.7.6.

6.8.6 Field Inspection Procedure. Isolated power and equipotential ground systems are unique. It is recommended to have these systems tested and certified before use. This is one way to insure proper installation and operation. Manufacturers of isolated power systems are generally equipped to test the installed equipment. The testing should preferably be done with the electrical contractor present.

All tests on the isolated system, equipotential ground network, and the line isolation monitor should be in accordance with ANSI/NFPA 70-1984 (Article 517) [2] and ANSI/NFPA 99-1984 [3].

The test and certification procedure covers the following:

(1) Operational check of all equipment.

(2) Inspection of the complete installation for applicable code conformance.

(3) In depth testing of the isolated power system.

    (a) Line voltage measurements

    (b) Line-to-ground impedance measurements

    (c) LIM calibration

(4) Recording of initial system hazard current readings from the LIM for hospital records. Initial hazard current readings represent predicted current leakage with no devices connected to the isolated system.

(5) Testing of the equipotential ground network.

    (a) All power receptacle grounds

    (b) All ground receptacles

    (c) All permanently exposed building metal

    (d) All permanently installed equipment

(6) Complete dissertation on the isolated power system to the hospital personnel including:

    (a) Basic theoretical concept and benefits of isolated power

    (b) Proper use

    (c) Proper maintenance procedure

(7) Periodic testing and record keeping. A log book with initial hazard current readings is supplied to the hospital with a letter of certification, including all recorded test data.

6.9 References

[1] ANSI/AAMI SCL 12-78, Safe Current Limits for Electromedical Apparatus.[24]

[2] ANSI/NFPA 70-1984, National Electrical Code.

[3] ANSI/NFPA 99-1984, Standard for Health Care Facilities. (Contains standards formerly identified as NFPA 76A, NFPA 76B, NFPA 56A, as well as others in the Health Care Facility series.)

[4] UL 544-1976, Standard for Medical and Dental Equipment.[25]

[5] UL 1047-1976, Standard for Isolated Power Systems Equipment.

[6] *Accreditation Manual for Hospitals*, by Joint Commission for the Accreditation of Hospitals, 1984.

[7] *Guidelines for Construction and Equipment of Hospitals and Medical Facilities*. US Department of Health and Human Services, Oct 1981.

---

[24] This publication is available from the Sales Department, American National Standards Institute, 1430 Broadway, New York, NY 10018 or from the Order Department, Association for the Advancement of Medical Instruments, Suite 602, 1901 North Fort Myer Drive, Arlington, VA 22209.

[25] UL publications are available from Publication Stock, Underwriters Laboratories, Inc, 333 Pfingsten Rd, Northbrook, IL 60062.

7. Lighting for Health Care Facilities

7.1 General Discussion. The term "health care facilities" covers a wide variety of facilities whose primary concern is the maintenance of good health or the improvement of health. The term normally assumes physical health, but also encompasses mental health facilities.

This chapter cannot hope to explore all the various and technologically diverse lighting needs of the health care facility at any one time. Medical advances and the introduction of more sophisticated medical equipment and techniques will date this document as it is being written. However, the fundamental principles of good lighting design encouraged in this document should serve to provide guidelines sufficient to the intelligent and studied application of lighting as the new medical needs, equipment, and techniques present themselves. As new research increases our knowledge of visual requirements, the lighting industry must be responsive in providing both the equipment and the application of the equipment to take maximum advantage of scientific and technological advances in the science and art of illumination.

While the obvious primary purpose of lighting in the health care facility is to serve the demands of the medical and nursing staff, it should also be suited to the emotional and psychological needs of the patient.

Peculiar to lighting, most of our outside stimuli come from what we perceive and, to a lesser extent, what we hear, feel or smell.

It then becomes incumbent on the lighting engineer to provide lighting and lighting facilities which will maintain and improve the patient's mental feeling and outlook.

Fundamental to this chapter are the often-repeated phrases "patient comfort" or "patient's personal needs." Health care patients are frequently unable to adjust their position or surroundings to avoid discomfort, and since sight is the primary outside influence on the patient, discomfort in lighting is particularly objectionable.

Finally, this chapter shall be used in concert with available literature (see 7.6).

7.2 Lighting Objectives. As alluded to in 7.1, the objective of health care facility lighting is two-fold.

(1) It should provide the seeing environment required to successfully perform the various tasks.

(2) It should provide psychological and physiological support to the patient.

Modern concepts of lighting are "task oriented," that is, lighting is provided which is required to perform a task efficiently. The task should be evaluated in terms of its inherent difficulty, who performs the task, and the necessity for speed and accuracy.

Most health care tasks are inherently difficult, and require great accuracy and speed, and they are performed by a wide variety of people who have varying degrees of visual ability. Conversely, many health care tasks such as routine clerical, accounting, managerial, and office-related tasks, food service, maintenance, auto parking, and other tasks may be treated in the same manner as similar tasks in commercial and industrial buildings. The reader is directed to other references for such considerations, and this volume will necessarily treat only those tasks which may be considered to be unique to health care facilities.

The patient in the health care facility, as well as his family and friends, is emotionally vulnerable. Patients are to some degree frightened or apprehensive. Strange, often painful, uncomfortable, or embarrassing treatments add to the challenge of producing a lighting environment which supports the patient's comfort, well-being, emotional stability, and presumed recovery. At the very least, the lighting environment should not detract from the patient's condition, whether physiological or psychological.

Flexible wiring systems, easily relocatable fixtures, easily replaceable fixtures, easily maintainable fixtures, directional lenses, "low brightness" lenses, dimming and flexible switching should be incorporated into the final design to facilitate the lighting objectives. Many of these features will also provide for flexible systems which can be altered to fit new and unforeseen medical or space requirements, allowing the lighting equipment to be moved or changed as a part of the furniture.

Lighting equipment in health care facilities should be selected to provide optimum serviceability, reliability, and sanitation. Fixtures are frequently subjected to wash-downs using corrosive cleaning compounds and agents. Sanitation and the resultant frequent cleaning require fixtures without crevices or cracks which may harbor dirt or other unsanitary miscellanea. Heavy duty "hospital grade" outlets and switches should be standard components of lighting equipment. Lenses, particularly those frequently subject to cleaning or to patient contact, should be gasketed to prevent entry of cleaning agents or patient care fluids. Gasketing should be cleanable; that is, hard or, if foam type, closed cell foam with a smooth exterior surface.

The subject of lighting cannot be discussed without proper reference to the energy consumed. One hardly needs to state that health care facilities should receive the highest priority for lighting energy consumption. Sound principles of lighting energy management such as found in ANSI/ASHRAE/IES 90A-1980 (Section 9) [1] [26] should be observed.

---

[26] The numbers in brackets correspond to those references at the end of this chapter.

Connected lighting loads, as well as the diversity which can be assumed, will vary widely within the hospital. For instance, in a patient room of 120 ft^2, a total of 700 W (5.8 W/ft^2) connected load may normally experience a diversity of 15% or 100 W (during daylight hours), while the adjacent nurses' station load of 4 W/ft^2 will experience a 100% diversity during the same time. The lighting engineer should consider these factors in the branch circuit design and in the feeder and panelboard design to present wider utilization of electrical facilities, as well as providing for future growth and rearrangement of facilities.

Lastly, the lighting engineer must not design in a vacuum. The entire environment should be evaluated and planned in concert with the interior designer, the architect, and the appropriate medical staff. The success of the lighting design cannot be measured in footcandles (fc), but must be measured in the intangibles of comfort, task efficiency and overall satisfaction.

7.3 Design Criteria

7.3.1 Luminaire Requirements and Distribution. A luminaire is a complete lighting unit consisting of lamp(s) together with lamp-holders to position the lamp, parts to direct and distribute the light, a ballast when discharge lamps are employed and a provision for connection to an electric power supply.

Luminaires are essential for providing light of a quality which makes tasks more visible and to control light source brightness in order to minimize discomfort glare. Their distribution of light may vary from totally direct to totally indirect with many variations between the two extremes. Luminaire mounting on ceilings varies from recessed to surface-mounted to suspended. However, luminaires today are also mounted on walls, partitions, office furniture and on freestanding units located on the floor.

A great variety of shielding media are used in and on luminaires to control light distribution and glare. These include reflectors, louvers, lenses, polarizers and diffusers of many different materials.

Certain luminaire characteristics should be reviewed before specifying or purchasing the units. These include:

(1) Lumen output of each unit which affects:
    (a) Spacing of luminaires
    (b) Quantity of light delivered
    (c) Uniformity or non-uniformity of light delivered

(2) Control of light suitable for the specific visual tasks and activities encountered
    (a) Diffusion or directional quality of light delivered
    (b) Creation of shadows, modelling effects
    (c) Effect on veiling reflections with specular tasks
    (d) Uniformity or non-uniformity of light delivered
    (e) Visual comfort of the luminaire system installed

(3) Efficiency of the light sources employed and of the luminaire in delivering the light
    (a) Utilization of direct, indirect and intermediate light distribution types
    (b) Effect on power requirements

(c) System voltage utilization

(4) Maintenance characteristics of the lamps and luminaire

  (a) Maintenance of lamp light output through life

  (b) Susceptibility of luminaire to dirt collection

  (c) Ease of cleaning

  (d) Ease of relamping

  (e) Characteristics of glass, plastics, paint, metals used

  (f) Durability

(5) Flexibility of installation

  (a) Troffers laid into suspended grid ceiling

  (b) Use of approved plug-in power connectors for luminaires

  (c) Luminaires installed on furniture (desks, beds)

  (d) Luminaires mounted on shelves

  (e) Luminaires installed on free-standing bases for positioning on floor or furniture

(6) Coordination with mechanical system

  (a) Luminaires for air supply

  (b) Luminaires for air return (assessment of their effect on air changes, fan horsepower, duct size)

  (c) Lighting contribution to building heat

  (d) Heat redistribution system

  (e) Heat storage/recovery systems

(7) Architectural considerations

  (a) Size and proportions of space

  (b) Size/scale of luminaires and layout pattern

  (c) Layout of furnishings

  (d) Structural and mechanical features

7.3.2 Special Light Distributions from Luminaires. Many visual tasks have specular characteristics which make their illumination critical in order to achieve good visibility. Materials inhibiting such specularity include pencil writing, most printing inks, print from office copying machines and even ballpoint pen writing, to some extent.

Certain kinds of lighting control materials have been developed and include polarizing materials, batwing and radial batwing lenses, and special controlling reflectors on luminaires to produce a batwing distribution. Indirect lighting which produces a uniformly bright ceiling may also be utilized. The veiling reflection effect can be most effectively minimized if one can control the location of task and luminaires with respect to the eye of the person viewing so there are no veiling reflections (no luminaire at the mirror angle for the eye with respect to the task). Since it is not always possible to have this kind of control, especially with many work stations in a room, the special distributions may prove to be helpful.

It is recommended that comparisons of the effectiveness of various shielding materials be made using the ESI metric to determine which will be more effective in a particular application.

7.3.3 Light Sources. A number of light sources are available to the lighting designer having a broad range of important characteristics such as efficiency (lumens per watt), color, size, brightness, diffusion, lumen maintenance, starting and restarting properties and economics. Many of these will need evaluation in deciding which source to use in particular applications. Computer programs, experience and good engineering judgment will help insure that the correct source is selected.

(1) *Daylight.* There is much interest in the application of daylight in buildings in view of the potential for reducing energy consumed in electric lighting systems. The use of skylights, windows, optical devices and various configurations of building facades are being explored with this end in view.

However, it must be remembered that windows have other energy implications besides lighting, including heat loss in winter and heat gain in summer. To reduce energy requirements for space heating and cooling, buildings are being designed with smaller windows, with insulating glass, with low transmission glass and with glass having heat reflecting coatings. These cut down on daylight transmitted to building interiors.

In an energy-efficient building, windows should be evaluated on their overall energy implications and should be effective on a *net* saving of energy. Energy saved in electric lighting should be balanced against heat gains and losses through the windows to determine their overall impact on energy use.

Assuming that windows are energy-efficient in the overall in a particular building with a specific orientation and climate, then controls should be employed to switch off or dim down the electric lighting when daylight is adequate.

Daylighting quantity varies over a wide range. In full sunshine outdoors 5000 to 10 000 fc can be measured. Under cloudy conditions anywhere from a few hundred to a few thousand fc are available, depending on the thickness of the cloud cover. Thus, the illumination which penetrates a building interior varies over a very broad range and depends not only on the weather and time-of-day, but also on the shielding media used at the windows and their position at a particular time. Daylighting also falls off rapidly as distance from the window increases.

Work stations within a building should be positioned so that, as occupants face their visual tasks, the windows are at their side or behind them. It is usually not desirable to face windows directly while working, and the high brightnesses sometimes presented outdoors may provide visual discomfort or raise the eye's brightness adaptation level to a point that may make the visual tasks indoors less visible with their much lower luminance level.

(2) *Incandescent Lamps.* This is the oldest form of electric light source. It depends on a tungsten filament heated to incandescence for its light. Lamp wattages used for general illumination usually range from about 17 to 24 lumens per watt (lm/W) in that range. Higher wattage lamps have the higher efficacies.

Because of their simplicity and good optical properties, incandescent lamps are suitable for many types of supplementary and local task lighting. However, since they are less efficient than the other electric lamp sources, they are not suitable for general lighting of sizable work areas having long burning hours.

Filament temperature, lamp life, and luminous efficiency are closely related in incandescent lamps. The higher the temperature, the more lm/W are generated and the shorter the lamp life. With lower filament temperatures lamp life is greatly extended, but luminous efficacy is considerably reduced, making it necessary to increase lamp wattage to provide a desired level of illumination.

The lamp variables, together with energy cost, capital investment in luminaires and power distribution systems, and labor costs, are related in an economic equation to determine optimum lamp life. For typical applications, economic lamp lives range from a few hundred to a few thousand hours. Manufacturers supply lamps of various life ratings to account for some of the variables among users.

If high energy costs are a consideration, the more efficient incandescent lamps should be used. Extremely long-lived lamps waste considerable energy. It is frequently possible to get the desired light for a task using the next lower wattage of a standard lamp compared with higher wattage necessary with the long-lived lamps.

(a) *Voltage*. Since the efficiency, light output, life and wattage of incandescent lamps are significantly affected by their operating voltage, they should be operated at or near their design voltage for best value. The majority of incandescent lamps are designed for 120 V distribution systems. However, some lamps are available, designed for 115, 125, and 130 V operation. Higher voltage lamps are available for 230, 250, and 277 V operation.

The higher voltage lamps are, in general, less efficient (except for the tungsten-halogen types) and have more fragile filaments than 120 V lamps. There is also greater hazard in replacing these higher voltage lamps in luminaires and such maintenance should be performed only by qualified personnel who are familiar with the system voltage and the lamp requirements.

(b) *Color*. Incandescent lamps are warm in character compared with most other electric light sources and with daylight. They are approximately 3000 K color temperature, having a preponderance of red and yellow wavelengths and much less green and blue. Colors can be created by applying enamel coatings to the glass bulbs or color filters over the luminaires. This creates the color by absorbing the unwanted wavelengths and is an inefficient process, especially in green and blue. Nevertheless, it is a convenient, simple process and widely used where color is needed.

(c) *Tungsten-Halogen Lamps*. These incandescent lamps employ tungsten filaments in compact quartz bulbs with a small amount of halogen gas in the bulb's atmosphere. The tungsten-halogen regenerative cycle operates between the bulb wall and the filament, preventing any accumulation of evaporated tungsten from being deposited on and blackening the bulb surface. As a result, these lamps maintain a high percentage of their initial light output throughout life. Lamp life is, typically, about double that of standard incandescent lamps, while lamp efficiency is somewhat higher.

(d) *Dimming*. Incandescent lamps can be dimmed easily by reducing voltage at the lamp socket. Variable auto transformers and solid-state devices are most often used for this effect. Dimming may be desirable for certain special effects or where more than one level of illumination is necessary. However, it should be remembered that light output drops much more rapidly than wattage as incandescent lamps are dimmed and lamp efficacy is greatly reduced.

(3) *Fluorescent Lamps.* Fluorescent lamps are electric arc discharge sources which depend on a two-step process for generating light. The electric arc discharge through low pressure mercury vapor generates short wave ultra-violet which, in turn, excites phosphors deposited on the bulb wall of the lamp, thereby generating light. The phosphor is vitally important, determining the efficacy, color and lumen maintenance of the light produced.

Fluorescent lamps generate light more efficiently than incandescent or mercury, though there is great variation in fluorescent lamp efficacy, due principally to color. Fluorescent lamps also have characteristics of low brightness and diffusion, making them excellent for many lighting applications where high brightness specular reflections should be avoided and luminaire discomfort glare controlled.

Fluorescent lamps have tubular bulbs, are made in a variety of lengths and for a number of operating currents. For example, 430 milliamperes (mA) is the typical operating current of rapid start and slimline fluorescent lamps. Ballasts can be selected, however, which will operate these lamps at 200 mA or 300 mA for reduced wattage and similarly reduced light output.

High output fluorescent lamps are operated at 800 mA and these have about 45% higher light output per unit of length than the 430 mA lamps. There are also extra-high output fluorescent lamps operated at 1500 mA which generate 60% to 70% more light per unit length than even high output lamps. The more highly loaded lamps have applications where higher levels of illumination are needed or where higher mounting heights are involved and the number of lamps/fixtures can be reduced for economic reasons.

(a) *Reduced Wattage Fluorescent Lamps.* Fluorescent lamps of specific lengths and tube diameters have individual electrical characteristics to which their ballasts must be designed for fairly close tolerances. Consequently, substitutions of different lamp types in sockets designed for a particular lamp can rarely be done satisfactorily, even if the lengths allow a physical fit. However, in recent years due to rising energy costs, lamp manufacturers have made reduced-wattage fluorescent lamps available which fit in the existing sockets of particular lamps. They will operate satisfactorily on the existing ballasts and reduce the lamp/ballast system watts by 10% to 20%, depending on the lamp type and luminaire type. These are available for the 3 ft and 4 ft rapid start lamps, and for slimline, high output and extra-high output types.

The "first-generation" of these reduced wattage lamps reduced light output in about the same proportion as wattage. If less light were acceptable, this was satisfactory. However, if lighting maintenance procedures were improved, such as cleaning luminaires every year or two and replacing all lamps in groups every three or four years, the average lighting level maintained might be equal to, or even greater than that maintained with the standard, higher wattage lamps with typical maintenance procedures.

A second generation of reduced wattage fluorescent lamps has been developed employing a newly created more efficient fluorescent phosphor. This has made it possible to provide the same reduction in wattage achieved with the original lamps, yet provide virtually as much light as with standard lamps. Though the choice of colors is limited, this second-generation lamp provides light at lowest cost and least energy use in new lighting installations as well as being suited for retrofit in existing systems where energy reductions are desired but reduced light is not.

The reduced-wattage fluorescent lamps of both types, first and second generation, are more sensitive to temperature than standard lamps. Consequently, they are not recommended for use in areas where ambients will be less than 60 °F. (Standard lamps are satisfactory down to 50 °F.) In addition, these lamps are not recommended for use on low power factor ballasts, or reduced current/reduced light output ballasts, for use on dimming systems or for use in emergency lighting units. Standard lamps should be used for these applications.

(b) *Fluorescent Lamp Color.* A great variety of fluorescent lamp colors are available as it is a simple matter to change phosphor components and achieve new colors. Specification of lamp color involves, principally, matters of efficiency and aesthetics.

Much of the early history of fluorescent lamp colors involved trade-offs in lamp efficacy with color rendition. Lamps high in lumens per watt were only fair in color rendition, while those which provided excellent color rendition were substantially lower in lm/W.

Currently, however, there are lamp colors available which combine high color rendition with high efficacy, due to improved phosphor technology. Such lamps are considerably higher in price than the high color rendering lamps of lower efficacy, but analyses show they are cost-effective.

For applications of fluorescent lighting where good appearance of people, food, furnishings or other objects is essential, high color rendering fluorescent lamps should be used. In pathology labs, for example, where color appearance of tissues is of concern, high color rendering lamps of good spectral balance with color temperature ranging between 4000 K and 5000 K are usually employed.

Several saturated colors are available in fluorescent lamps such as pink, blue, red, gold, green. These are obtained through the use of fluorescent phosphors in the lamp which generate the color of light desired. In a few cases, a colored filter is employed integrally with the lamp's glass tube to increase the color's saturation.

(c) *Fluorescent Lamps and Temperature.* The starting and operating characteristics of fluorescent lamps are significantly affected by temperature. Rated light output from most fluorescent lamps is achieved with ambient temperatures of 70 °F to 80 °F. Above this temperature range light output is reduced as in many enclosed commercial luminaires. For example, at 120 °F the light output may be between 75% and 90% of rated depending on whether the air is still or circulating. In high ambient temperatures, circulating air improves the light output.

Light output of fluorescent lamps also drops rapidly at temperatures below 60 °F. For satisfactory outdoor operation in cold weather, ballasts for fluorescent lamps should be used which supply sufficient voltage to ensure reliable lamp starting and should be of a design which will withstand low temperatures.

In very cold weather regular fluorescent lamps may not reach their full rated light output, particularly if subjected to air currents. However, if the lamps are used in a closed fixture or shielded from drafts, the ambient temperature around the lamp should build up during operation and light output will increase nearer to rated values.

The fluorescent lamps which operate at higher current (800 and 1500 mA) will, in properly designed multiple-lamp enclosed luminaires, maintain light output better than lamps of lower current. In addition, certain fluorescent lamps which operate at 1500 mA have been designed especially for outdoor application. One type is intended for use in single-lamp enclosed fixtures. Another is provided with a clear-glass outer jacket gasketed to the lamp and is intended for use in open fixtures. In typical outdoor environments the light output of the jacketed lamp is at its maximum in an ambient of –10 °F. Due to the variation in outdoor conditions under which fluorescent lamps may be expected to operate, such as temperature, wind, and equipment, it may be desirable to seek the advice of lamp or luminaire manufacturers regarding the best choice of lamps and equipment for a specific application.

(d) *Dimming of Fluorescent Lamps.* Equipment for dimming is presently available for 40 W and 30 W rapid start fluorescent lamps. This broadens their possible applications to auditoriums, classrooms, conference rooms, offices and patient rooms. It also provides an opportunity to tie electric lighting systems in with daylighting to maintain constant levels of task lighting indoors as daylight varies in quantity.

Various electronic systems have been devised for dimming fluorescent systems. Manufacturers should be consulted for information on characteristics of their equipment such as dimming range, starting reliability at various brightness levels, cost, etc.

(e) *Fluorescent Lamp Ballasts.* Fluorescent lamps (and other discharge lamps) must have ballasts to perform several functions: to provide the appropriate voltage to start the lamp; to maintain the appropriate voltage and current to the lamp during operation; and to provide power factor correction (usually).

Ballasts may consume from 5% to 20% of a lighting system's energy. They may also have an effect on the life, light output and lumen maintenance of the lamps in the system. Hence, specification of an appropriate ballast is highly important to the satisfactory performance and economy of a lighting system. Since there are so many different types of ballasts with a variety of characteristics, it is recommended that manufacturers' literature be consulted for more details.

The rapid start ballast is the predominant type in use today. It provides a low voltage source of heat for the fluorescent lamp cathodes (in addition to the functions mentioned above) and this allows the lamp(s) to start within one to two seconds after voltage is applied.

Rapid start lamps are available operating at 430 mA, 800 mA (high output) and 1500 mA (extra high output). The most popular and economical type ballast available operates two rapid start lamps in series. The power factor is corrected to in excess of 90%, leading. This slightly leading power factor can help improve the system power factor for a building, since other loads are, typically, lagging.

(f) *Grounding.* ANSI/NFPA 70-1984 (Section 410-17) [8] requires that all fixtures and lighting equipment (including ballasts) be grounded. Rapid start ballasts require a starting aid consisting of a grounded metal strip running the full length of the lamp. The metal of the fluorescent fixture when grounded can act as a starting aid.

(g) *Slimline Lamp.* Slimline lamps are a lamp type that start instantly due to the high open circuit voltage available from the ballast when the switch is closed. They may be operated at any of several currents (200 mA, 300 mA, 425 mA, for example) by selection of the appropriate ballast. The most popular and economical ballast available for slimline lamps is the two-lamp series type. However, a lead-lag ballast is also available which operates a pair of lamps in parallel, one leading and one lagging, so the net result is a high power factor circuit. The lead-lag ballast is more costly than the series type.

(h) *Low Watts Loss Ballasts.* Within recent years, manufacturers have developed fluorescent lamp ballasts that reduce ballast losses by almost half with respect to conventional ballasts. Ballasts run cooler due to the lower watts loss and last considerably longer. Though somewhat higher in cost than conventional ballasts, they are cost-effective and should be used in all new lighting and as replacements for ballast failures in existing installations.

(i) *Voltage.* Ballasts are available for the standard distribution system voltages. Ballasts should be operated close to their rated voltage, but no more than 5% higher or 10% lower than the rating. Higher voltage will overheat ballasts and shorten life. Lower voltage will reduce lamp life and lamps may fail to start.

(j) *Temperature.* Extremes of hot or cold can be damaging to ballast life and performance. Ambient temperature of the areas where ballasts are installed will affect the ballast operating temperature. Fixture design will also have an effect. The ballast case hot spot should not exceed 90 °C during operation.

Thermally protected ballasts (Class P) will cut out if their case temperature exceeds 90 °C, or cause the lights to cycle off and on if the factor causing the excessive temperature persists. Ballasts without thermal cutouts will have their lives shortened with operation above 90 °C.

Most ballasts designed for indoor operation of fluorescent lamps provide voltage for satisfactory starting of the lamps at 50 °F (60 °F for the reduced wattage fluorescent lamps). Low temperature ballasts are available which can provide higher voltage to start lamps as low as –20 °F.

(k) *Lamp Burnouts.* Some ballasts may overheat with lamps flickering near the end of life or if one of a pair of lamps is removed from the lamp holders. Prompt replacement of flickering or burned out lamps should be performed.

(l) *Lamp Removal.* When lamps are removed from fixtures which remain energized, a small amount of energy is consumed by the ballast at very low power factor (except for slimline fixtures having circuit interrupting lamp holders). This is due to the "magnetizing" current flowing through the ballast primary. A ballast for a pair of 4 ft rapid start lamps will consume 6.5 W with the lamps removed. If the fixture will not be relamped within a short period of time, it should be disconnected from its power source by qualified personnel.

(m) *Sound.* Ballasts are electromagnetic devices operating on alternating current which generate sound. The loudness of the sound created depends on the ballast, the luminaire in which it is mounted and the sound characteristics of the room in which the luminaires are installed. Whether or not the ballast sound is audible depends on the background noise level of the room. Most manufacturers provide a sound level rating for their ballasts which can be used in a standard sound rating system to determine if ballast sound will be inaudible or not.

(4) *High Intensity Discharge (HID) Lamps.* The mercury, metal halide and high pressure sodium lamps make up this family. These are electric arc discharge lamps, requiring ballasts, but distinguished from fluorescent lamps by higher pressure (a little more than one atmosphere) in their arc tubes.

(a) *Mercury Lamps.* Mercury lamps have been widely applied for indoor and outdoor applications for many years. However, they are largely obsolete in new installations since the advent of the substantially more efficient metal halide and high pressure sodium lamps. Applications for mercury lamps that would presently be justified would lie in the lower wattages, say, 175 W and lower, where the more efficient metal halide lamps have no equivalent "lumen package." For example, in rooms with lower ceilings and relatively low requirements for illumination level, mercury lamps might be an appropriate choice.

Mercury lamps have long lives, usually in excess of 24 000 hours. However, they are also characterized by poor lumen maintenance, especially on constant wattage (CW) or constant wattage autotransformer (CWA) ballasts. Practical economic life is generally more of the order of 12 000 to 16 000 hours. Used in the sockets for longer hours they waste a great deal of energy with their greatly reduced light output.

(b) *Self-ballasted Mercury Lamps.* These lamps are characterized by extremely long lives and mean lm/W no better than incandescent lamps over their rated lives. They use an incandescent tungsten filament in series with the mercury arc tube as a ballast during start-up and steady-state operation. The filament consumes about 60% of the total lamp watts during operation, substantially reducing the overall lm/W efficacy of this source. Further, the extremely long lamp life works to the disadvantage of the lighting system efficiency due to the fairly rapid depreciation of light output from the mercury arc tube. At the end of life, lm/W may be lower than that of typical incandescent lamps. Their principal virtue is long life and reduced labor cost for lamp replacement. However, conventional mercury lamps with their separate ballasts would be far more cost-effective. Metal halide and high pressure sodium lamps would be even more so.

(c) *Metal Halide Lamps.* Metal halide lamps are substantially more efficient than mercury lamps and should be employed where an HID lamp is appropriate and color is important. These lamps are made with both clear outer bulbs and phosphor-coated outer bulbs.

The phosphor-coated lamp's color rendering is superior to the clear lamp, though that of the clear lamp is good. The clear lamp would provide for better optical control in a lighting fixture than the phosphor-coated bulb. Therefore, the clear lamp would be preferred in outdoor floodlighting equipment where the best beam control is desired—projecting light over long distances, restricting light to a specific target area with minimum spill, etc.

Electrically, two types of metal halide lamps are available. One type has characteristics requiring its own ballast for starting and operating. The other type is electrically interchangeable with mercury lamps on most of the commonly used mercury ballasts (about 80% of existing types). Only the 400 W and 1000 W metal halide lamps are available in the interchangeable types. This makes it possible to upgrade existing mercury lighting systems that may not provide adequate lighting simply by changing lamps in existing fixtures without increasing the connected load or energy consumption.

More recently, metal halide lamps interchangeable with mercury lamps have been made available at reduced wattage. For example, there is a 325 W metal halide lamp that can be used in 400 W mercury lamp sockets. This allows for a substantial reduction in energy use, and an increase in the delivered light at the same time.

The technology of metal halide lamps is still evolving rapidly and there appear to be significant opportunities for developing lamps with performance much improved over that currently achieved. At present, however, there are certain limits with some of the lamps as to burning position, or significant differences in lamp performance in one position compared with another. Certain lamps also have requirements for operation in enclosed luminaires only. Users are advised to consult published manufacturer's data for current information on lamp operating conditions.

1) Mercury and Metal Halide Self-extinguishing Lamps. Both mercury and metal halide lamps produce considerable ultra-violet energy in their arc discharge. This energy is very useful with phosphor-coated outer bulbs, reacting with the phosphor to generate light that improves the color rendition of the total light from the lamp. None of this type of ultra-violet gets out of the lamp as the glass outer bulb will not transmit it.

However, in a few instances, the outer bulbs of mercury lamps have been broken during service where the arc tube continues to operate. If people are in the area for some period of time, they experience a temporary reddening of the skin or irritation of the eyes due to the erythemal action of the ultra-violet coming directly from the arc tube.

Consequently, lamp manufacturers are now making a line of lamps having a "disconnecting" feature that will deactivate a lamp within a short, specified time interval after the outer bulb has been broken. These are available for new or existing installations employing open fixtures where the lamps could be broken. Of course, use of enclosed fixtures that would not permit foreign objects to break the bulbs would allow standard lamps to be used.

Glass lenses in fixtures also prevent or block the ultra-violet radiation, and may be employed to both prevent lamp breakage and ultra-violet radiation. Acrylic plastic lenses do not afford ultra-violet protection.

Starting Characteristics—Mercury and Metal Halide. Both mercury and metal halide lamps require 5 to 8 minutes of starting time (warm-up) before they reach full light output. This is because the vapor pressure of the light-generating arc tube materials is quite low at the start and takes several minutes to vaporize into the arc stream.

If mercury or metal halide lamps experience a momentary power interruption during normal operation or a voltage dip low enough, the arc tube will extinguish and a 5- to 15-minute period of "cool-down" will be required. With the lamp "off" but the arc tube "hot," the vapor pressure in the arc tube is too high for the available voltage from the ballast to restart the lamp. As the lamp cools, the vapor pressure drops and the voltage required to start the arc decreases and, eventually, the available ballast voltage is sufficient. Higher ballast voltage would allow faster restart, but would also increase ballast cost. This limitation appears not to have been a deterrent to the widespread use of mercury or metal halide lamps.

(d) *High Pressure Sodium (HPS) Lamps.* These lamps are characterized by a relatively high pressure electric arc discharge (slightly over one atmosphere) in a special ceramic arc tube containing a small amount of sodium in an amalgam form. When the lamp is first started, there is very low pressure in the arc tube and the sodium generates its characteristic monochromatic color. However, at the operating pressure involved with this lamp, the spectral output broadens, and all visible light wavelengths are present, though in different proportions compared with other familiar sources. The color appears as light yellow or pink. Lumen per watt efficacy is quite high and since source size is quite small, control of light distribution is good.

High pressure sodium lamps have three characteristics quite different from other high intensity discharge lamps—fast warm-up, fast restrike and much better lumen maintenance. Warm-up to full light output generally occurs within 2 minutes, restrike within 1 minute. Ballasts for the HPS lamps have a high voltage/low current starting circuit generating a pulse of about 2500 V. This provides the fast restrike time, usually within less than 1 minute after a power interruption. Ballasts are available (at higher cost) that will provide instant restrike for certain wattage HPS lamps, should that be necessary. High pressure sodium lamps provide mean lumen maintenance near 90% over their approximately 24 000 hours rated life, substantially better than metal halide and mercury lamps.

A high pressure sodium lamp has also been developed providing better color than the standard lamps. This is accomplished by changes in the electrical characteristics of the lamp's arc tube. The improved color involves some sacrifice in lm/W efficacy and lamp life.

(e) *HID Lamp Ballasts.* Most of the previous comments on ballasts for fluorescent lamps apply to ballasts for high intensity discharge lamps. Their functions are the same and since most are electromagnetic devices, their characteristics are similar.

Ballasts for high pressure sodium lamps differ from other high intensity discharge lamp ballasts in that they have a high voltage pulse to aid in starting the lamp. This pulse also aids in restarting hot lamps within about 1 minute if the voltage dips, or a momentary power interruption occurs that extinguishes the lamp.

With older high pressure sodium ballasts, it was necessary to change burned-out lamps promptly, and not remove lamps from sockets for an appreciable period of time (several days) without taking the fixture off the line, or the pulsed starting aid would be damaged. At present, some of the ballasts available do not have such limitations.

1) Grounding. HID ballasts shall be grounded in a manner complying with ANSI/IEEE 70-1984 [8] or local codes where appropriate.

2) Fusing. It is sometimes desirable to use a line fuse with high intensity discharge ballasts. This will prevent branch circuit breakers from opening in case there is a defective ballast on the line.

3) Noise. High intensity discharge ballasts are designed to allow for the operation of HID lamps in commercial buildings without objectionable sound. It is possible in very quiet spaces with a low background noise level to hear ballast hum. For most applications, the sound would be inaudible. In most "open plan" offices, the use of "white noise" introduced over a public address system is common practice. This is a low-frequency, usually unobjectionable sound intended to mask sound transmission from one work station to another. This would also help to mask ballast sound if high intensity discharge lamps are used to provide the ambient lighting.

4) Radio Interference. A small amount of interference may be detected during lamp starting. There should be no objectionable interference during operation.

Voltage—Lag and reactor type ballasts should have a supply voltage within ±5% of their design voltage. For constant wattage autotransformer (CWA) ballasts, the voltage should be within ±10% of their design voltage.

(f) *Low Pressure Sodium (LPS) Lamps.* These lamps are characterized by high lm/W efficacy and monochromatic yellow color. Most of the spectral energy output is concentrated between 589 and 590 nanometers (nm). The arc discharge takes place in a tube containing vaporized sodium in the free state. Low pressure sodium lamps are more like fluorescent lamps in physical size than high intensity discharge lamps. Fluorescent lamps are also low pressure discharge lamps employing mercury vapor instead of sodium in the arc.

Low pressure sodium lamps available in North America are made by European manufacturers. The lamps available have two different characteristics. One has the typical light depreciation of most lamps with light dropping off as operating hours increase. The other type has a wattage that may vary with hours of operation. Any wattage change will affect light output and also the capacity of the power distribution system. Suppliers should be contacted for data on watts throughout life, light output, etc.

If lamp color is not a deterrent to application, economic comparisons may be made with other lamps such as high pressure sodium. Such comparisons will involve assumptions for utilization of light with typical luminaires in order to determine how effectively each lamp/fixture combination delivers lumens to the task(s) and their relative (or absolute) costs. Computer programs are available for such comparisons.

Care should be taken in disposing of these lamps since, when they are broken, the free sodium in the lamp in contact with water can create a fire hazard. The manufacturers' specific instructions should be followed in disposing of burned-out lamps.

7.3.4 Room

(1) *Reflectances.* The reflectance of room surfaces is an important factor in the efficient utilization of light and, therefore, the efficient utilization of lighting energy. It is also important to visual comfort because brightness should be within certain well-established limits (ratios) in areas where demanding visual tasks are performed.

For best utilization of light, the ceiling should be painted white. The walls, floor and equipment finishes should be within the recommended reflectance ranges of Table 12.

To get even higher utilization of light, proposals are sometimes made to employ finishes on walls, floors and furniture with reflectances even higher than those in Table 12. Specifiers are cautioned against such experiments, as the recommended reflectance values have been well established over several decades of practice. Even lighter finishes could cause legitimate complaints about glare and upset the brightness relationships necessary for visual comfort.

The lighting engineer should include a specification for room reflectances as part of his design or ensure that he is consulted by those having the responsibility for color specifications.

Certain portions of walls or trim surfaces or room appointments may have higher or lower reflectance than the limits of the ranges of Table 12 if these areas are thought of as accents and restricted to no more than 10% of the total visual field.

(2) *Color.* Color is a complex subject involving both physical parameters that can be expressed in mathematical terms and psychological factors that relate to individual interpretations of color.

Certain colors seem to be warm in character while others are considered cool. Light sources have such characteristics and their color may sometimes be a factor in source selection in order to complement a warm, cool or neutral color scheme. Warmth or coolness in color scheme and light source may also be a factor in perceived temperature by occupants of a space. (This could have energy implications for space heating or cooling, winter and summer.)

Certain light sources may have high efficacy of light production with fair or poor color rendition. Others may have excellent color rendition with only moder-

Table 12
Recommended Surface Reflectances

Surface	Reflectance Equivalent Range (%)
Ceiling finishes*	80–90
Walls	40–60
Furniture and equipment	25–45
Floors	20–40
Surgical gowns, surgical drapes	less than 30

* Reflectance for finish only. Overall average reflectance of textured acoustic materials may be somewhat lower.

ate efficacy. In recent years, phosphor developments have resulted in fluorescent lamps with excellent color and good-to-excellent efficacy. These are factors that must be weighed, along with many others, in light source specification for particular applications.

There are two terms that can provide useful color information about lighting: one is chromaticity or apparent color temperature, sometimes called correlated color temperature; the other is color rendering index, symbolized as CRI in color literature.

Chromaticity is the measure of a light source's "warmth" or "coolness" expressed in the Kelvin temperature scale. It describes the appearance of the theoretical "black body" of physics, a perfect absorber and emitter of radiation, if it were heated to incandescence. At the first phase of incandescence, the object is a ruddy red. At higher temperatures the color changes from a range of warm, yellowish-white colors to white, and then to cool blue-white colors at still higher temperatures.

Some of the general service incandescent lamps and warm white fluorescent colors have 3000 K correlated color temperature. Cool white fluorescent lamps are at 4200 K. Chromaticities of sun and skylight vary over a broad range through the day.

Chromaticity provides no information about how well a light source will render various object colors. Natural daylight has excellent color rendition, though the appearance of colors under daylight will vary with time of day, season, latitude, weather and other atmospheric conditions. Many of the electric light sources also have excellent color rendition, others not as good. An incandescent lamp emits relatively small amounts of blue and green light relative to red, so it tends to mute or gray cool object colors such as blue.

A measure of how well a light source renders colors is the color rendering index (CRI). This is a number that compares a specific light source of interest against a reference source on a 0 to 100 scale. The system is limited and sometimes misunderstood, because a comparison of two sources is meaningful only if the two sources being compared have the same chromaticity. It would not be meaningful to compare the CRI of an incandescent lamp with a cool white fluorescent lamp because the chromaticity of incandescent is 3000 K while cool white is 4200 K. A comparison could be made between cool white (CRI=66) and deluxe cool white (CRI=89) because both have the same chromaticity.

From a design viewpoint, if the appearance of colors is important, one approach might be to select a chromaticity for its warmth or coolness that is suitable for a particular application. Then find a source with a high CRI in that chromaticity.

Sometimes an interior designer or colorist is called upon to select the color scheme for a health care facility. The lighting engineer must ensure that the color specifications are reasonable for good visual comfort in areas where critical seeing is performed, and that his assumptions about ceiling, wall, and floor reflectances were realistic in terms of the installed materials. Otherwise, his lighting calculations may not be reliable.

(3) *Other Considerations.* There is a great deal that is subjective about how individuals may react to a space. Nevertheless, in recent years, studies of the psy-

chology of lighting have provided statistically significant data as to how groups of people would react to various kinds of lighting. Criteria have been developed that would allow one to use lighting to create impressions of a "public" or "private" space, for example. These criteria could be helpful in applying lighting in such areas as entrance lobbies, patient rooms, eating areas, conference rooms, corridors and offices.

References [11] and [12] provide information on the psychology of light that would be helpful to users of this handbook.

7.3.5 Some Quality Factors in Lighting

(1) *Visual Comfort.* In many lighted rooms, it is desired to provide illumination without annoyance or discomfort due to luminaire or window brightness. Reference to Visual Comfort Probability (VCP) data, available from luminaire manufacturers, is helpful in the selection of luminaires that will not present discomfort glare. The VCP data is calculated by means of an empirically derived formula that assesses the brightness characteristics of individual fixtures, the room finishes, and lighting level, together with a statistical data base of brightness tolerances of people. The Illuminating Engineering Society of North America (IES Lighting Handbook [14]) recommends a VCP of 70, or higher, for spaces of concern.

Many types of shielding materials are available, including a variety of lenses, polarizers and louvers. One material may differ significantly from another in its brightness properties, so it is necessary to have a manufacturer's VCP data to properly evaluate each material being considered.

Windows can sometimes present a source of discomfort with a direct view of the sun, clouds, sky, or bright buildings. For this reason, windows should have shades, blinds, draperies, low transmission glass or other suitable shielding to reduce the brightness in the field of view. Room occupants should not face windows, normally, in performing their work, but have the windows at their sides or backs.

(2) *Veiling Reflections.* Veiling reflections in tasks reduce visibility by lowering the contrast between details of the task (a specular reflection from a graphite pencil stroke, for example) and its background. They occur when a light source and the eye of a worker are at the mirror-angle of reflection with the specular detail of a visual task. They are often difficult to "dodge" by shifting the viewing angle with the task since luminaires (or windows) that produce the effects are of substantial area and there are frequently many of them that can be reflected.

The most important single tactic for minimizing the veiling reflection effects is geometry. If the sources that light the task can be positioned out of the mirror-angle of reflection with respect to the task and worker's eyes, task visibility will be greatest. This is frequently practical in single occupancy rooms where the work location is known. It is also possible with built-in work station lighting, if lights are located to illuminate the task from both sides. Unfortunately, on many such work stations the sources are positioned under a shelf or cabinet directly in front of the task, often the worst location.

In some spaces, it is best to position work stations in between rows of ceiling luminaires, with occupants facing parallel to the rows so that most of the light on

the tasks comes from the sides and not from luminaires on the ceiling immediately in front of the work station.

Certain lighting distributions may also reduce the effect of veiling reflections
such as polarizing lighting panels, bat-wing lenses, bat-wing reflectors on luminaires, and indirect lighting.

Indirect lighting works best in large rooms with low furniture and little or no
use of screens or "room dividers." The veiling effects are least when the ceiling is
uniformly lit and the tasks are lit by a large area of ceiling. This begins to
approach a reference condition known as "sphere lighting." However, even in
large open-plan spaces, if high furniture or many screens, or both, are used to
partition the space, the utilization of the indirect lighting is greatly reduced and
the effect of veiling reflections is substantially increased.

Progress has been made in predicting, measuring and evaluating the effects of
veiling reflections. The term "Equivalent Sphere Illumination" (ESI) has resulted
from this new technology. It allows the lighting effectiveness of one or more practical lighting systems to be compared with the sphere reference condition and
with each other. This is conveniently expressed as ESI.

For example, if the measured (or predicted) ESI at a point in a room is 50 ESI,
then the practical lighting system is providing task visibility equal to 50 fc of
sphere lighting. However, if it requires 75 conventional fc to achieve 50 ESI at the
task location, the Lighting Effectiveness Factor (LEF) is 0.67 and considerable
energy is being wasted. On the other hand, if the 50 ESI are being achieved with
only 30 conventional fc supplied, the LEF is 1.67 and the energy conserving
potential is significant.

At this time there is no scientific basis for translating specific IES illuminance
recommendations into ESI. However, the ESI concept is useful in comparing
practical lighting systems for their effectiveness in reducing veiling reflections.

7.3.6 Illuminance Design Procedure

(1) *Illumination Quantity.* The Illuminating Engineering Society of North America changed the basis for its recommended levels of illumination in 1979 [14]. The
previous system involved single number target values of fc (or ESI) for tasks (that
represented an averaging of assumptions about user eyesight, age, task demand,
etc). The new system involves illuminance ranges that correlate with recommendations in the International Commission on Illumination (CIE) Publication
29-1975. These are summarized in Table 13.

To determine the nominal design illuminance from the range, Table 14 should
be consulted and weighting factors assessed. The selection of weighting factor
depends on the age of the workers, the reflectance of the task background and
the demand for speed and accuracy of task performance. All of these factors are
identified as significant variables affecting task performance by recent research.

The individual designer will be required to make more specific decisions with
the new IES system than in the past and more responsibility will reside with him
for the performance of the lighting system installed.

There are a considerable number of illuminance values for various tasks and
areas of health care facilities in the Application Volume of [14].

Table 13
Illuminance Categories and Illuminance Values
for Generic Types of Activities in Interiors*

Type of Activity	Illuminance Category	Ranges of Illumination		Reference Work-Plane
		lx	fc	
Public spaces with dark surroundings	A	20–30–50	2–3–5	General lighting throughout spaces
Simple orientation for short temporary visits	B	50–75–100	5–7.5–10	
Working spaces where visual tasks are only occasionally performed	C	100–150–200	10–15–20	
Performance of visual tasks of high contrast or large size	D	200–300–500	20–30–50	Illuminance on task
Performance of visual tasks of medium contrast or small size	E	500–750–1000	50–75–100	
Performance of visual tasks of low contrast or very small size	F	1000–1500–2000	100–150–200	
Performance of visual tasks of low contrast and very small size over a prolonged period	G	2000–3000–5000	200–300–500	Illuminance on task, obtained by a combination of general and local (supplementary lighting)
Performance of very prolonged and exacting visual tasks	H	5000–7500–10 000	500–750–1000	
Performance of very special visual tasks of extremely low contrast and small size	I	10 000–15 000–20 000	1000–1500–2000	

*Adapted from the *International Guide on Interior Lighting*, Table 1.2, CIE Pub 29-1975, International Commission on Illumination, Paris.

(2) *Illuminance Calculations.* There are two principal approaches to the calculation of illuminance: One involves situations where uniform distribution of illuminance is desirable, as in densely occupied spaces, such as nurseries; the other is where nonuniform illuminance is desirable as a more energy-efficient way of providing for task performance.

The uniform illuminance method involves the use of coefficients of utilization supplied by luminaire manufacturers, together with maintenance factors applied in a formula to determine the number of luminaires necessary to maintain the desired illuminance in a space. Then it is necessary to arrange the luminaires appropriately so as to provide the desired distribution of illuminance or minimize veiling reflections in tasks, or both.

Table 14
Weighting Factors to Be Considered in
Selecting Specific Illuminance within Ranges of Values for Each Category

For Illuminance Categories A through C			
	Weighting Factor		
Room and Occupant Characteristics	-1	0	+1
Occupants' Ages	Under 40	40-55	Over 55
Room Surface Reflectances	Greater than 70%	30-70%	Less than 30%

For Illuminance Categories D through I			
	Weighting Factor		
Task and Worker Characteristics	-1	0	+1
Workers' Ages	Under 40	40-55	Over 55
Speed and/or Accuracy	Not important	Important	Critical
Reflectance of Task Background	Greater than 70%	30-70%	Less than 30%

The computation of nonuniform illuminance is more complex since it involves a calculation for the direct contribution of each luminaire at a particular point in a room plus the contribution of inter-reflected light from room surfaces to the point of interest. This process is repeated for each point in the space where illuminance information is desired. This is called the "point-by-point" method of calculating illuminance.

Because of the great many individual calculations required, computer programs have been developed to perform them. These are available through various computer services and from manufacturers.

The IES Lighting Handbook [14] contains considerable information on the calculation of both uniform and nonuniform illuminance. Reference to this document is suggested rather than repeat such information here.

7.4 Functional Design Consideration

7.4.1 Nursing Unit (Adult Medical, Surgical and Postpartum Care)

(1) *Patient Rooms*

(a) *General.* The patient's room lighting involves the consideration of many factors and its design is more involved than is generally thought. Not only are the patient's personal needs to be considered, but the varying requirements of the medical staff, and of the housekeeping and maintenance personnel. The patient may be required to lie in positions that are marginally comfortable at best and every effort should be given to the lighting design to see the patient is not forced to view objectionable brightness. The range of illumination tasks includes floor level night lighting, unobtrusive observation of the patient, examination of the patient, reading by the patient, and general illumination for staff, visitors and housekeeping. Lighting color rendition is important for patient examination purposes, and should be equivalent to color rendition required elsewhere in the hospital. (See Table 15.)

(b) *Night Lighting.* The floor is the principal surface to be illuminated so that staff members can adequately circulate within the room, and so ambulatory patients can safely see their way about. It is difficult to provide both functions from a single-level light source. The patient whose eyes are accustomed to the dark room needs less illumination than the nurse entering from a lighted corridor.

The luminaire should be mounted on the wall 14 in to 16 in above the floor and should have a louvered cover to direct the light down and across the floor. There should be no direct illumination above the horizontal. The louver should be backed with clear glass or a lens for cleanliness. Placement in the room is important. A location near the door is recommended for single rooms. In multi-bed rooms the positioning of the light should be such as to best serve all the bed locations. Two night lights may be necessary for four-bed rooms such as might be required for spinal cord injury patients and their conveyances.

Some prefabricated headwall units include night lights as a standard item. Their location adjacent to the bed is not generally the best location and their use in such a location should be discouraged.

Night lights should be powered by a dedicated night light circuit and controlled locally from inside the room door. As an energy conservation measure, a master switch or time clock located at the nurses station or in an electric closet can be used to insure that the night light circuits are not energized during daylight hours. To best accommodate the needs of both nurse and patient without compromise, the fixture can be selected to provide the higher lighting level needed by the nurse and the room control equipped with dimming capability. The IES [14] recommends illuminance category A (see Table 13), 2-5 fc (20-50 lx) measured at the floor 3 ft from the wall and having corresponding maximum luminances of 20 and 60 fL visible from the fixture or as reflected by the floor.

(c) *Patient Controlled Lighting.* The in-bed patient should be given the control of lighting used for general lighting and reading in the bed area. In multi-bed rooms the general illumination in each bed area should be separate and locally controlled. The principal bed lighting task is reading. The reading zone is considered to be approximately 3 ft 9 in above the floor, and the area of the zone will depend on whether the fixture is fixed in position or adjustable. Because the patient may move about the bed, a larger illuminated area is necessary when fixed luminaires are used. Fixed luminaires should cover approximately a 6 ft^2 pattern while adjustable units need only cover a 3 ft^2 pattern. The lighting pattern edge illumination should not be less than two-thirds of the center lighting level.

It is important to provide control of the luminance in the surrounding bed area to avoid a harsh contrast with the reading zone. Daylight controlled by blinds and drapes serves this purpose well in the daytime. After dark, fluorescent bedlights that provide a soft up-light component to wash the wall and ceiling are most commonly used for this purpose. Located on the headwall above and behind the patient's head, this type of bedlight usually includes a separately controlled down-light component as a fixed reading lamp. Both up- and down-light components

Table 15
Illuminance Selection and Lighting Design Considerations

#	Activity	Illuminance Category	Target Illuminance Range fc To Obtain lx Multiply by 11 (approx.)			Design Considerations								Remarks
			Low	Mid	High	Occupant	Worker	Speed/ Accuracy	Room Surface Reflectance	Task Background Reflectance	Visual Comfort	Control Dimming/ Switching Multiple Levels	High Color Rendering Index	
						Age	Age							
1	Ambulance (Local)	E	50	75	100		X	X		X				—
2	Anesthetizing	E	50	75	100		X	X		X	X	X	X	—
	Autopsy and Morgue													
3	Autopsy, General	E	50	75	100		X	X		X	X		X	—
4	Autopsy Table	G	200	300	500		X	X		X	X		X	—
5	Morgue, General	D	20	30	50		X							—
6	Museum	E	50	75	100	X	X	X		X	X			—
7	Cardiac Function Lab	E	50	75	100		X						X	—
	Central Sterile Supply													
8	Inspection, General	E	50	75	100		X	X		X	X			—
9	Inspection	F	100	150	200		X	X		X	X			—
10	At Sinks	E	50	75	100		X	X		X	X			—
11	Work Areas, General	D	20	30	50		X							—
12	Processed Storage	D	20	30	50		X							—
	Corridors													
13	Nursing Areas — Day	C	10	15	20	X			X					—
14	Nursing Areas — Night	B	5	7.5	10	X			X					—
15	Operating Areas, Delivery, Recovery, and Laboratory Suites and Services	E	50	75	100	X			X		X	X	X	—
	Critical Care Areas													
16	General	C	10	15	20	X	X		X			X	X	—
17	Examination	E	50	75	100	X	X	X	X	X	X	X	X	—
18	Surgical Task Lighting	H	500	750	1000		X	X		X	X	X	X	Supplementary Task Ltg.*
19	Handwashing	F	100	150	200		X							—
20	Cystoscopy Room	E	50	75	100		X	X		X	X	X	X	—
	Dental Suite													
21	General	D	20	30	50		X	X		X	X	X	X	—
22	Instrument Tray	E	50	75	100		X	X		X	X	X	X	—

*May require levels in excess of 2500 fc (27 000 lx). See text.

Table 15 (Cont'd)
Illuminance Selection and Lighting Design Considerations

	Activity	Illuminance Category	Target Illuminance Range fc — To Obtain lx Multiply by 11 (approx.)			Design Considerations									
			Low	Mid	High	Age — Occupant	Age — Worker	Speed/Accuracy	Room Surface Reflectance	Task Background Reflectance	Visual Comfort	Control Dimming/Switching Multiple Levels	High Color Rendering Index	Remarks	
23	Oral Cavity	H	500	750	1000	—	X	X	—	X	X	X	X	—	23
24	Prosthetic Lab, General	D	20	30	50	—	X	X	—	X	X	—	X	—	24
25	Prosthetic Lab, Work Bench	E	50	75	100	—	X	X	—	X	X	—	X	—	25
26	Prosthetic Lab, Local	F	50	75	100	—	X	X	—	X	X	—	X	—	26
27	Recovery Room, General	C	10	15	20	X	X	X	X	X	X	X	X	—	27
28	Recovery Room, Emergency Examination	E	50	75	100	—	X	X	—	X	X	X	X	—	28
29	Dialysis Unit, Medical	E	50	75	100	—	X	X	—	X	X	X	X	—	29
30	Elevators	C	10	15	20	X	X	X	X	X	X	X	—	—	30
31	EKG and Specimen Room — General	B	5	7.5	10	X	—	—	X	—	—	—	—	—	31
32	On Equipment	C	10	15	20	X	—	—	X	—	—	—	—	—	32
33	Emergency Outpatient — General	E	50	75	100	—	X	X	—	X	X	—	X	—	33
34	Local	F	100	150	200	—	X	X	—	X	X	X	X	—	34
35	Endoscopy Rooms — General	E	50	75	100	—	X	X	—	X	X	—	X	—	35
36	Peritoneoscopy	D	20	30	50	—	X	X	—	X	X	—	X	—	36
37	Culdoscopy	D	20	30	50	—	X	X	—	X	X	—	X	—	37
38	Examination & Treatment Rooms — General	D	20	30	50	—	X	X	—	X	X	—	X	—	38
39	Local	E	50	75	100	—	X	X	—	X	X	—	X	—	39
40	Eye Surgery	F	100	150	200	—	X	X	—	X	X	X	X	—	40
41	Fracture Room — General	E	50	75	100	—	X	X	—	X	X	—	X	—	41
42	Local	F	100	150	200	—	X	X	—	X	X	X	X	—	42
43	Inhalation Therapy	D	20	30	50	—	X	X	—	X	X	—	X	—	43
44	Laboratories — Specimen Collecting	E	50	75	100	—	X	X	—	X	X	—	X	—	44

251

Table 15 (Cont'd)
Illuminance Selection and Lighting Design Considerations

#	Activity	Illuminance Category	Target Illuminance Range fc — To Obtain lx Multiply by 11 (approx.)			Design Considerations — Age		Speed/ Accuracy	Room Surface Reflectance	Task Background Reflectance	Visual Comfort	Control Dimming/ Switching Multiple Levels	High Color Rendering Index	Remarks
			Low	Mid	High	Occupant	Worker							
45	Tissue Laboratories	F	100	150	200	—	X	X	—	X	X	—	X	—
46	Microscopic Reading Room	D	20	30	50	—	X	X	—	X	X	X	X	—
47	Gross Specimen Review	F	100	150	250	—	X	X	—	X	X	—	X	—
48	Chemistry Rooms	E	50	75	100	—	X	X	—	X	X	—	X	—
	Bacteriology Rooms													
49	General	E	50	75	100	—	X	X	—	X	X	—	X	—
50	Reading Culture Plates	F	100	150	200	—	X	X	—	X	X	X	X	—
51	Hematology	E	50	75	100	—	X	X	—	X	X	—	X	—
	Linens													
52	Sorting Soiled Linen	D	20	30	50	—	X	—	—	—	—	—	—	—
53	Central (Clean) Linen Room	D	20	30	50	—	X	—	—	—	—	—	—	—
54	Sewing Room, General	D	20	30	50	—	X	—	—	—	—	—	—	—
55	Sewing Room, Work Area	E	50	75	100	—	—	—	—	X	X	—	X	—
56	Linen Closet	B	5	7.5	10	—	—	—	—	—	—	—	—	—
57	Lobby	C	10	15	20	X	—	—	X	—	—	—	—	—
58	Locker Rooms	C	10	15	20	X	—	—	X	—	—	—	—	—
59	Medical Illustration Studio	F	100	150	200	—	X	X	—	X	X	X	X	—
60	Medical Records	E	50	75	100	—	X	X	—	X	X	—	X	—
	Nurseries													
61	General	C	10	15	20	X	—	—	X	—	—	—	X	—
62	Observation and Treatment	E	50	75	100	—	X	X	—	X	X	X	X	—
	Nursing Stations													
63	General	D	20	30	50	X	—	—	X	—	—	X	—	—
64	Desk	E	50	75	100	—	X	X	X	X	X	X	X	—
65	Corridors, Day	C	10	15	20	X	—	—	X	—	—	—	X	—
66	Corridors, Night	A	2	3	5	X	—	—	X	—	—	—	—	—
67	Medication Station	E	50	75	100	—	X	X	—	X	X	X	X	—
68	Obstetric Delivery Suite Labor Rms. General	C	10	15	20	X	—	—	X	—	—	X	X	—

Table 15 (Cont'd)
Illuminance Selection and Lighting Design Considerations

#	Activity	Illuminance Category	Target Illuminance Range fc (To Obtain lx Multiply by 11 (approx.))			Age		Speed/ Accuracy	Room Surface Reflectance	Task Background Reflectance	Visual Comfort	Control Dimming/ Switching Multiple Levels	High Color Rendering Index	Remarks	#
			Low	Mid	High	Occupant	Worker								
69	Local	E	50	75	100	—	X	X	—	X	X	X	X	—	69
70	Berthing Room	F	100	150	200	—	X	X	—	X	X	X	X	—	70
	Delivery Area														
71	Scrub, General	G	200	300	500	—	X	X	—	X	X	X	X	—	71
72	General	G	200	300	500	—	X	X	—	X	X	X	X	—	72
73	Delivery Table	G	200	300	500	—	X	X	—	X	X	X	X	Supplemental Task Ltg.*	73
74	Resuscitation	G	200	300	500	—	X	X	—	X	X	X	X	—	74
75	Postdelivery Recovery Area	E	50	75	100	—	X	X	—	X	X	X	X	—	75
76	Substerilizing Room	B	5	7.5	10	—	X	—	X	—	—	—	—	—	76
	Occupational Therapy														
77	Work Area, General	D	20	30	50	X	—	—	X	—	—	—	—	—	77
78	Work Tables or Benches	E	50	75	100	—	X	—	—	X	X	—	—	—	78
	Patients' Rooms														
79	General	B	5	7.5	10	X	—	—	X	—	—	X	—	—	79
80	Observation	A	2	3	5	X	—	—	X	—	—	X	X	—	80
81	Critical Examination	E	50	75	100	—	X	X	—	X	X	X	—	—	81
82	Reading	D	20	30	50	X	—	—	X	—	—	X	—	—	82
83	Toilets	D	20	30	50	X	—	X	—	X	X	—	—	—	83
	Pharmacy														
84	General	E	50	75	100	—	X	X	—	X	X	—	—	—	84
85	Alcohol Vault	D	20	30	50	—	X	—	—	—	—	—	—	—	85
86	Laminar Flow Bench	F	100	150	200	—	X	X	—	X	X	X	—	—	86
87	Night Light	A	2	3	5	X	—	—	—	—	—	—	—	—	87
88	Parenteral Solution Room	D	20	30	50	—	X	X	—	X	X	—	—	—	88
	Physical Therapy Departments														
89	Gymnasiums	D	20	30	50	X	—	—	X	—	—	—	—	—	89
90	Tank Rooms	D	20	30	50	X	—	—	X	—	—	—	—	—	90
91	Treatment Cubicles	D	20	30	50	X	—	—	X	—	—	—	—	—	91

*May require levels in excess of 2500 fc (27 000 lx). See text.

Table 15 (Cont'd)
Illuminance Selection and Lighting Design Considerations

#	Activity	Illuminance Category	Target Illuminance Range fc To Obtain lx Multiply by 11 (approx.) Low	Mid	High	Age Occupant	Age Worker	Speed/Accuracy	Room Surface Reflectance	Task Background Reflectance	Visual Comfort	Control Dimming	Switching Multiple Levels	High Color Rendering Index	Remarks
92	Postanesthetic Recovery Room — General	E	50	75	100	—	X	X	—	X	X	X	X	X	—
93	Local	H	500	750	1000	—	X	—	—	X	X	X	X	X	Supplemental Task Ltg.*
94	Pulmonary Function Laboratories	E	50	75	100	—	X	X	—	X	X	—	—	X	—
	Radiological Suite / Diagnostic Section														
95	General	A	2	3	5	X	—	—	—	—	—	—	—	—	—
96	Waiting Area	A	2	3	5	X	—	—	—	—	—	—	—	—	—
97	Radiographic/Fluoroscopic Room	A	2	3	5	—	X	—	—	X	X	X	X	X	—
98	Film Sorting	F	100	150	200	—	X	X	—	X	X	—	—	X	—
99	Barium Kitchen	E	50	75	100	—	X	X	—	—	—	—	—	—	—
	Radiation Therapy Section														
100	General	B	5	7.5	10	X	—	—	X	—	—	—	—	—	—
101	Waiting Area	B	5	7.5	10	X	X	X	X	X	X	—	—	—	—
102	Isotope Kitchen, General	E	50	75	100	—	X	X	—	X	X	—	—	—	—
103	Isotope Kitchen, Benches	E	50	75	100	—	—	—	—	—	—	—	—	—	—
	Computerized Radiotomography Section														
104	Scanning Room	B	5	7.5	10	—	X	X	—	X	X	X	X	X	—
105	Equipment Maintenance Room	E	50	75	100	—	X	X	—	X	X	—	—	—	—
	Solarium														
106	General	C	10	15	20	X	—	—	X	—	—	—	—	—	—
107	Local for Reading	D	20	30	50	X	—	—	X	—	—	—	—	—	—
108	Stairways	C	10	15	20	X	—	—	—	—	—	—	—	—	—
	Surgical Suite														
109	Operating Room, General	F	100	150	200	—	X	X	—	X	X	X	X	X	Supplemental Task Ltg.*
110	Operating Table	—	—	—	2500	—	X	X	—	X	X	X	X	X	—
111	Scrub Room	E	50	75	100	—	X	X	—	X	X	—	—	X	—

*May require levels in excess of 2500 fc (27 000 lx). See text.

Table 15 (Cont'd)
Illuminance Selection and Lighting Design Considerations

	Activity	Illuminance Category	Target Illuminance Range fc — To Obtain lx Multiply by 11 (approx.)			Design Considerations								
						Age		Speed/ Accuracy	Room Surface Reflectance	Task Background Reflectance	Visual Comfort	Control Dimming/ Switching Multiple Levels	High Color Rendering Index	Remarks
			Low	Mid	High	Occupant	Worker							
112	Instruments and Sterile Supply Room	D	20	30	50	—	X	—	—	X	X	—	—	—
113	Clean Up Room, Instruments	E	50	75	100	X	X	—	—	X	X	—	—	—
114	Anesthesia Storage	C	10	15	20	X	—	—	—	—	—	—	—	—
115	Substerilizing Room	C	10	15	20	—	X	X	—	X	X	X	X	—
116	Surgical Induction Room	E	50	75	100	—	X	X	—	X	X	X	X	—
117	Surgical Holding Area	E	50	75	100	X	—	—	—	—	—	—	—	—
118	Toilets	C	10	15	20	—	X	—	—	—	—	—	—	—
119	Utility Room	D	20	30	50	—	—	—	—	—	—	—	—	—
	Waiting Areas													
120	General	C	10	15	20	X	—	—	X	—	—	—	—	—
121	Local for Reading	D	20	30	50	X	—	—	X	—	—	—	—	—

should be restricted to the respective bed area. The patient (or staff) can easily select up, down, or both lighting functions by a local fixture mounted pull-cord control. Control buttons or switches that are mounted on the headwall are generally difficult to reach and should be avoided because when beds are raised or lowered, or the head portion tilted forward, the wall (and switch) may be out of patient's reach. Pull-cords are unsightly, a maintenance problem and unsanitary, but they prove to be convenient and the initial cost is low. Alternate methods of controlling these fixtures include remote switch control in the nurse call remote unit. For this same reason the downward light distribution should be coordinated with the fixture mounting height on the wall to provide reading light over the bed back and the patient's shoulders.

Adjustable extending arm type reading lights are often used as an adjunct to the above fixed fluorescent type, providing extra flexibility with respect to the positioning of the bed and patient. These units, which are either wall or bed mounted, are often used by patients as handles for repositioning themselves, causing a continuing maintenance problem. Unless their hardware is properly enclosed, their lamps provided with adequate heat shields, and their motion appropriately limited, the patient could be subject to injury when he is groping for the light behind his head. When used alone the adjustable unit can be operated selectively as a reading light or aimed elsewhere as general illumination. As with all headwall mounted devices, projecting bedlights should be mounted above the bed's headboard travel to prevent damage to the light when the bed is raised. Conversely, the mounting of adjustable reading lights and other apparatus on the headboard may damage fixed projecting bedlights. Up-light and down-light surfaces of fixed headwall units should be enclosed with lens covers to prevent the entrance of dust and foreign objects.

Other less common approaches to bed lighting include fixed ceiling mounted lighting fixtures mounted at the headwall and designed to both wash the wall for general illumination and to provide light for reading; and side lights mounted in special prefabricated headwalls which partially enclose the head of the bed. Floor lamps or side table lamps are not generally acceptable because they are not suitable for all patient in-bed positions; they are only practical in single rooms because of their spill light; and they often add to housekeeping problems.

The unique servicing requirements of bedlights must be considered when units are specified. Fixed or adjustable units should be designed for rapid replacement of either the whole fixture or the main electrical components as a unit, through plug-in devices. This requirement minimizes inconvenience to the patient and staff by relegating fixture repair to the electrical shop.

The IES has recommended [13] that the luminances of lighting fixtures and of the patient's room surroundings should not exceed 90 fL as viewed from the patient's normal in-bed positions, and that the general illumination level maximum-to-minimum ratio not exceed 1 to 5 in a horizontal plane 30 in above the floor within a radial distance of 8 ft from the maximum lighting level on the plane. All general lighting impinging on the patient should be of the color improved type.

(d) *Housekeeping and General Illumination.* There is a need for general illumination in all bedrooms over and above that provided by the patient's lights, to facilitate efficient housekeeping functions and to quickly furnish light for nursing functions. The dropping of small objects, the spilling of liquid and patient related accidents require additional light in order to clean hidden floor areas around beds and other furniture. Such lighting should be controllable by the nurse or other staff personnel as they enter the room. Direct fluorescent illumination from the ceiling area outside of the patient's curtain tracks is preferred since the angle of the light cast into the bed areas will improve the seeing of objects beneath furniture and between beds. In single- or two-bed rooms an appropriately placed over-mirror light at a lavatory may double for this function. Depending on the room layout a three-way switch arrangement at the lavatory and room door may be necessary.

A relatively low level of lighting is required, and when necessary the patient's bedlights can be used to provide additional illumination. Many hospital bedrooms are designed with an entrance vestibule which also connects with a bathroom, or sink and locker alcove. Where these are single- or two-bed rooms a ceiling mounted fluorescent fixture located at the room entrance can serve as both general bedroom light and vestibule light.

(e) *Patient Observation and Routine Nursing.* The nursing staff, without disturbing the patient, should be able to observe the general condition and directly related medical apparatus during sleeping hours. For this purpose the IES recommends lighting of good color rendering quality in the bed area. The patient's bedlight up-light component is generally used for this purpose because of its relatively good color and availability; however, at its maximum setting it may disturb the patient's sleep. A local dimmer or switch may be utilized for the bedlight up-light components. A small ceiling mounted fluorescent unit provided back of the plane of the patient's head may also be used for this purpose. If the nurse needs additional light to read charts or instruments, the patient's reading light may be used; or a small louvered light, locally switched, can be mounted on the headwall between 3 and 4 ft above the floor.

(f) *Examination Lighting.* Lighting for examination of the patient rooms can be provided through portable fixtures or through permanently mounted fixtures, depending on the requirements of the nursing unit and the policy of the facility. In either case, illumination of relatively shadowless light is required at the center of a 2 ft diameter area where the peripheral intensity is at least 50% of maximum intensity when measured no closer than 2 ft from the lamp enclosure. There are numerous types of permanently mounted commercially available fixtures ranging from incandescent wall and ceiling mounted retractable arm units, to adjustable ceiling mounted units, to fixed incandescent and fluorescent ceiling mounted units, and high intensity indirect headwall mounted types. Arm type incandescent units should employ heat shields, and similar high intensity indirect wall units should be enclosed and shielded from paper materials inadvertently placed in or on the units. Caution is advised in the selection of examination lights that by protruding excessively from the ceiling or wall may injure patients or staff.

The patient is only under examination briefly and the uncomfortable glare from the examination light will not be particularly important to him; however, every effort should be made to select a fixture that, when properly used, will confine its light to the respective bed area.

(2) *Service Areas*

(a) *Administrative Centers or Nurses Stations*

1) General. It is customary for each nursing unit of the hospital to have a central nurses station where the coordination of staff functions for the unit is concentrated. A higher countertop is usually used to delineate the area of the station from the central corridors of the unit, and may be partially enclosed to the ceiling with glazed window areas. A desk area backing the counter is the location for nurse call system consoles, telephones, patient registers and other equipment; and the site of most nursing function paperwork.

2) Desk. The desk should be uniformly illuminated through a combination of undercounter lights and ceiling fixtures. This task requires relatively high illumination on the task area, and a lesser level for general area illumination. The undercounter lights should be shielded from direct view and positioned to minimize reflected glare as viewed from a seated position. The overhead lighting, while principally illuminating the counter, serves to illuminate the general area of the station. Generally fluorescent luminaires placed parallel to and centered approximately over chair edge of the desk will produce good uniform lighting in the task area. In large stations additional luminaires may be necessary for other functional locations.

3) Corridors. Illumination of 10–20 fc (100–200 lx) should be provided in the nursing corridors of the unit with a cut-back of 2–5 fc (20–50 lx) at night. Means for dimming or multi-level switching of the nursing station lights should be provided to reduce the contrast with the corridor lighting at night. Reduction to a lower level at the desk top is suggested when switching is employed. It is also essential to select luminaires which confine their light to the station are particularly when patient rooms are in the immediate vicinity. If an enclosing glass wall intervenes between the station counter and adjacent nursing corridors, the placement of ceiling mounted lighting fixtures and the selection of light controlling elements become more critical. Glare from the glass can obstruct the nurses' view of the corridors. Louvered lighting fixtures that have a low luminance at the high angles are generally preferred in such situations. A system of task-oriented incandescent down-lights to serve the night illumination function may be more suitable in certain station designs. However, fixture placement is crucial in such a system to maintain visual comfort.

4) Controls. The general illumination in the nursing station should be controlled near the entrance to the station. This may require a dual control location where the station serves two corridors at either side. Some or all of the ceiling lighting should be powered from an emergency power circuit and can often be designated for the night illumination.

(b) *Nursing Offices, Utility and General Purpose Areas.* Illumination of these areas requires little special consideration and should be lighted with conventional fluorescent ceiling luminaires in accordance with standard recommended practices for the task involved. Supplemental under-cabinet lighting may be required.

(c) *Drug Distribution Station.* This area may be an open portion of the nurse station area or a separate adjoining room. There is a countertop with sink, wall cabinets and usually a narcotic vault and small refrigerator. The countertop area illumination is important. Medicine preparations must be examined closely, and good color rendition is required. Placement of lighting fixtures over the front edge of the counter to provide the recommended illumination on the top is desired. The light control and placement of the fixtures should also satisfy the illumination requirements of cabinet shelves and also include the narcotic cabinet vault illumination.

7.4.2 Intensive Care Unit

(1) *General.* These areas are designed for people who for one reason or another are extremely ill. This may include serious medical illness, recovery from major critical surgery, coronary care, and other similar type care. In these areas, both the psychological and functional aspects of the lighting design are extremely important.

(2) *Patient Rooms.* The patient in a critical care area may vary in physical condition from a degree of illness that calls for a normally low level of ambient light to accommodate patient comfort, to a patient physically well enough to engage in activities such as reading. Lighting levels in the patient bed area should be variable through the use of a dimmer with a separate reading light desirable. The reading light, if not integral in the wall, should be easily removable from the work area to avoid interference during emergency care.

A much higher level of lighting will be required in the patient area during time of examination and treatment so that tissues, vascular system details, etc, may be clearly observed by the medical staff. This level of light will vary from levels of 50–100 fc (500–1000 lx) to levels of 1000–2000 fc (10 000–20 000 lx). While the lower range of these values may be achieved by the general lighting, the higher levels necessitate some provisions for additional lighting for emergency tasks, up to and including surgical lights.

General lighting for the patient area should be located so that no visual discomfort is experienced by the patient in either a prone or sitting position. Due to the critical diagnostic requirements of this area and to aid the patient psychologically, when viewing his own skin tones, etc, the color rendering quality of the lighting should be good.

While it is required by various codes to provide windows to enable the patient to view the outdoors, this lighting should not be used when evaluating the task or ambient light to be provided in the patient area.

(3) *Service Areas*

(a) *Nurses Station.* General lighting in the nursing unit areas of an intensive or critical care area should be of sufficient level to allow the reading of handwritten charts, monitoring equipment, etc. This lighting should be arranged so as not to impose itself on the patient areas in a detrimental way. The lighting in the area of the monitoring devices should be carefully laid out so as to eliminate harmful glare on glass faces yet provide adequate lighting for reading both non-illuminated and internally illuminated devices.

7.4.3 Newborn Nurseries Unit

(1) *General.* Seeing tasks in the nursery room center on the cribs and incubators. As in critical patient areas there is a need for lighting both for general illumination and close observation, with provision for reducing the general illumination to provide a subdued environment for sleeping. A moderately high level of illuminance is required for close observation and a moderately low general lighting level adjustable within the range. The luminance of the luminaires should not exceed 90 fL as viewed from the bassinet locations which will require careful selection of the general lighting system.

Good color rendition is required. Slight changes in skin color must be discernible. Sources in the higher kelvin ranges having relatively even spectral power distribution such as deluxe cool white fluorescent are recommended. Certain infant therapy involves the use of special fluorescent light treatment, and ultra-violet light is often used for bacteriological purposes. The reader should refer to literature dedicated to these specialized subjects for specific considerations.

The placement of fixed light sources for both examination and general illumination is critical. Disability glare from the specular surfaces of bassinet or incubator covers may obscure the infant. Indirect fixtures, large low-brightness luminaires, or luminous ceilings are preferable.

Table 16
Color and Color Rendering Characteristics of
Common Light Sources

Lamp Design	Correlated Color Temperature (°K)	CIE General Color Rendering Index (CRI)
Fluorescent		
Warm White	3020	52
Warm White Deluxe	2940	73
Cool White	4250	62
Cool White Deluxe	4050	89
Simulated D50	5150	95
Simulated D65	6520	91
Simulated D75	7500	93
Mercury		
Color Improved	4430	32
Metal Halide Clear	3720	60
High Pressure Sodium	2100	21
Tungsten Halogen DXW	3190	100

NOTE: Manufacturers' current data should be consulted for most recent and up-to-date information.

7.4.4 Pediatric and Adolescent Unit

(1) *General.* Children can generally be separated into four age groups when considering their lighting needs. Up to 1 year, 1 to 6 years, grade school and adolescent years. In many areas such as corridors, waiting rooms, and lobbies, all ages may be present. A light and airy atmosphere with occasional familiar contact with the outside is desirable and, where practical, windows should have low sills to permit small children to see outside.

Variety is important for the young child because of his shorter interest span. Good, diffuse general illumination is necessary because the floor is the child's realm, and toys unobserved can become a tripping hazard; yet, the highlighting of certain room and corridor locations will provide new areas of interest and exploration. Because the floor is the predominant "task" area for the young child, illumination requirements should include the floor plane.

Children's "tasks" are often similar to those of adults. Drawing, coloring, painting and even reading should be anticipated. Color matching of objects may be part of a child's projects. The use of diffuse light of a moderate level of good color quality is recommended. Quality lighting minimizes glare that can contribute to child frustration. Soft lighting introduced by curtained windows will provide a more home-like atmosphere during the day, helping to dispell the apprehensions children feel about large institutional buildings.

The observation of children by the staff is also to be considered. Improved-color light sources let the nurses accurately observe the patient's condition. Luminaires should be well shielded or located to minimize direct and reflected glare at observation windows. Where the nurse must observe the children from the nursing station the lighting should not prevent her from seeing the children, or them from seeing her. The control of lighting through the switching or dimming of specific curtained-off areas will allow their being darkened for napping purposes. General lighting in crib areas should be moderately low.

The adolescent child will require much the same considerations as an adult. To provide privacy they should be given control of their own bed area lighting, similar to that recommended under General Patient Rooms.

Medical considerations are of the greater importance in examination and treatment areas. However, switching should be provided to lower the lighting level. A lower intensity, when considered adequate, will lessen the apprehension of the child.

7.4.5 Psychiatric Nursing Unit

(1) *General.* There is a considerable range in the type of facilities having to do with the mentally ill. Some general psychiatric hospital areas are similar in design to the standard hospital nursing areas. The patients may require some particular treatment and would be considered only slightly disturbed. At the other extreme are the facility areas where highly emotionally disturbed patients may be found. Here stringent security measures are necessary to prevent patients from injuring themselves or others.

(2) *Patient Rooms.* In the hospital's general psychiatric areas, bedrooms can usually be illuminated in the same manner as standard nursing bedrooms utiliz-

ing conventional wall mounted fluorescent bedlights. Extendable arm reading or examination lights should be avoided, however. The use of floor lamps, table lamps, and desk lamps may, in some cases, be permitted to help provide a home-like atmosphere. There should be an effort to avoid the "institutional" appearance so often associated with this type of patient and he should be made to feel relaxed and assured. Where patients share rooms, the variety of luminaire types will allow individual selection and encourage communication and cooperation between patients. The inclusion of portable lamp types will also allow the staff to vary the room according to the type of patient. A security room (or rooms) is usually included in each psychiatric nursing ward for special cases. These rooms should be illuminated in a similar manner to those in facilities reserved for the more violent or unpredictable patient.

Where the facility must house patients requiring higher security, careful evaluation should be given the degree of security needed. The lighting fixtures should not reflect a prison-like atmosphere except where the most violent or destructive patients are housed. Along with ceiling lights, wall mounted bedlights of the security type may be employed in areas where patients are not destructive. In the bedrooms of violent patients, utilize ceiling mounted security type fixtures which are out of reach of the patient and which are indestructible with respect to thrown objects. Nightlights that provide approximately 0.5 fc at bed level, may be incorporated in the ceiling mounted lighting fixtures. Controlling switches should be placed outside of the room door.

Adequate daylight should be included in patient rooms and in most other patient areas such as dining rooms, dayrooms and therapy rooms. General warm tone light sources are preferred because of their soothing effect, and fluorescent fixtures should utilize deluxe type lamps to improve the appearance of flesh tones. The designer should consult with the user to determine the extent to which special lighting effects can be employed. The use of color, texture and highlighting to define spaces or tasks, while usually desirable, may be unsatisfactory when applied with respect to certain types of patients. In such cases even illumination is more desirable because it doesn't produce exaggerations of form that can alarm the patients. The system should be flexible enough to conform, through switching, with either requirement. The safety of both patient and the staff must be considered as well.

It is extremely important in these areas of health facilities that the engineer consult with hospital authorities to coordinate the complete design of the areas, including the lighting system design.

7.4.6 Surgical Facilities

(1) *General Operating Room.* The coordination of room surfaces, equipment locations, the variety of procedures, variety in location of the task, physiological aspects (tissue exposure to heat, etc.), and variety of size of the task are some of the variables that must be balanced.

Proper lighting design in the operating suite of the hospital is extremely complex.

During surgical procedures the surgical light should be capable of providing approximately 2500 fc within very strict color and size restrictions to accommodate the surgical team's visual comfort and reduce eye fatigue. Various recommendations exist for wound-to-surgical field, surgical-field-to-instrument-tables, and surgical-field-to-room-surface ratio of light levels. Meeting these requirements dictates a high general room lighting level.

The general room light should also have a good color rendering index. When fluorescent lighting is used, its color temperature should be closely matched to the surgical light. The most often used types are deluxe cool white (approximately 4000 K) and the 5000 K or 7500 K color improved lamps. This enables patient colors to appear the same under both general and surgical lighting. It is also desirable to control the general lighting level so as to provide maximum flexibility over the range of services from surgery in a major cavity to X-ray of the patient. This may be accomplished by some type of dimming or step control (for example 0 percent – 50 percent – 100 percent). Because of the sensitive electronic instruments involved, circuit filtering, RF shielding lenses or other special constructions may be required for discharge type lighting in order to reduce the radio frequency interference.

Surgical suite room reflectances are approximately as follows: ceiling 90 percent, walls 60 percent to 70 percent, floors 10 percent to 30 percent, gowns and surgical drapes 15 percent to 30 percent. Instruments and other supplies in the operating room are normally of a matte type finish to suppress glare and thus present no particular problem in the lighting design.

The general arrangement of lighting to obtain the desired footcandle level will require particular attention and coordination since the ceiling space also contains medical gas equipment and hose drops, ventilation and air conditioning equipment, radiology tracks and equipment, and other specialized items such as closed circuit television equipment.

Generally, the surgical light should be ceiling mounted. For many procedures, lighting is needed from more than a single angle to properly illuminate the surgical field and eliminate unwanted shadows. (Some shadowing, however, is necessary to give depth of field to the surgeon). Therefore, multiple head units should be used in general operating rooms. This is usually a dual-head unit. Each head should be capable of separate positioning and separate lighting level control.

When closed circuit television equipment or other specialized equipment such as microscopes for microsurgery are to be used, special attention is required to the color temperature of the lighting and to the heat produced to ensure true color rendition without posing any additional hazards to the patient.

(2) *Special Operating Rooms.* The requirements for operating rooms in which eye, ear, nose, throat, orthopedic surgery and neurosurgery are performed, is basically the same as that for general operating rooms.

Special lighting requirements can be met by the use of microscopes and of headlamps worn by the surgeon. Reduced lighting levels, even darkened rooms, are often necessary during these special procedures. This may be obtained by the switching arrangement previously discussed for the general operating room.

There may be various pieces of specialized equipment in the room including floor or ceiling pedestal mounted items such as surgery microscopes, CCTV cameras and monitors, and lasers. The general illumination should be diffuse enough to minimize shadows from these pieces of equipment and prevent obscuration of monitor images.

The anesthesiologist and other peripheral personnel may require local task lighting during periods of room darkening.

It is necessary to coordinate the surgical light for rooms using laminar air-flow devices so that minimal disruption of air flow due to heat convection may be achieved.

(3) *Surgical Cystology and Other Endoscopic Procedures.* Cystology is normally carried out in a darkened room, however, preparatory procedures such as introduction of the cystoscope must be carried out in a room with an ambient lighting level similar to a general operating room. Therefore, general room lighting of a high level is necessary with switching or dimming controls to lower the level to any point including total darkness.

It is often necessary to have a surgical light for some procedures. This light should be located at the lower end of the table and if possible, it should be capable of being directed over the urologist's shoulder.

When providing capability for room dimming, it should be remembered that the anesthesiologist must at all times be capable of seeing the color of the patient's skin and blood and of reading all dials and monitors.

(4) *Recovery Rooms.* In the recovery room the patient is monitored by a variety of devices and by visual observation. Lighting should be arranged to provide a range of lighting from low level for rest to a fairly high level for any emergency procedures which may be necessary. It may be necessary to provide this high level by means of an additional light at the bed. The lighting should be arranged so that it is not directly in the patient's eyes and so that all monitors may be read without glare.

(5) *Service Areas*

(a) *Scrub Facility.* Scrub areas are typically alcove type areas adjacent to main surgical corridors. While in these areas, the surgical team must not only do a thorough job of scrubbing, but their eyes should become adjusted for a moderately high lighting level that approximates the general lighting level in the operating room itself. The corridors adjacent to operating rooms should also contain the same lighting levels as this scrub area.

If the scrub area is to be used only for surgical areas where procedures requiring only low ambient levels are to be performed, this same lower level should also be obtainable in the scrub area.

(b) *Patient's Holding Area.* The patient is usually brought to this area prior to surgery and is held in waiting for typically one-half hour or less. Since the patient has generally received some sedative as preparation for surgery, it is desirable to have a low level of lighting. This lighting should be arranged so as to be out of the patient's line-of-sight as much as possible.

In many facilities, this area is used to begin surgical induction instead of the operating room. If this is to be true, it will be desirable to adjust the level of lighting to a moderately high level to aid the anesthesiologist in the task of placing needles in the vein of the patient. Typically, the anesthesiologist wishes to begin this procedure under a lower lighting level (roughly that of the reduced level used for patient holding) and then increase it to satisfy his needs. If the anesthesiologist wishes to insert a tube into the trachea by means of a lighted laryngoscope, a reduced lighting level will again be necessary.

7.4.7 Obstetrical Facilities

(1) *Delivery Room.* The general lighting for the delivery room is the same as for a general operating room with a high level and good color rendition a necessity. There are not, however, the problems of ceiling mounted X-ray or special air conditioning/ventilation openings causing the space problems experienced in an operating room ceiling.

There should be a ceiling mounted delivery light which can be positioned over the obstetrician's shoulder. This light should be capable of providing approximately 2500 fc at the work area.

It is also desirable to have a high level of lighting in the area of the delivery room in which initial clean-up, resuscitation, and evaluation of the newborn infant is to take place. As jaundice and cyanosis are typical problems, good color rendition will be necessary in this area.

(2) *Labor Room.* Labor room lighting is basically the same as for a typical patient room. Good color rendition is essential in the observation of the patient as skin tone is an important diagnostic aid. It is also important to be able to read the various dials and monitors used without glare problems. It is necessary in a labor room to provide a high level of lighting in the area of the lower abdomen and perineum for examination purposes. This level is often provided by portable or adjustable examination lights.

(3) *Scrub, Corridor, and Recovery Areas.* The lighting for the delivery scrub, corridor, and recovery areas are the same as those for the general operating suite. It is necessary that the exam light in recovery be capable of providing high levels in the lower abdoment and perineum area.

7.4.8 Outpatient and Emergency Suite. The outpatient or ambulatory care facilities may encompass a large and varied number of specialized areas which parallel similar facilities in the hospital. The facility may include Emergency Evaluation and Treatment, Clinical, Educational, Laboratory, Radiology, and other hospital type units. The most frequently utilized room is the Multipurpose Examination and Treatment Room.

(1)*Emergency Patient Care Services.* This is actually a group of specialized rooms grouped near the emergency entrance. Usually included is a Staff Working and Charting Station, a Minor Operating Room, Life Support Room, Observation and Treatment Room, Security Examination Room, and support areas.

   (a) *Treatment Rooms*

     1) A Minor Operating Room when provided, should have a general illumination layout similar to that required for general operating rooms in surgery suites. Refer to the "Surgical Lighting" section of this chapter for additional requirements. A small surgery light(s) capable of providing illumination of 1000 to 2000 fc (10 000 to 20 000 lx) is required. The unit should include a wall or fixture mounted intensity control, be track or single-point mounted and articulated to cover the operating table. Requirements for optics, color temperature

and controls should be as provided in the "Surgical Lighting" section of this chapter.

2) The Life Support Room is in fact a small intensive care unit. Patients are in bed and closely supervised. Local physiological monitoring is generally employed at bedside, and emergency procedures may be required at any time. The local illumination at each bed should be individually controlled and should provide adjustments in light level through dimming or multi-level lamp switching. A 2 ft × 4 ft luminaire, with lens closure, mounted over each bed is suggested. It should provide a moderately high lighting level at maximum output. The color of the light source should provide a CRI of 90 or above to insure accurate color rendition of the patient's complexion. A ceiling or wall mounted examination light similar to the unit described for Examination and Treatment Rooms is required for each life support bed.

(b) *Staff Working and Charting.* This station is similar to a standard hospital Nurses Station, providing the control point for the emergency unit. Lighting of the station should be as prescribed elsewhere in this chapter for Nursing Stations. Corridor lighting levels in the Emergency unit should be in keeping with the higher room lighting levels in the unit and thus reduce adaptability problems.

(2) *Outpatient Clinic Services.* Besides the basic Examination and Treatment Rooms, the Consultation Rooms, Offices, and the utility spaces, there may be such areas as the Eye, Ear, Nose and Throat Clinic, Satellite Pharamacy, Radiology, a small Laboratory, and other hospital related departments. Specific illumination requirements for these departments are covered elsewhere in this chapter.

(a) Examination Rooms General. This room which is found to the greatest extent in clinical areas, usually is coupled with a doctor's office or consultation room. A moderately high lighting level is recommended for examinations and should be provided at the examination table. Ideally, 50 fc for local examination is recommended. However, it is advantageous to use three-lamp and four-lamp fluorescent luminaires for the general illumination, switched or dimmed to allow reduction of the light level during certain procedures. Because these rooms often change in furniture layout to suit personnel preferences, and to provide an economical installation, some facilities will be better served with a general illumination level supplemented with a portable or fixed examination light. The general light source should be of the color improved type. For cleanliness, enclosed luminaires should be used, preferably with low-brightness lens closures.

The examination light may be a special portable unit for a specific purpose; however, each examination room should have a general purpose examination light. This flexible arm fixture should be wall or ceiling mounted, and positioned to adequately cover the examination table area. The lighthead should be large enough to direct the light in a relatively shadowless manner. The lamp (or lamps) should be of good color rendering quality which will not distort flesh tones.

(b) *Consultation Room.* This room, which is usually located adjacent to an Examination and Treatment room (or rooms) is primarily an office, and the illumination should be as recommended for offices. Because this room may be used for both relaxed consultation and conventional desk work, a means should be provided to reduce the light level when appropriate.

(c) *The Observation and Treatment Room* provides beds for persons recovering from minor surgery or other treatment given in the clinic or emergency unit vicinity. Patients are observed and evaluated here prior to their release or admittance into a hospital nursing unit. The room is usually configured as an open ward area with curtained bed spaces. As in the Life Support unit, each bed should have its own over-bed fluorescent lighting. Local multi-level control should be provided. A ceiling or wall mounted examination light similar to the unit described for Examination and Treatment rooms should be included at each bed. A wall mounted fluorescent bedlight, the same as that used in general nursing bedrooms, may also be appropriate since, in some facilities, patients may be capable of reading or visiting, and the subdued light is more suitable.

When a patient is in a mental state where he may be a threat to the safety of himself or others, a Security Examination Room is necessary. The general illumination in this room should be the same as recommended for Examination and Treatment Rooms. The examination light however, should be portable so it can be removed from being accessible to the patient.

(d) *Ophthalmic Areas.* The principle rooms in the Ophthalmic Area are the Examination and Treatment Room, Refraction Room, Visual Field Room, and Darkroom Adaptation Room. The Examination and Treatment Room may often double for the Refraction Room by including the eye lane. An Examination and Treatment Room should be illuminated the same as other general medical examination rooms. The general illumination should be as uniform as practicable and of the deluxe improved color, fluorescent type. For cleanliness, enclosed luminaires should be employed, preferably with low-brightness lens closures. Dimming or multi-level lamp switching should be included to allow partial or complete darkening of the room.

The Refraction Room requires a moderately low level of light. The two halves of the eye lane should be switched separately, controlled from the examiner's position near the patient. This same switching feature should be integrated into the lighting when the eye lane is located in an Examination and Treatment Room.

The Visual Fields and Darkroom Adaptation Rooms may be separate or combined. The lighting requirements for these rooms are similar to those of the Examination and Treatment Rooms. A moderate level of general illumination is recommended with provisions for dimming the light to complete darkness.

(e) *Dental Suites.*

1) General. The dental suite offers the designer a variety of special illumination challenges. From a beginning in the treatment and operatory rooms at the patient's mouth, through the hygiene units, laboratories, and X-ray rooms, the lighting design is of special nature. Where tasks actually involve work with teeth or dentures the color of the light should be of high quality white light with a CRI above 90. This not only helps the dentist discern tooth problems, but insures that false teeth will match their companions under all lighting conditions.

2) Examination and Treatment Operatories. These rooms are the most frequently used patient rooms and include hygiene maxillofacial, general treatment and oral surgery rooms. The principal task area is the patient's mouth (oral cavity). The dental examination light (two in Oral Surgery) should provide a min-

imum of 1000 fc in the mouth. Higher levels may be used but provision should be made to switch or dim the light to the minimum value. The illumination in the mouth must come from a convergent beam to provide a shadow-free light at the task, and the resultant light pattern should be small enough to exclude light from the patient's eyes. With these parameters the directional lighthead should be located approximately 4 ft from the patient's head within easy reach of the dentist. Track mounting of the light assembly at the ceiling can be included to increase the articulating function of the unit.

The ambient light level in the area of the patient's head and the instrument tray should be high, and maximum to minimum luminances in the area should not vary more than 3 to 1. The examination and treatment operatories are usually small in size so that the general lighting fixtures can serve both the chair area and the surrounding work bench tops. One suggested fixture arrangement positions 2 ft $\times$ 4 ft fluorescent fixtures in a horseshoe pattern with the open end toward the patient's footwall, and the closed end consisting of a fixture mounted crosswise just back of the patient's head line. This generally places the fixtures in position to serve both the patient area and work surfaces near the walls. The center of the horseshoe is available to mount a track or post mounted examination light(s).

To acquire the intensities recommended, the general luminaires may have to operate six lamps apiece because most lamps currently available with the required high color rendering index are nearly $\frac{1}{3}$ less in lumen output than standard lamps.

3) Dental Recovery Room. Patients are brought to this room following extensive dental work for follow-up observation and to gain their equilibrium after anesthesia. A restful atmosphere is required and subdued general illumination is recommended. Since emergency treatment may be necessary from time-to-time, there should be provisions to raise the general illumination level. The fluorescent lamps should be of the deluxe type.

4) Dental Laboratories. These laboratories differ from non-dental laboratories in that fine inspection and speed are emphasized. At laboratory bench locations a minimum lighting level of 700 fc is recommended in pathology or clinical labs. A higher level is usually required in prostheses and maxillo-facial labs; higher illuminance levels should be provided at certain specific bench locations. The general lighting of benches can be accomplished through the use of fluorescent luminaires, run in continuous rows, approximately over the front edge of wall mounted benches and crosswise to double sided island or peninsula benches. The use of the three-lamp or four-lamp fixtures having lens closures are recommended, with multi-level lamp switching included. As in the operatories, the light source should have a CRI of 90 or above and designs should be based on the generally lower lumen output of these special lamps.

Where plaster impressions and modeling is performed in the Prosthetics Laboratory, a high level of directional light is required to detect imperfections and blemishes on the dark shiny surfaces. Where these operations are performed, provide a ceiling light track over the front edge of the bench. Include two adjustable spot lights per task location on track. The track should include sufficient circuits to allow local switching at each task location.

5) X-ray Rooms. Unlike most non-dental radiology rooms, the seeing task is small and higher illuminance levels are necessary to accurately position the patient and equipment. Provision for switching or dimming to lower levels should be included.

6) Preventive Dentistry. Patients are taught oral hygiene selfcare in this area. Usually individual booths or carrels are provided, each with a sink and mirror. Fluorescent lighting fixtures with an enclosing diffuser should be mounted vertically at both sides of each booth mirror. The lamp should be of a deluxe type for reasonable color rendition of mouth and facial tones. The units should provide moderately high illuminance on the facial area.

The general lighting in the room should be positioned over the booth area or other work table space, and located to minimize their reflection in the patients' mirror.

7) Other areas of the dental suite are of a nonspecial nature and their illumination requirements are covered elsewhere. The anticipation of dental work can be traumatic for some patients so corridors and waiting areas should be lighted comfortably to provide a restful and calming atmosphere.

7.4.9 Radiology Suite

(1) *General.* The radiology suite generally contains a wide variety of very complex operations. Typically, these may include radiology/fluoroscopy room, radiation therapy room, computerized tomography (body scan) room, special procedures room, and various support areas.

It is important that the patient view himself psychologically as pleasing as possible. Therefore, incandescent or color improved fluorescent lighting is normally recommended. It is also necessary in all types of radiology rooms to be able to dim the lighting level for various procedures and individual preferences. Typically, these rooms are served by separate control areas, therefore separate dimming capability should be provided for this area in each room.

(2) *Radiology/Fluoroscopy Room.* Radiology/fluoroscopy rooms formerly required total darkness; however, with the advancement of image intensification, a low illuminance level is now preferred. It is desirable that a fairly high level of light be available in these rooms for cleanup. There is a large amount of ceiling rails and apparatus that compete with the lighting and air conditioning for the available ceiling space. In addition, the designer should consider that the patient should not be forced to look directly into the lighting. It is also necessary to consider the structural mounting above the ceiling for the X-ray equipment. This often will make it difficult if not impossible to consider fluorescent lighting units. The frequent on-off nature of fluoroscopy, the desire by some radiologists for extremely low ambient light levels, and the competition for ceiling spaces make incandescent lights an excellent option. However, if all other conflicts are resolved, fluorescent lighting is an acceptable choice.

(3) *Special Procedure Room.* Special procedure rooms are similar to radiology/ fluoroscopy rooms except that more complex, often invasive, procedures are used. A higher level of lighting should be provided than is required for the radiol-

ogy/fluoroscopy rooms. A combination of low level incandescent units on dimmer control and high level fluorescent units, multi-lamp switched, is recommended to give a wide range of lighting flexibility. The special procedures room is generally larger than other radiology rooms, and with careful design, continuous rows of flourescent fixtures can usually be worked into the ceiling grid. An incandescent level of 0–10 fc (0–108 lx) and a fluorescent maximum of 50 fc (538 lx) is suggested. Special examination or task lighting units may be required by some facilities to provide a local level of 200 fc (2152 lx).

Isolated power is used to reduce the possibility of microshock during invasive procedures and because some procedure rooms (vascular) are considered as "wet" locations. If this is to be true, an isolated power system may be used and the designer should adjust switching arrangements accordingly.

(4) *Radiation Therapy Room.* In radiation therapy rooms, the psychological considerations make some type of unobtrusive type of dimmable lighting desirable. These considerations are the dominant considerations for this type of room as the ceilings are generally clear of obstructions allowing a greater variance in the location of lighting. This lighting should be positioned to provide no direct glare to the patient's eyes. If the upper wall areas are clear of equipment, indirect lighting from the wall-mounted fluorescents should be given consideration as a comfortable solution to the glare problem.

(5) *Computerized Tomography Room.* In computerized tomography rooms, the treatment area should have dimming capability for its lighting as low levels are generally used during treatment and high levels for equipment maintenance. Lighting for the control area should be placed to miminize glare on the screens of the control devices.

(6) *Film Processing.* The darkroom has a requirement for two types of lighting. A fairly low level of "white" light is needed for cleanup, and a safelight is required to prevent fogging the film during processing. These two types of light should be switched separately in separate physical locations to prevent accidental exposure of the film. A two-pole switch mounted near the work counter can be circuited to energize the safelight while simultaneously disabling the white light, and if a rotary light-lock entrance is not employed, an "in use" sign outside the door can be energized with the safelight. The filter for this safelight should be matched to the film type. There should be a switch on the film storage bin located within the darkroom which will extinguish the "white" light if the bin is inadvertantly opened while the light is on and thus avoid damage of the film. New developing systems may no longer require a darkroom; processing of the film is being done automatically internally within a machine.

(7) *Viewing and Administration.* General lighting is typically needed only for cleanup and circulation in the viewing rooms. The basic purpose of this room is to provide viewing boxes to read and evaluate X-ray films. During use of these boxes, all general lighting is normally turned off. In some instances, a desk may be provided in these spaces for a secretary or other use. If this is true, task lighting must adequately be provided for typing, transcription, and reading of material. This lighting should not interfere with the viewing of X-ray films and therefore tends to be rather directional. Desk lighting is often used.

(8) *Waiting and Holding Area.* Waiting areas in the radiology suite should provide lighting that is warm and pleasing for the patient's comfort and ease. Use of windows, table lamps, and indirect lighting are some techniques which aid in calming the patient. If the waiting area has an area for holding of patients on gurneys, the lighting should be planned not only to soothe, as previously mentioned, but also coordinated to avoid direct light in the patient's eyes.

7.4.10 Laboratory

(1) *Laboratory Work Counters.* The basic pathology laboratory can be properly illuminated utilizing rules that apply to all such areas where work benches or tables predominate. It is important to limit reflected glare from surfaces of bench tops and equipment. A moderately high level of diffuse lighting is desirable to reduce shadowing that can be disabling to laboratory personnel.

Orienting rows of fluorescent luminaires properly to suit bench and table locations can provide very satisfactory results. The designer should position the rows or fixtures in any configuration relative to the furniture layout without constraints being introduced by the ceiling system design or the location of other utilities. Such constraints may lead the designer into the use of surface mounted luminaires, a practice which may not be appreciated by the architectural designer who often favors recessed luminaires.

Fixture rows should be run parallel to and approximately centered over the front edge of wall-mounted benches, and run at right angles to double-sided island or peninsula benches. In large rooms logical work areas should be separately controlled to allow shutdown of lighting for energy conservation, when appropriate. Under-cabinet lights may be required at specific equipment locations to compensate for cabinet shadowing or for the unavoidable interrupting of the general lighting system design. Such under-cabinet luminaires should be well shielded from direct view and positioned as far forward as practicable to prevent veiling reflections.

Large fume hoods and similar permanent equipment may force the omission of portions of the ceiling lighting layout. If lighting within this equipment is not supplied, the designer should provide appropriate compensation for the loss of general illumination in the area.

Certain laboratory tests require good color rendering light. Tissue, gross specimen, and bacteriology laboratories are examples. Lamps providing a CRI of 90 or above are recommended, and their generally lower lumen output should be considered in the lighting design.

Tissue and gross specimen laboratories will require a general illumination on the table surfaces of 200 fc and, where microscopes are used in luminaires, should be positioned to minimize glare on surrounding surfaces. Background surfaces for microscopes should be dark in color and of low reflectance. When a separate Microscope Reading Room is provided, a moderate illuminance level is sufficient with dimming or lamp switching provided.

Bacteriology rooms require additional lighting in specific areas where culture plates are read. At these locations additional fixtures or lamps can be operated to raise the illumination level from a moderate general level of illuminance to a higher level. Local control should be provided as an energy conservation measure.

(2) *Specimen Collection and Blood Donor.* Specimen collecting and blood donor rooms usually are part of the laboratory area. Moderately high illumination should be provided at locations where venipuncture is performed. To aid in the location of veins, this lighting should be partially directional rather than uniform and diffuse in character. This may be accomplished through the use of a supplemental adjustable examination light or through the careful positioning of the ceiling luminaires with respect to the bed or couch, providing oblique illumination on the subject. Shadowing due to the location of staff personnel should be avoided in the selection of luminaire locations.

(3) *Electron Microscope Room.* This room (or suite of rooms) should be located with great care to minimize vibration and magnetic interference. Because of the sensitivity to magnetism, fluorescent ballasts should be kept at least 10 ft from the instrument. This will affect the lighting design in the scope room and possibly in the rooms below. Incandescent light sources may be employed in lieu of fluorescent to avoid the above interference problem.

A high light level is not required and usually a subdued level is most desirable. However, sufficient light should be provided for maintenance and set-ups. Illuminance should be controlled by a nonmagnetic, electronic dimmer. The dimmer control should be located near the electron microscope with a 3-way switch located at the room door.

7.4.11 Dialysis. The dialysis area is the site of many varied activities. The staff must have adequate illumination to perform the many duties involved in preparing equipment and attaching it to the patient, monitoring the procedures, cleaning up afterwards, and seeing to the orderly operation of all functions in the area. The patient must be confined to the dialysis couch or bed for many hours, and his comfort is very important. The illumination in the dialysis area must be compatible with all these needs.

A high illuminance is required for insertion of the cannula. This function may take place with the patient in a regular dialysis bed or in an examination and treatment room. A portable spotlight or a narrow beam downlight for supplemental light is recommended. Downlights over either side of the bed or examination table, locally controlled, can provide additional versatility. The color quality of the light must be adequate to detect abnormalities in skin coloring. A locally controlled fluorescent lighting fixture should also be included over each bed, providing a moderately high general illuminance level for general staff functions in the patient vicinity. The light source should be of the deluxe type to give reasonably accurate color rendition of skin tones.

During dialysis the patient may wish to read or perform some simple task to occupy the time. A standard hospital bedlight should be provided for this purpose which can be controlled by the patient. A deluxe or warm tone lamp is recommended for the bed lamp to improve the appearance of the patient's complexion, an important psychological consideration. The selection of wall finishes can also help provide a calming atmosphere.

Over-bed luminaires and general luminaires over the circulation areas should be selected considering the comfort of the patient during his restricted stay. Spill light from areas adjacent to each patient should be well controlled to prevent irritation and to promote a restful environment. This same environment should be provided in patient waiting areas to lessen the apprehension associated with anticipation of dialysis procedures. Floor or table lamps in conjunction with comfortable furniture will aid in establishing a home-like atmosphere.

There will be areas for storage of equipment, a nurses station or control office, a biochemistry laboratory, toilets and locker facilities. Such areas should be illuminated in accordance with standard recommended practice. Equipment servicing and dialysate preparation should be provided with moderately high illumination.

7.4.12 Autopsy. Although there is a similarity to surgical procedures in the autopsy process, the seeing task is not as difficult because the cutting cavity need not be as carefully restricted, hence deep cavity lighting is unnecessary. In lieu of surgery lights, large area fluorescent luminaires located directly over the table area should provide a moderately high illuminance. This local general illumination should be supplemented with either small portable surgery lights or several adjustable ceiling mounted spotlights in combination with the general fluorescent illumination. A spot located just beyond the head end of the table should include infrared filtering for observing delicate tissues in the brain area. Scales or other work counter areas may require highlighting, and general luminaires should be positioned accordingly.

7.4.13 Pharmacy

(1) *Dispensing Area.* The tasks performed in most areas of the pharmacy involve the reading of labels and the reasonably accurate recognition of colors. A moderately high level of illuminance is required in the compounding and dispensing areas where the more exacting tasks are performed. Surfaces on counters and in the surrounding areas should be light in color with a matte finish to reduce reflected glare.

Enclosed fluorescent fixtures utilizing light controlling lenses are recommended, oriented to suit task locations. If practicable, continuous rows of fixtures should be run parallel to, and approximately centered over, the front edge of wall-mounted work counters, and cross-wise to double-sided island or peninsula work counters. Row spacing and lamps-per-fixture should be efficiently selected to provide the required illumination at the counter work stations.

Moderately high illuminance level is recommended for manufacturing and solution rooms with fixtures also oriented to suit task locations.

In general, emphasis should be on both reducing shadowing from large areas of light and the brightness of the fixture sources. The working environment as viewed from the prescription window should be one of cleanliness and efficiency.

At busy times, patients may be required to wait for their prescriptions to be filled. The waiting area should be comfortable, allowing sufficient illumination for light reading or viewing of television. Ideally, low level general illumination with high-lighted areas is preferred, and may be accomplished with downlights or table lamps placed to avoid obscuration of television viewing or the reading of a pharmacy patient-call tote board.

(2) *Storage Area.* In the active storage area, fixture rows should be placed to effectively direct light into shelves and bins. Where the top shelves are well below the ceiling or near head height, fixture rows may be run at right angles to the

shelves and bins. Where the top shelves are close to the ceiling, rows should be centered on the aisles parallel to the shelves or bins. In the latter case, stack lighting fixtures similar to those employed in libraries are effective in directing light into lower shelves.

7.4.14 Long Term Care Facilities.

(1) *Nursing Home Care, General.* The nursing home bedroom generally differs from the standard hospital bedroom in that there is less medical paraphernalia on the walls, and the room is decorated to be more in keeping with a home environment. There may be floor and table lamps to go with the comfortable chairs provided. Curtained windows should control daylight and provide the resident with a restful view. Both daylight and artificial illumination should be coordinated with the placement of wall or ceiling mounted TV sets. Bedlight and nightlighting should be the same as recommended for the general patient rooms in hospitals.

Corridors should be colorful, bright and airy, both to give a pleasing environment, and for safety. Some residents will have impaired vision, and good lighting should clearly define obstacles in the passageways. Cove lighting, downlighting or luminous ceiling areas can be used in corridors to enhance and define areas such as lobbies, vestibules and nurse stations. Illumination of a moderately low level is recommended for corridors during the day with a cut-back at night.

Dining rooms, recreational areas, and dayrooms should be given special lighting consideration keyed into the architectural treatment of the rooms. There may be skylights, a pool table, a projection screen, a food service line, tables, couches and similar features to be considered. A provision of dimming may be required for dining, or for watching TV or motion pictures. In large rooms with dividers, selective switching of lighting levels by logical areas may be appropriate. The luminaires should be pleasing in appearance, differing in some degree from the stereotype institutional fixtures found in the hospital environment. Table and floor lamps help to give a homelike atmosphere to the dayrooms.

The brightness of luminaires should be well controlled to maximize patient comfort and promote safety. The maximum recommended general lighting levels may be selected from the lower levels of illuminance for dining areas, and upper levels for recreation rooms and dayrooms. In each case, dimming or switching should be included to provide means for appropriate reduction in lighting levels.

As in the nursing areas of hospitals, an examination and treatment room is provided to allow examination with some degree of privacy. The general illumination should be as uniform as praticable and of the improved color, fluorescent type. For cleanliness, enclosed luminaires should be used, preferably with low brightness lens closures. Dimming or multi-level lamp switching should be included to facilitate the use of any instruments which function best in low ambient light levels. Note, the three lamp fluorescent fixture provides the option of three light levels with only two switch controls. The provision of a uniform light level also recognizes that the examination and treatment room typically changes some of its furniture configuration from time to time.

The examination light may be a portable specialized unit for a specific purpose; however, each examination room should have a general purpose examination light. This flexible arm fixture should be wall- or ceiling-mounted, and positioned to adequately cover the examination table area. The lighthead should be large enough to direct the light in a relatively shadowless manner. The lamp (or lamps) should be of good color rendering quality that will not distort flesh tones.

(2) *Convalescent Facilities.* Requirements vary depending on condition of the patients. Some bedrooms will need to be designed the same as those in nursing homes where initial help or supervision is necessary. When the patient is fully ambulatory or essentially self-sufficient, the bedroom areas should resemble hotel rooms or apartments. Except for special conditions, lighting should come from night table lamps, floor lamps and desk lamps. An electrical receptacle switched at the door can control one of the lamps for entrance convenience.

Considerations for corridor, dining and recreational areas requirements are similar to those of nursing home care except for the greater degree of freedom enjoyed by most patients. Livelier activities than found in a nursing home will be appropriate, and the lighting for such areas must be planned accordingly.

(3) *Geriatric Facilities.* These facilities should have a lighting design essentially the same as that recommended for nursing homes. The tasks are similar, involving persons who often have impaired vision and slow reflex action time, and who may be confined to a bed. The need is for good lighting for safety and to provide a cheery environment.

7.5 Emergency Lighting

7.5.1 Codes. The minimum requirements for emergency lighting are found in the Codes of the National Fire Protection Association (NFPA). These codes are often adopted by state and local construction codes which may provide additional requirements. The following specific NFPA documents apply:

ANSI/NFPA 101-1985 [10]
ANSI/NFPA 99-1984 [9]
ANSI/NFPA 70-1984 [8]

(1) *Code for Safety to Life from Fire in Buildings and Structures.* ANSI/NFPA 101-1985 [10], Sections 5 and 10, outline requirements for "means of egress" lighting, and lighting requirements for Exit and Exit Directional signs. Chapter 10, Health Care Occupancies, covers the subjects of Illumination of Means of Egress, Emergency Lighting, and the Marking of Means of Egress. The reader is referred to ANSI/NFPA 99-1984 [9] and ANSI/NFPA 70-1984 [8] for emergency power requirements. Generally, the floor of egress ways shall be illuminated to not less than 1.0 fc, and the failure of any electrical lamp in a fixture shall not leave the area in darkness. The power for "means of egress" emergency lighting shall be provided by the Life Safety branch of the Essential Electrical System of the health care facility. The power system shall automatically provide power for the emergency lights within 10 s of failure of the normal power system.

The rules for locations of exit signs and their lettering are outlined in ANSI/NFPA 101-1985 [10]. Their illumination, whether internal or external, should be a minimum of 5 fc on the illuminated surface. Exit sign illumination should also be connected to the Life Safety branch of the Essential Electrical System.

(2) *Standard for Health Care Facilities.* ANSI/NFPA 99-1984 [9] and ANSI/

NFPA 70-1984 [8] describe the emergency power systems for hospitals. Basically, the essential system is divided into three distinct branches: Life Safety, Critical, and Equipment. There is lighting operated from each of the three branches. Circuits of the Life Safety branch should not have switch controls available to other than maintenance personnel. In addition to the requirements of ANSI/NFPA 101-1985 [10], the Life Safety branch shall provide illumination at the emergency power generator set. Often battery operated emergency lights are also located at the generator to aid in emergency repairs.

The Critical branch of the essential system provides power for task illumination at specific listed areas such as Nursing Stations, Surgery, Intensive Care, etc, which may be crucial to the care of patients during a failure of the normal power system.

The Equipment branch includes power to elevators. Here, cab lighting is necessary to prevent panic during emergencies. The designer is encouraged to thoroughly familiarize himself with the latest requirements of the above codes.

It may also be desirable in such areas as operating rooms to provide battery powered "instant on" lighting to supplement the Emergency Generator lighting which may take 10 s to start.

(3) *National Electrical Code.* ANSI/NFPA 70-1984 [8], Article 517, "Health Care Facilities," includes requirements for designs and design options for the Essential Electrical Systems for various health care facilities. Acceptable methods are outlined for applying the requirements of ANSI/NFPA 101-1985 [10] and ANSI/NFPA 99-1984 [9].

7.5.2 Other Considerations. Within the health care facility there are numerous areas, not on the Life Safety branch, where considerable inconvenience may arise with the failure of lighting on normal power. Selected luminares or groups of luminaires may be included on the Critical branch and switched as appropriate to the function of the area. If the facility is to operate for an extended length of time under disaster conditions the critical lighting layouts should be carefully planned to allow near normal functioning of portions of essential departments.

Corridor "white lights" (select luminaires of the Life Safety branch) should be appropriately arranged to serve as night lighting when luminaires of the normal power system are switched off. In patient areas such luminaires should be positioned to avoid casting light into doors of patient bedrooms.

Stair tower lighting, required to be on the Life Safety branch, should have alternate landings on separate circuits to prevent total darkness in the event of an individual circuit failure. At points of discharge the exterior lighting should also be on the Life Safety branch to aid personnel in getting clear of the building.

7.6 References

[1] ANSI/ASHRAE/IES 90A-1980, Energy Conservation in New Building Design.

[2] ANSI/IEEE Std 142-1982, Recommended Practice for Grounding of Industrial and Commercial Power Systems.

[3] ANSI/IEEE Std 241-1983, Recommended Practice for Electric Power Systems in Commercial Buildings.

[4] ANSI/IEEE Std 399-1980, Recommended Practice for Industrial and Commercial Power System Analysis.

[5] ANSI/IEEE Std 446-1980, Recommended Practice for Emergency and Standby Power Systems for Industrial and Commercial Applications.

[6] ANSI/IEEE Std 493-1980, Recommended Practice for the Design of Reliable Industrial and Commercial Power Systems.

[7] ANSI/IEEE Std 739-1984, Recommended Practice for Energy Conservation and Cost-Effective Planning in Industrial Facilities.

[8] ANSI/NFPA 70-1984, National Electrical Code.

[9] ANSI/NFPA 99-1984, Standard for Health Care Facilities.

[10] ANSI/NFPA 101-1985, Code for Safety to Life from Fire in Buildings and Structures.

[11] IEEE Std 141-1976, Recommended Practice for Electric Power Distribution for Industrial Plants.

[12] IEEE Std 242-1975, Recommended Practice for Protection and Coordination of Industrial and Commercial Power Systems.

[13] Health Care Facilities Subcommittee of the Institutions Committee of the IESNA. *Lighting for Health Care Facilities*, CP-29. New York: Illuminating Engineering Society (IES), January 23, 1978.

[14] IES Lighting Handbook. New York: Illuminating Engineering Society (IES); Application Volume, 1981; Reference Volume, 1984.

[15] Committee on Office Lighting of the IES. American National Standard Practice for Office Lighting. *Journal of the Illuminating Engineering Society*, vol 1, no 1, October 1973.

[16] Committee on Residence Lighting of the IES. Design Criteria for Lighting Interior Living Spaces. RP-11, *Lighting Design & Application*, vol 10, no 2 and vol 10, no 3, February–March 1980.

[17] Committee on School and College Lighting of the IES. American National Standard Guide for School Lighting. *Lighting Design and Application*, vol 8, no 2, February 1978.

[18] FLYNN, J.E. and SPENCER, T.J. The Effects of Light Source Color on User Impression and Satisfaction. *Journal of the Illuminating Engineering Society*, vol 6, no 3, April 1977, p 167.

[19] FLYNN, J.E., SPENCER, T.J., MARTYNIUK, O., and HENDRICK, C. Interim Study of Procedures for Investigating the Effect of Light on Impression and Behavior. *Journal of the Illuminating Engineering Society*, vol 3, no 1, October 1973, p 87.

7.7 Bibliography

ASHRAE/IES 100.5-1981, Energy Conservation Existing Buildings — Institutional.[27]

Committee on Industrial Lighting of the IES. American National Standard Practice for Industrial Lighting. *Journal of the Illuminating Engineering Society*, vol 2, no 4, July 1973.

Committee on Kitchen Lighting of the IES. Lighting for Commercial Kitchens. *Journal of the Illuminating Engineering Society*, vol L1, no 7, July 1956.

Committee on Library Lighting of the IES. Recommended Practice of Library Lighting. *Journal of the Illuminating Engineering Society*, vol 3, no 3, April 1974.

---

[27] This publication can be obtained from Publication Sales, American Society of Heating, Refrigerating, and Air Conditioning Engineers, 1791 Tullie Circle, NE, Atlanta, GA 30329 or from Publication Sales, Illuminating Engineering Society, 345 East 47th Street, New York, NY 10017.

8. Communication and Signal Systems

8.1 System Design Considerations

8.1.1 Introduction. Communication and signal systems make possible the efficient and timely operations of health care facilities. The ever-increasing cost of health care, together with the accelerating levels of technological sophistication of the equipment, mandate that these systems be planned with a thorough understanding of the operational and engineering requirements, as well as the economics of their implementation.

Each of the major categories of current communication and signal systems, together with its nominal physical plant space and installation requirements, is included in this section. This section treats the systems as separate and distinctive. Although some of them can be integrated with others, it is possible to design them as separate entities. When designing a health care facility for new construction or remodeling, it is necessary to consider all systems and to plan accordingly.

8.1.2 Programming. Advanced technologies, a large number of combination possibilities, and a wide range of different available functions, make it difficult to evaluate the different systems. It is not the number of functions listed that determines the efficiency of a system, but the way each function can assist the user of the system in improving his daily communication. Functions have to be logical and simple to operate, otherwise they will have only theoretical interest. Before deciding upon a system it is imperative to check the following points:

(1) *Analysis.* Properly integrated communications in a facility should be one of the key factors in analyzing and designing spaces, equipment, and personnel requirements for each health care function. Properly designed total communications can help reduce recurring expenses and can increase the effectiveness of staff—all of which may be translated into improved patient care.

What is required, in the earliest preplanning stages of a project, is an analysis of the current and future communication needs—a master plan for communications. In preparing such a plan, the design team should take into account the current operating techniques of the facility as well as new techniques that can be applied in the future. They should also consider possible changes in the organization during the next five to ten years. These might include university affiliation, mergers, feeder hospitals, extended care facilities, psychiatric facilities, day centers and other factors and developments which may affect the total plan.

A study of this type involves both the in-house planning team—the administrator, the medical staff, the nursing staff—and the design team.

Factors that should be considered include the movement of supplies, communication and traffic flow, the number of inpatients and outpatients handled each day, number of emergencies, surgical procedures, coronary care provided, etc.

(2) *Communication and Signal Systems Plan.* When the preliminary communication study has been made, a communications program may be developed. This program will outline the specific communication requirements in the various departments of the facility and will suggest possible ways of satisfying these communication needs.

To prepare this program, an in-depth study of the internal communication system should be made by the design team. These people may be staff members of the facility's architectural or engineering organization or may be outside communications specialists. The results of this study are then translated into a narrative program matrix, including grid sheets showing total communications.

The planning team should prepare a detailed evaluation of the internal and external communications network, including traffic and feasibility studies for each and every department. These studies will show how each department communicates, with whom it communicates, why it communicates, where it communicates, and what is accomplished by the communication.

(3) *Economic Analysis.* Comparative analysis should be made of alternatives, including cash flow and life cycle cost analysis.

(4) *System Supplier Qualifications.* It is recommended that communication and signal system suppliers be established companies that maintain a staff of competent technicians qualified to assume proper installation of the systems specified, and capable of providing maintenance and repair for these systems on a contract or job order basis. The supplier should have the capability of dispatching a maintenance or repair truck with a qualified repairman to the job site within four hours of a request for service on the equipment.

8.1.3 Communication and Signal Facilities. There are three basic elements of health care communication and signal systems that should be planned for in advance. The first is user apparatus, which broadly includes telephones, speakers, nurse call buttons, doctors register stations, radio pagers, two-way radios, and a host of other devices. Second, communication systems require a large quantity of on-premises communication central equipment that must be properly located in the facility. Thirdly, a network of communication paths (cable plant) should be provided to connect this apparatus and communication equipment. In a broad sense, these three elements should be combined to afford the staff and patients communication and signal capabilities. These systems should meet their original needs, and should also be capable of being changed and expanded most efficiently and most economically as those needs change, as they almost certainly will.

8.1.4 Communication and Signal Control Centers

(1) *General.* The engineer must pay very careful attention to design considerations and layout of the control centers within the health care facility. It is imperative that these critical areas be carefully planned in order to facilitate efficient operation of the staff using them. In order to do this, the engineer must have a good knowledge of the procedures to be carried out in these control centers. This knowledge is easily gained through conferencing with the staff who will occupy the area. The staff can be quite helpful in suggesting design considerations or layouts which would work well in their particular facility. The engineer must also have a knowledge of the communication systems needed in a particular center of control. The following will serve as a checklist:

(2) *Central Control Center*
  (a) Telephone operator console
  (b) Staff register annunciator
  (c) Voice paging system microphone
  (d) Radio paging system encoder
  (e) Fire alarm fan control for smoke control
  (f) Emergency generator annunciator
  (g) Fire alarm annunciator
  (h) Medical gas alarm annunciator
  (i) Emergency elevator control and annunciator
  (j) Code blue annunciator
  (k) Patient management computers
  (l) Blood bank alarm
  (m) Clock on system
  (n) Radio control systems
  (o) Security and administrative control communication systems

(3) *Nurse Station*
  (a) Telephone
  (b) Intercom
  (c) Nurse call annunciator
  (d) Nurse assist annunciator
  (e) Code blue annunciator
  (f) Medical gas alarm annunciator
  (g) Patient management computer terminal
  (h) Clock on system
  (i) Patient physiological monitors

(4) *Emergency Room Control Center*
  (a) Telephone
  (b) Intercom
  (c) Nurse call annunciator
  (d) Nurse assist annunciator
  (e) Code blue annunciator
  (f) Emergency medical service communication radio control
  (g) Patient management computer terminal

(h) Clock on system

(i) Patient physiological monitors

(5) *Operating Suite Control Center*

(a) Telephone

(b) Intercom

(c) Nurse call annunciator

(d) Nurse assist annunciator

(e) Code blue annunciator

(f) Medical gas alarm annunciator

(g) Patient management computer terminal

(h) Clock on system

(i) Patient physiological monitors

8.1.5 Cable Plant

(1) *Introduction.* The cable plant provides the signal path between the user terminals and the central control equipment of all communications and signaling systems. The term covers not only the insulated conductors themselves, but also the methods and materials used to support and protect the conductors.

The choice of conductors used for the signal path is usually dictated by the signal characteristics of the communication system under discussion. Conductor size and number, insulation type and color, shielding and jacketing are essentially system dependent (as is discussed elsewhere in this section). The choice of methods for support and protection of these conductors is also dependent on system characteristics; but the engineer should give attention to classifying the physical spaces where the cable plant is installed before making this choice. The following discusses the three basic methods for support and protection of communications conductors in health care facilities.

(2) *Cable in Raceway.* As the engineer lays out the route for installation of communication conductors, he must classify the physical spaces along the route. The classifications are:

(a) Indoors

1) exposed to physical damage

2) in ducts or plenums

3) in noncombustible ceiling blind spaces

4) concealed spaces

5) in shafts

6) in hoistways

(b) Outdoors

1) aerial

2) aerial, over roofs

3) underground

4) on buildings, exposed to physical damage

(c) Indoors or Outdoors

1) locations which are hazardous due to the presence of flammable or explosive materials.

Raceways will almost always be required for the following:

- Ducts or plenums used for environmental air
- Concealed spaces
- Hoistways
- Shafts
- Aerially
- Underground

Refer to ANSI/NFPA 70-1984 (Articles 725, 760, 800, and 820) [3][28] for exceptions to the requirements for raceways. Raceways will be required for communications systems that are nonpower-limited and for life safety systems. For communication circuits that are power-limited raceways are not required. Refer to ANSI/NFPA 70-1984 (Article 760) [3].

The communications system should be further classified under one or more of the following articles of ANSI/NFPA 70-1984 [3].

Article 640 Sound Recording and Similar Equipment

Article 725 Class 1, Class 2, and Class 3 Remote-Control, Signaling, and Power-Limited Circuits

Article 760 Fire Protective Signaling Systems

Article 800 Communication Circuits

Article 810 Radio and Television Equipment

Article 820 Community Antenna Television and Radio Distribution Systems

Wiring methods for each category of communications system are discussed in the appropriate article. The engineer should be familiar with these articles.

Where communications conductors are installed without raceway, they are considered to be open cabling, and they shall be installed as described below.

(3) *Open Cabling.* Open cabling is a wiring method for communications conductors that allows insulated conductors to be installed without the use of an enclosing raceway. Open cabling may be installed within a building, aerially between buildings, or underground.

The installation of open cabling shall comply with state and local codes governing these wiring methods. The decision to use cable in raceway or open cabling shall be made by the engineer, and the criteria used in making this decision will usually be installed cost and system requirements.

Any communications system under consideration for open wiring should be analyzed from the following standpoints:

(a) Is raceway required to insure protection of conductors from impact or other physical damage? These requirements are established by the articles of ANSI/NFPA 70-1984 [3] listed in 8.1.5(2).

(b) Is raceway required to provide shielding from electromagnetic interference?

If the answer to these questions is no, then open cabling should be considered for the system. This method of cable support will often be less expensive to install and easier to maintain and modify.

---

[28] The numbers in brackets correspond to those in the references at the end of this chapter.

Open cabling should be installed so as to minimize physical stress on the cables, and maintenance will be much easier if the cables are neatly trained and supported.

Indoors, these goals may be met by supporting the cable from the building structure at regular intervals. The most common methods for cable support are nylon ties, bridle rings, and cable tray. Nylon ties are the least expensive method initially, but they become the most expensive methods if frequent cable rerouting is required. Cable tray provides the most accessible and continuous support but is initially expensive. Outdoors, open cabling will be either direct buried cable, messenger supported aerially, or supported from the building structure in the same manner as indoor runs.

Whenever open cabling is used the engineer should be familiar with the specific article of ANSI/NFPA 70-1984 [3] covering the communications system. The open cable installation methods allowed by these articles contain restrictions on installation adjacent to power and lighting conductors, vertical cable runs, penetration of fire barriers, aerial conductors exposed to lightning, etc.

(4) *Open Cabling in Plenums.* Where open cable wiring methods are selected for installation in air-handling ducts or plenums, the methods for supporting the cables will be the same as previously discussed, but the cable insulation must be specified to meet special code requirements. Such cable is frequently referred to as plenum cable.

The installation of open cabling in air-handling plenums must comply with state and local codes governing this wiring method. The choice between cable-in-raceway and open cabling should be made by the engineer, and the criteria used in making this choice will most likely be installed cost and required system reliability.

Limiting the spread of fire and products of combustion is of great concern in health care design, and the design of communications systems requires special attention to this area. Communications cabling is frequently insulated with combustible materials, and the cabling usually extends throughout the building, concealed in hollow spaces, above ceilings, and in return air plenums.

ANSI/NFPA 70-1984 [3] addresses this potentially hazardous situation in Article 300, Sections 300-21 and 300-22. Section 300-21 requires the engineer to design electrical installations in "hollow spaces, vertical shafts, and ventilation or air-handling ducts" so that the possible spread of fire or products of combustion will not be substantially increased. This section also requires approved firestops at openings in fire barriers. Section 300-22 specifically discusses four different hollow spaces where electrical installations are restricted. The following sentences paraphrase these code restrictions:

(a) *Ducts for Dust, Loose Stock, or Vapor Removal.* No wiring of any kind is allowed in these ducts.

(b) *Ducts or Plenums Used for Environmental Air.* Spaces in this category are "ducts or plenums specifically fabricated to transport environmental air." The code allows certain types of wiring in raceway to be installed in such ducts, but open wiring is not permitted.

(c) *Other Space Used for Environmental Air.* ANSI/NFPA 70-1984 [3] clarifies "other space" as "other spaces such as spaces over hung ceilings which are used for environmental air handling purposes." Again, the code allows wiring in certain types of raceway, and in addition, "other factory assembled multiconductor control or power cable which is specifically listed for the use."

(d) *Air-Handling Areas Beneath Raised Floors, Data Processing Areas.* Open wiring is allowed in such spaces under certain conditions. These conditions are listed in Article 645.

It is important to be familiar with Article 300-22, because it defines potentially hazardous "hollow spaces" in a clear way, and broadly states what wiring methods, if any, are allowed in each type of space. However, the engineer should also be familiar with the articles pertaining to the specific communication system that is to be installed, before reaching a full understanding of ANSI/NFPA 70-1984 [3] wiring requirements for such spaces (see 8.1.5.2).

Each of these articles contains the following exception to Article 300-22, referenced to the class of conductor covered by the Articles:

"...cables...listed as having adequate fire-resistant and low smoke producing characteristics shall be permitted for ducts, hollow spaces used as ducts, and plenums other than those described in Section 300-22(a)."

This exception allows the engineer to install certain listed cables as open wiring in air-handling ducts and plenums, as long as the duct does not handle dust, loose stock, or vapor. The "listed" requirement refers to inspection and testing of the cable by a listing organization.

Two other Articles in ANSI/NFPA 70-1984 [3] refer to Article 725 for code requirements governing wiring (Article 640 Sound Recording and Similar Equipment, and Article 810 Radio and Television Equipment), and therefore the cabling installations governed by these articles may also be located in air-handling plenums under the conditions of the exception to 300-22.

Cable manufacturers can supply single and multiconductor cables which are listed to be applied under one or more of the Articles in ANSI/NFPA 70-1984 [3] which contain the exception. Cables are available in either shielded or non-shielded construction.

8.1.6 Communication and Signal Closets. The following design considerations should be kept in mind while planning the location and size of communication and signal closets:

(1) *Location Requirements*

(a) Locate main closets within 50 ft of the center of the building or within 50 ft of the center of the area to be served. Locate satellite closets near the center of the area they serve. Satellite closets will be fed from the main closets.

(b) Locate the closets such that they do not inhibit future renovations. Suitable locations include corridor walls or the core area of the building.

(c) Locate the closets so that mechanical ducts or pipes are not above or below the space.

(d) Locate the closets in a "stacked" arrangement.

(e) Locate the closets such that each floor has a separate communications closet and electrical power closet.

(2) *Space Requirements*

(a) Allow sufficient space to accommodate all communication equipment, keeping in mind any plans for future expansion.

(b) Allow sufficient space to conform with all codes for minimum clearances.

(c) Use, as a general guideline for communication panels, the following dimensions: 18 in wide by 30 in high by 6 in deep for a typical one-door communications cabinet needed for each manual nurse call system (serving 60 stations), 48 in wide by 36 in high by 6 in deep for a typical two-door communications cabinet, or 24 in wide by 36 in high by 6 in deep for each of two typical one-door communications cabinets needed for each microprocessor-based nurse call system (serving 80 stations).

8.1.7 Equipment Spaces

(1) *Main Equipment Spaces.* These spaces should be located where space is less valuable to the function of the facility and as close as possible to the center of the facility to minimize cable plant costs.

Give the room design careful consideration. The layout process is a function of the space available. The following items should be considered:

(a) *Lighting.* Provide 50 fc task illumination at maintenance locations. Provide controls to decrease light levels over diagnostic CRT (Cathode Ray Tube) screens.

(b) *Water Leaks.* Avoid this potential problem by ensuring pipes do not enter the space except as required for fire extinguishing systems and water-cooled air conditioning units.

(c) *Raised Floor.* If required, 12 to 18 in is recommended.

(d) *Floor Finish.* Provide a dust-free finish to minimize equipment malfunctions. If the floor is concrete ensure it is sealed.

(e) *Ventilation.* Provide adequate ventilation. Most equipment is a heat source and will malfunction above certain limits.

(f) *Room Finish.* Avoid spray-on fireproofing of any exposed structure to minimize equipment malfunctions.

8.1.8 Power Supply

(1) *General.* All electrical communications and signaling systems require at least one connection to the building power distribution system to obtain operating power. The manner in which this connection is made in health care facilities is governed by code requirements and good design practice. The goal of these requirements and practices is to insure the reliability of communications and signaling systems essential to patient safety. The codes directly applicable to this area are:

(a) ANSI/NFPA 70-1984 [3]

(b) ANSI/NFPA 99-1984 [6]

(c) ANSI/NFPA 101-1985 [7]

(2) *Design Considerations—Clinics, Medical and Dental Offices, and Outpatient Facilities.* The only code requirements established for communications and signal-

ing systems in these occupancies govern the fire alarm system. Where the system is a local energy type, the ac power source should comply with ANSI/NFPA 72A-1985 [4], which requires two sources of supply and a dedicated circuit for the fire alarm system. Wiring methods must comply with Article 517-C of ANSI/NFPA 70-1984 [3], which in the case of a fire alarm system are no different than Chapters 1 through 4 of that standard.

If a building in these occupancies contains elevator controls, security, radio paging, voice paging or visual paging systems, it is good design practice to provide a second source of supply for each system.

(3) *Nursing Homes and Residential Custodial Care Facilities*

(a) Occupancies in these categories must first be examined for code applicability:

1) Are patients at any time sustained by electrical or mechanical life support devices?

2) Are patients at any time subjected to surgical procedures requiring general anesthesia?

If the answer to both of these questions is no, and if the occupancy is provided with a four hour alternate power source complying with Article 517-40 Exception of ANSI/NFPA 70-1984 [3], then the engineer must insure that lighting in communications areas and all alarm systems within the building are connected to the alternate power source.

Where the answer to either of these questions is yes, the occupancy must be provided with an essential electrical system, as described by Article 517-44 of ANSI/NFPA 70-1984 [3].

(b) In these occupancies, the life safety branch of the essential electrical system shall provide power to the following communications and signaling systems (and only these systems):

1) Fire alarm

2) Medical gas alarm

3) Communications systems used for issuing instruction during emergency conditions

(c) In addition, the following systems shall be connected to the critical branch

1) Elevator communications

2) Control systems and alarms required for operation of major apparatus

Wiring methods for connection to the essential electrical system shall comply with Chapters 1 through 4 of ANSI/NFPA 70-1984 [3], except that life safety branch wiring must be kept entirely independent of all other wiring (see Article 517-44 of ANSI/NFPA 70-1984 [3]).

It is recommended that the remaining communications and signaling systems not already mentioned be connected to the critical branch.

(4) *Hospitals.* The code requirements for connection of ac power to hospital communications and signaling systems are as follows:

(a) Life safety branch (no other systems may be connected)

1) Fire alarm

2) Medical gas alarm

3) Communications systems used for issuing instructions during emergency conditions

(b) Critical branch

1) Telephone

2) Nurse call system

3) Nurse assist system

4) Code blue system

(c) Equipment branch

1) Control systems and alarms required for safe operation of major apparatus

2) Controls for compressed air systems serving medical and surgical functions

3) Elevator controls and communications for selected elevators (see Article 517-64 of ANSI/NFPA 70-1984 [3])

Under both the critical branch and equipment branch headings, the code will allow connection of equipment necessary for effective hospital operation. It is recommended that all communications and signaling systems not already mentioned be connected to the critical branch.

Article 517-60(b)(1) and 60(b)(3) require that both the life safety and critical branch wiring be kept entirely independent of other wiring and each other. Equipment branch wiring may be installed with nonessential (normal) power wiring. All provisions of Chapters 1 through 4 of ANSI/NFPA 70-1984 [3] apply to wiring methods in hospitals, with the exception that life safety and critical branch wiring shall be installed in metallic raceway.

8.1.9 Computer and Combination Systems. Microcomputer prices are dropping steadily. This fact, coupled with increasing knowledge and sensitivity in the development and utilization of the required software, promises cost-effective, "user friendly" solutions to communications problems.

The primary difference between the microcomputer systems and all others centers around the functional flexibility and adaptability of the system as controlled by the stored program data processor. Functions; instructions; user terminology, nomenclature and vocabulary; display formats; message content and many other variables can be customized for each installation. State-of-the-art systems allow most of this flexibility to be in the hands of the user. Capable and responsible suppliers can provide extensive in-service training in system operation, set-up, modification and testing.

Microcomputers allow many systems to be combined, with such functions as bed status, dietary programs, automatic paging terminals, patient and staff directories, etc. Although this combination will work, the overall complexity of the resulting system may render it unusable. It may be prudent to purchase separate stand-alone systems so that the user may depend upon several systems (and operators) in a critical emergency. Also, beware of the mainframe information supplier who may offer you an add-on program for the staff register or other supplementary functions. These are highly specialized areas that may be best handled by noncomputer staff members.

8.1.10 Future Outlook. In the longer view, there is no question that the individual communications functions of present-day systems will in the future be accomplished by a single integrated system. The technology of digital computers and broadband cable links provides the opportunity for this integration, and the pressure of health care costs and advanced medical technology provides the incentive.

The engineer should be aware of direction and intensity of this trend, because the design of current health care installations should incorporate the greatest possible compatibility with future systems. This capability should be based on a recognition of the physical and electrical basis for the integrated system of the future. The cable plant will no longer consist of many different types of cables and outlets, but rather one or two cable types with common outlets located in almost every room of the facility. The central control center will no longer contain many different system displays and inputs, but rather mainframe computers. Every user terminal will contain some sort of computer, and the quality of the electrical power supplied to these terminals will be critical. Allowing space for fiber optics, television cable and data lines at a central building location may be wise since buildings built today will still be standing when the next generation of communication systems appears. In any case, space must be allowed for system growth in all riser and distribution networks, since most facilities will experience growth, and an on-line system may be replaced with a parallel system before it is cut over. New systems may be added in existing communication network space. The space allowed will always pay for itself in future capability in communication dependent health care facilities.

The trend to centralization and integration of the communications functions will place increasing importance on the reliability of the basic system components, and therefore on the design, installation, and maintenance of those components.

8.2 Telephone Systems

8.2.1 Introduction. A telephone interconnect system is an extension of an international telephone communication network that links building telephones to telephones throughout the world. A telephone system serves telephones at stations throughout a building and consists of a cable plant and terminal board network, a switcher (often a Private Branch Exchange–PBX), service cable and connections to the telephone utility.

8.2.2 Design Criteria. Telephone communications are necessary to every health care facility for normal daily operation. Telephone systems should provide efficient and immediate contact between people in each facility and the community it serves. A major design consideration is the level of service that the institution wishes to provide patients. For example, some will choose to resell WATS service to them. This requires more sophisticated billing equipment.

8.2.3 System Types and Selection

(1) *Key Telephone Systems.* Small installations of up to 50 telephones may be

handled using key telephone sets. Large key systems are available but PBX systems become competitive for installations of over 20 telephones and offer advantages for all systems.

A key telephone system utilizes telephone instruments with pushbuttons, each of which may choose access to outgoing or intercom lines. Technically, the switcher in a key system is included in each of the instruments. Several features available with key systems are:

(a) *Telephonic Intercom.* One or more intercom lines may be used as an interoffice system.

(b) *Call Annunciator.* A tone burst, light or both announce waiting calls when a pushbutton at the attendant's console is pushed or an intercom code is dialed.

(c) *Station Ringing.* Station ringing may be provided at selected stations.

(d) *Hold.* Calls may be put on hold.

(e) *Voice Paging.* Any station may initialize paging at a public address system.

(f) *Radio Paging.* Any station may initialize radio paging through a dial interconnected radio paging system.

(g) *Conference.* Conference calls may be made from one station.

Key telephone systems may include several simultaneous talking paths; however, each link (line out, tie line or intercom line) requires a dedicated button at each phone. Thus, large key systems are cumbersome.

(2) *Private Branch Exchange Systems.* PBX systems have historically been available as manual, electromechanical, or electronic devices. Current technology favors an automatic system generally known as an EPABX (Electronic Private Automatic Branch Exchange). An EPABX will feature everything that a key system features. It may also include the following features:

(a) Direct inward dialing to preselected stations. This allows persons outside the facility to reach any or all telephones inside the facility without intervention of the facility operator.

(b) Direct outward dialing subject to restrictions applied on a station-by-station basis.

(c) Call transfer from station to station without operator assistance.

(d) Auto redial feature which provides for automatic call-back when station called is no longer busy.

(e) Abbreviated dialing of frequently called numbers including short codes for dialing special system connections (e.g., public address paging, radio paging, dictation systems, etc).

(f) Do-not-disturb feature that prevents incoming calls from ringing the station.

(g) Call-forwarding (automatic) to transfer received calls to other stations.

(h) Station hunting (automatic) to an alternate telephone if the called number is busy.

(i) Record keeping and printout for management or billing purposes of long distance and local calls outside the facility.

(j) Automatic route selection of outgoing calls via WATS, foreign exchange, long distance and alternate facilities.

(k) Tandem switching (automatic rerouting of calls from one PBX system to another PBX system) to control privately owned transmission lines and maintain central cost-accounting in large building complexes.

Current EPABX systems consist of a centralized electronic switcher with a microprocessor-based control unit. The microprocessor architecture is similar to current data processing systems and will usually include memory, memory backup, programming and printout facilities. The computing power of the microprocessor and its software capabilities allow for complete system flexibility for the features listed above.

(3) *System Supplier.* Historically, the telephone companies owned and operated telephone systems throughout the business world including those in health care facilities. Currently, many manufacturers are providing telephone systems of all sizes for both lease and sale. The engineer may become involved in choosing or specifying a telephone system, and the issues discussed in 8.2.3(4) , (5), (6), and (7) should be analyzed.

(4) *Economic Analysis.* Communication costs are a substantial portion of every health care facility budget. Telephone system prices, trunk charges, and maintenance and operator costs all bear on communication costs. Features of modern systems are designed to minimize user costs. Both direct cost savings (for example, least cost call routing) and indirect cost savings (for example, reduced calling time by automatic call-back) may be substantial in any facility. Identification of those features that will minimize time and expense to the user is the engineer's goal. Often, selection of a sophisticated system, with a greater initial cost, results in the least long-term cost to the user.

(5) *Capacity.* System cost increases with increased system capacity and it is not appropriate to pay for capacity that will not be used in the future, so system selection should include an analysis of immediate and future needs.

The basic capacity of a PBX system is described using several parameters. The number of station lines corresponds to the stations required to serve the facility. Attendant consoles are counted separately from other stations. The number of trunks must support the volume of calls to and from the outside world, whether local, long distance or other. Services like public address paging, radio paging, and dictation have specialized interfaces to the system. The number of simultaneous communication paths determines how many telephones and data terminals may use the system at the same time. This number is usually less than 35% of the number of stations.

The growth capacity is the single most important factor in choosing a telephone system. It has three components.

(a) The number of stations working on the system at cutover (initiation of service).

(b) The number of stations which can be added by plugging in printed circuit boards without adding expansion cabinets. This is normally 15% or more of the number of stations at cutover.

(c) The maximum number of stations which can be installed on the system. This should cover growth for the expected useful life of the system (7 to 10 years).

(6) *Features.* The features needed for an installation vary and may include those listed in 8.2.3(1) and 8.2.3(2). The system features listed herein are not exhaustive, but represent those most useful in any installation. Each feature serves to aid the user and is recommended for all systems specified. Other features may be included. The engineer should consider both the present and future needs of an installation when specifying system features (for example, a facility may require billing records 5 years after the system is installed).

(7) *Software.* EPABX system flexibility is the result of software engineering. The ease with which a software system is changed, especially in a growing facility, is the measure of its usefulness. Many systems are equipped with user interfaces to allow changes to all station parameters and addition of stations. The engineer should specify those control elements needed for changes.

Software changes, though they are the basis for system flexibility, require storage elsewhere than volatile semiconductor memory. Three types of memory are available for software storage in EPABX systems. Recorded magnetic material, on tape or disc, is readily changed and easily stored, but is subject to dirt and wear because these devices are electromechanical in nature. Storage in devices known as EPROM (erasable programmable read only memory) or PROM (programmable read only memory), which are solid-state devices, avoid the physical problems of magnetic material. EPROM and PROM devices require special equipment, not normally part of EPABX electronics, to initialize their circuits; therefore, on-site changes to an EPABX system are more difficult with these devices. Magnetic core memories, the product of early computer technology, serve to keep permanent records without moving parts, but they consume a lot of power, are larger than other solid-state devices and are expensive.

The engineer may write a performance specification or explore the particular advantages of each memory system and specify one system, but most users do not "see" these differences. Typically, the problems of each type of system have been resolved by manufacturers so the system reliability is high in each case.

(8) *Speed.* Generally, all microprocessor-controlled EPABX systems are very fast, so that where system capacity is sufficient the user never notices a delay.

(9) *Voice Quality.* The voice quality of most EPABX systems on the market exceeds industry standards for frequency response. However, the maximum data rate will vary between systems. Special signal modulation, such as EKG transmission, may also vary. Exploration by the engineer should be done where special signals are required.

(10) *Reliability.* Many electronic telephone systems, especially those based on microprocessors, feature redundant circuits. Internal data is copied and checked by the software systems, and microprocessor hardware and power supply circuitry are duplicated. Battery backup systems may be integral to telephone switchers to add reliability to the required emergency source and to prevent momentary loss of communications during emergency switchover. Duplications

increase a system's price but must be considered for reliability needed in health care facilities.

8.2.4 Design Considerations

(1) *Installation.* The electronics and wiring of a telephone communication system requires space in each facility. The engineer must locate, size and equip each room, closet and raceway network required by the system.

(2) *Power.* Telephone equipment cabinets are generally fed individually with 20 or 30 A branch circuits. Attendant consoles may require a 20 A circuit at the attendant station. Disconnects may be required in the equipment room. Some systems are fed at one point so information from the system supplier is required for each installation.

(3) *Equipment rooms.* Required room dimensions vary over a wide range with system sizes and should be investigated by the engineer. The equipment room usually contains the switcher electronics and the main terminal board (battery backup equipment should be located elsewhere). A ground wire bonded to the building ground is required. The floor structure must be capable of supporting the telephone equipment cabinets. The room may require air conditioning (for cooling) and substantial ventilation (for battery gases), so the engineer must verify HVAC requirements of the equipment to be furnished. The door should be lockable for security. The equipment room should be centrally located to reduce cabling expenses in the facility. No piping or sprinkler heads should be located in the room and the floor should be above flood level.

(4) *Apparatus Closets.* When relay equipment is furnished for department key sets or when additional equipment is required outside the equipment room, it is located in apparatus closets. Apparatus closets should be lined with ¾ in thick fire-resistant plywood. Lighting, receptacles on a separate branch circuit and a ground wire bonded to the building ground are required. A walk-in closet should be at least 3 ft wide (4 ft for some installations). A shallow closet may be between 1½ and 2½ ft deep and should be provided with full width doors without center posts.

(5) *Satellite Closets.* Satellite closets are equipped like apparatus closets except they may not require receptacles. They will contain terminal boards and should be located near the center of the area they serve.

(6) *Cable Plant.* Cable risers may be contained in raceways or sleeves in smaller facilities. In larger facilities, the bulk of cable riser may require slots or riser shafts between floors. When practical, terminal rooms along a system riser should be aligned above one another. When this is not possible, raceway should be provided. Slots, shafts, and, to a lesser extent, sleeves require special attention for fire prevention. Policies of the telephone company and local fire codes determine the installation requirements for the cable riser.

Station cabling, between satellite closets and station instruments, may be exposed; exposed above accessible ceilings; enclosed in conduit, underfloor raceway or a combination of cable tray and conduit; or distributed below the floor slab via poke-thru devices. Underfloor raceway systems are highly flexible but are expensive in most installations. Poke-thru devices provide both low initial cost and system flexibility but changes require disturbances to two floors and structure problems may result from floor drilling. Both underfloor raceway systems and poke-thru devices are best suited to the needs of the open office layout. Health care facilities are usually served by a combination of cable tray and conduit located in the ceiling and walls of the floor served. Checking the national and local codes is required.

8.2.5 Telephone Company Facility Requirements. Many existing facilities, small new facilities and departmental areas in large facilities are served by key systems that are installed by the telephone company. The following are typical requirements for such systems. It is noted that these may be used for preliminary planning but that requirements of each system supplier may vary and that telephone company requirements vary across the country.

(a) Satellite closets used for terminating station cables and distribution cables require approximately 2 linear ft of wall space for each 2000 sq ft of floor area served. A satellite closet serves up to 6000 sq ft of floor space.

(b) Apparatus closets used for terminating cables and for key system equipment may require 10 ft of wall for 5000 sq ft, 14 ft of wall for 10 000 sq ft and 28 ft of wall for 20 000 sq ft of served area.

(c) Main Terminal Room or Equipment Rooms. The main equipment room should be planned with the help of the telephone company building industry consultant or system supplier or both.

(d) Station Cable Raceway. Raceway for key set cable shall be sized per ANSI/NFPA 70-1984 [3] and telephone company requirements. The cable size will vary with the key set size.

(e) Distribution and Riser Raceway. A typical guide for conduit or sleeve sizing follows:

Total Floor Area Served (sq ft)	Number of 4 in Raceways
below 50 000	2
to 100 000	3
to 200 000	4
to 400 000	6
above 400 000	add 1 for each 100 000 sq ft

(f) Service Entrance Raceway. The raceway cross section required depends on the number of utility lines required by an installation. For large buildings, one 4 in raceway should be installed for each 150 000 sq ft of floor space with two raceways minimum. The serving utility should be contacted to verify both minimum service entrance size and location.

8.2.6 EPABX Installations. EPABX systems are smaller than key systems and are wired to station instruments with two or three pair communication cable. Therefore, they require less space, less terminal backboard area and smaller raceway than key systems. If a system is specified before the facility is built, then provisions for that system may be trimmed to fit. When the telephone system is bid, space should be allotted for the largest system allowed by the specifications.

8.3 Intercom

8.3.1 Introduction. Intercom systems provide fast, efficient, internal verbal communication within the health care facility. In addition, loud-speaking intercom systems can provide voice paging capabilities.

8.3.2 Design Criteria

(1) *General.* Statistical investigations made by objective communication consultants have shown that 70% of communication in health care facilities is internal. Other studies have indicated that a loud-speaking internal call via an intercom system takes an average of 30 seconds to complete, whereas an intercom call via a telephone takes 3 minutes. The internal-external communication ratio may deviate from facility to facility, but even if the ratio in a specific facility should be much lower than the average, the need for a separate loud-speaking system for internal communication is justified by two reasons.

First, using the telephone for internal calls will block external calls, even though voice lines may be available, since a number of telephones will always be busy on internal calls. Internal consultation on a telephone during an external call is impractical or even impossible, and creates a blocking situation.

Second, using a separate loud-speaking intercom system will speed up and improve internal communication. People are short and precise when others may overhear what is being said. The quick and simple operation of an intercom system stimulates frequent use.

In summary, the installation of a loud-speaking intercom system can improve the overall efficiency of a health care facility. It can also provide a backup internal communications system in case of failure of the basic telephone system.

(2) *System Selection.* There are a number of factors that affect the type and size of an intercom system, including the facility's size, the traffic capacity required and whether the system will be localized by department or one large hospital-wide intercom system with stations located throughout the facility.

(3) *Local Intercom Systems.* Small localized intercom systems can provide paging and hands-free answer-back voice communications within each department. Local intercom systems are especially suited to areas where there is a central control point for the department, such as a reception desk. For example, in a radiology department a master intercom station could be located at the reception desk with staff stations located in each X-ray room. The master station can call each staff station, and each staff station could call the master station, but staff stations could not call each other.

Local intercom systems are usually installed in radiology departments, laundry, dietary offices, loading docks, surgery suites, physical therapy and other areas required by the facility. In some cases an audio-visual nurse call system can provide intercom capabilities within a department and both nurse call and intercom requirements can be provided by one system. See 8.4.

(4) *Hospital-Wide All-Master Intercom Systems.* Depending on the facility's communications requirements there may be several situations in which one inter-

com station has to be able to call several others located throughout the facility. A standard master-staff intercom system cannot easily satisfy this multiple-station calling requirement and an all-master intercom system should be installed. In this type of system each station is a master station with the capability of calling any other station in the system and conversing hands-free at both stations. If the facility has a number of localized intercom requirements with branches to other departments, it may become more advantageous to install one large intercom system to serve both localized and facility-wide intercom requirements.

8.3.3 System Types and Selection

(1) *Local Intercom Systems.* Local intercom systems usually consist of one central master station with several staff stations located throughout the department. Ceiling speakers can also be installed to provide local paging.

(2) *All-Master Intercom Systems.* These types of systems can be divided into two separate groups: hardwired systems and microprocessor-controlled systems. Hardwired systems operate like local intercom systems with the exception that there are more master stations on the system with the capability of each master station being able to call more than one location.

Microprocessor-controlled systems use a common cabling scheme that reduces the wiring requirements and costs over a hardwired system. Some of the system options available from most system suppliers include:

(a) *Restricted Access:* Any station can be restricted to receive calls, operate a limited number of functions, and call only certain other stations.

(b) *Automatic Queuing:* Busy lines. If all lines should be busy, automatic queuing (searching for free line) is implemented. This feature allows high traffic seen in relation to the number of communication lines available.

(c) *Camp-On-Busy:* Called station engaged. If the called station is engaged, the caller receives engaged signal, and the call enters automatically camp-on-busy for up to 60 s. As soon as the called station becomes free, the call is automatically set up with normal call tone.

(d) *Automatic Recall:* Called station engaged—low priority call. During camp-on-busy, the caller can request an automatic recall to free his own station for other calls while waiting for the first station to become free. The first call is then established as soon as both stations are free.

(e) *Break-in:* Called station engaged—high priority call. During camp-on-busy the caller (A) can break in on the engaged station (B) if the call is urgent. Both parties in conversation (B and C) will be warned by call tone, and overhear the break-in call. (A) can withdraw at any time, leaving (B) and (C) in conversation. (C) can also be asked to withdraw, leaving (A) and (B) in conversation.

(f) *Break-in Immunity:* Any station can be modified to have break-in immunity. Such stations can then not be broken in on. The break-in function can, of course, be completely removed from the total system, if required.

(g) *Automatic Transfer:* Number transfer. Any station number can be transferred to any other station. The instruction can be given from any station in the system. More numbers can be transferred to the same station. This feature can be used for two main purposes:

1) *Secretarial Transfer.* Persons who do not wish to be disturbed for a period, or who are not present, can ask a colleague or a secretary to take their calls. During a meeting a secretary can take calls for all members.

2) *Follow-me.* Persons who visit other offices can route their calls to any present location. During a meeting all members can route their calls to the meeting room.

(h) *Conference:* Additional stations can be interconnected.

(i) *Group Call:* Announcement to a group of stations. A predetermined group of stations can be called from any station in the system, for giving a one-way message. A group call has priority over other calls. Several groups can be formed in the system (standard up to 10), and each station can be a member of up to 3 different groups. The groups are formed by programming in the stations.

(j) *All Call:* Group call to all stations—emergency call. All stations in the system can be called for giving a short one-way message. This function can be used for paging people. However, this is not advisable, especially in larger systems. Why disturb the complete organization to get hold of one individual? "All call" should only be used for emergency calls.

(k) *Call-Forwarding:* Backup station. This function allows one station to act as backup for one or more other stations.

(l) *Short Call:* Single-digit call. A predetermined station can be called by pressing one button, for example, the reception desk.

(m) *Public Address Access:* Announcements via P.A. system. The system can be linked to a public address system for giving one-way messages.

(n) *Selective Paging Access:* Paging a person on the move. The system can be linked to a selective paging system for paging persons via intercom. A person paged can answer from any intercom station in the system.

(o) *Other Functions:* Tailor-made functions. For special projects and larger systems any function can be defined in accordance with specified requirements. Standard features cover most needs, and are, of course, less expensive to incorporate.

8.3.4 Design Considerations. After the engineer has talked with the facility staff and has determined the type and size of the intercom system that best satisfies the facility's needs, he or she can begin to lay out the final system.

(1) *Station Locations.* Master and staff intercom stations can be either desk or wall mounted. It is recommended that these stations be wall mounted whenever possible to provide as much desk space as possible. Avoid locating stations in adjacent rooms in the same stud cavity to prevent potential feedback problems. Handsets may be required in high ambient noise areas. Exterior stations should be of weatherproof construction.

(2) *Station Grouping in an All-Master Intercom System.* When stations are combined together into different paging groups, the groups should be determined during design so that the system supplier properly installs the system. For example, the intercom stations in the surgery department should be in a separate paging group from those in the laboratory to prevent laboratory intercom paging calls from disturbing the surgery staff.

(3) *Station Identification.* In an all-master intercom system with stations installed throughout the facility a master index of station extension numbers will be required. One idea is to have the intercom station number the same as the telephone extension number in the same room. This would save printing two separate in-house telephone and intercom directories.

(4) *Central Controller.* Central controller should be installed in a communications closet. See requirements for telephone system. If the intercom system will be used to provide communications during an emergency, it should be connected to emergency power.

8.4 Nurse Call Systems

8.4.1 Introduction. A nurse call system primarily provides a means for a patient to signal the nursing staff that he or she requires assistance. In addition to patient-nurse communication, a nurse call system can also serve to provide other signaling requirements such as signaling other departments that a nurse or other staff member needs additional assistance.

8.4.2 Design Criteria

(1) *General.* Nurse call systems are required in hospitals, nursing homes and psychiatric care facilities by health facility regulations. Usually these requirements are minimum standards and the facility's own communications requirements will dictate the type of system installed and the location of the different components to integrate the nurse call system throughout the facility. Nurse call systems are not required in medical and dental offices, medical clinics and residential care facilities (depending on local code requirements); however, some type of signaling system may be desired by the staff for more efficient operation. Also depending on local code requirement, the system may be required to be listed by Underwriter's Laboratories, Inc, under ANSI/UL 1069-1982 [9]. Nurse call systems are primarily divided into two basic groups: visual systems which utilize light and tone signals for annunciation of calls, and audio-visual systems which provide voice communication in addition to the light and tone signals. By utilizing the right components, an audio-visual system can satisfy the interdepartment intercom requirements and provide voice communications with other areas in the facility.

(2) *Programming.* Before an engineer completes the design, he should confer with the staff members to find out how the particular department will operate and determine their specific communications requirements. In order to effectively confer with the staff, the engineer should have a basic understanding of the different systems available and their limitations so he can help the facility choose the type of system that best meets the requirements. For example, one of the requirements in a radiology department may be to have a signal system from the dressing room to the X-ray room to indicate when the patient is ready for examination. A visual nurse call system would satisfy this requirement; however, if voice communication for each X-ray room to a central reception desk is also requested, both functions could be served by an audio-visual nurse call system. If each X-ray room needs to be able to call other rooms besides a central

location, a separate intercom system and a visual nurse call system would have to be installed because audio-visual nurse call systems are limited in the number of other locations each staff station can call.

Some of the basic questions that an engineer needs to answer before designing a nurse call system include:

(a) How large is the department? Will a visual nurse call system satisfy the requirements or would an audio-visual system be a better choice?

(b) Which rooms or areas need to communicate with each other? Can this communication be accomplished by telephone or would a loud-speaking intercom system be a better choice? Do rooms in the department need to be able to talk with each other or just to a central location? The intercom capabilities of an audio-visual nurse call system can satisfy the latter requirement provided each room does not need to talk with more than one master station.

(c) In a hospital, are there any swing rooms that have to be connected to different nurses stations at different times depending on the bed requirements in each nursing unit?

(d) In a hospital or psychiatric care facility, which areas require nurse assist or other emergency calls and where should these calls be annunciated?

(e) In a hospital, are other nursing stations to provide backup help in an emergency or when the primary nurses station is left unattended?

8.4.3 Visual Systems. A visual nurse call system provides audible signaling and visual annunciation of patient calls. Two call priority levels are possible: normal calls and emergency calls from toilet emergency stations. Visual systems are used primarily in hospital ancillary areas such as physical therapy, radiology, hydrotherapy and emergency departments or other treatment areas where patients may be left unattended, and voice communication to a central location is not required by the staff. A visual nurse call system can be utilized on small nursing units where a more expensive audio-visual system with intercom capabilities does not provide a distinct advantage. Visual nurse call systems can also be utilized in nursing homes and residential care facilities.

(1) *Patient Bed Station.* A patient can originate a call on the system by depressing a call button on a cord. These calls will continuously illuminate the white section of the corridor dome light and white section of any associated zone dome lights, illuminate the patient call light and sound a tone at all duty stations and illuminate the patient room number, bed number and sound a tone at the master station annunciator. The call can only be cancelled at the originating station.

(2) *Toilet Emergency Station.* A patient can originate an emergency call on the system by pulling a cord. Originating a call from these stations will flash the white section of the corridor dome light, flash the white section of any associated zone dome lights, flash the patient call light and sound a fast tone at all duty stations and flash the patient's room number and sound a fast tone at the master station annunciator.

(3) *Duty Station.* These stations provide audible and visual annunciation of calls placed from any other station in the system, but do not indicate the room

number originating the call. Duty stations are usually located in clean and soiled utility rooms, medication rooms, and other areas in which staff members are likely to be when not at the nurses station.

(4) *Master Station Annunciator.* When a call is placed on the system, the room number and bed number are flashed or steadily illuminated depending on the priority level of the call. A call tone is also generated with a distinct difference in signal rates between normal and emergency calls.

8.4.4 Audio-Visual Systems. An audio-visual nurse call system provides audible signaling, visual annunciation, patient-to-staff communication, staff-to-staff communication and intercommunication between master station annunciators. An audio-visual system has some distinct advantages over a visual nurse call system. Minor patient requests such as "What time is it?", can be answered much more quickly and it is more reassuring for a patient to be able to talk with the nurse at the nurses station.

Audio-visual systems can be divided into two basic groups, basic hardwired systems and microprocessor-controlled systems. Microprocessor-controlled systems can provide more levels of calls on the system, can be programmed for swing room and call transfer and have reduced cabling requirements over hardwired systems. The overall size of the system, number of swing rooms and number of master station annunciators required will determine which system is the most cost-effective to meet the hospital's needs.

(1) *Patient Bed Station.* A patient can originate a call on the system by depressing a button on a pillow speaker or cordset. Most systems have a call selector switch that determines the type of call that is placed on the system as follows:

Normal calls illuminate the white section of the corridor dome light and white section of any associated zone dome lights, illuminate the patient call light and sound a tone at all duty stations and illuminate the patient's room number, bed number and sound a slow tone at the master station annunciator. These calls are cancelled after they are answered at the master station.

Personal attention calls perform the same functions as a normal call except they are only cancellable at the patient bed station.

Priority calls flash the corridor dome lights and associated zone dome lights, flash the patient call light and sound a fast tone at all duty stations and flash the patient's room number, bed number and sound a fast tone at the master station annunciator. Priority calls can only be cancelled at the patient bed station. Voice communication is established upon answer of the call at the master station.

As an option, a privacy switch can be provided in the patient bed station that will prevent conversation within the room from being monitored from the master station. This switch does not interfere with the placement of a call to the master station and the master station can still speak to the bed station. Unless this option is desired by the nursing staff, it is not recommended that it be included because it can create some confusion for the patient if it is inadvertently activated.

(2) *Patient Station Cordset.* Several different interchangeable cordsets are available for the patient's use to place a call. The pillow speaker is the most

widely used device when television sets are located in each patient room because it also contains controls to turn a TV set off and on, change the TV channel and regulate the TV volume. Switches can also be provided to control the patient reading light via a low voltage relay, and control radio entertainment. If patient TV's are not provided, a standard call button and cordset should be used. A few pressure pad cordsets should be specified for those patients who are unable to use a pushbutton. Cordsets designed for use in oxygen atmospheres are also available.

(3) *Toilet Emergency Station.* These stations are annunciated the same as priority calls from a patient bed station. Voice communication to the master station is not included. These stations are equipped with a pull cord and are located in toilet, shower, tub and hydrotherapy areas.

(4) *Staff Station.* Calling facilities and two-way voice communication to the master station can be accomplished from the staff station. These calls are annunciated at the master station the same as normal calls from a patient station. Staff stations can be located in offices, staff lounges and other areas that need intercom capabilities to the nurses station.

(5) *Duty Stations.* Calling facilities and two-way voice communication can be accomplished from a duty station. Calls are annunciated at the master station in the same manner as calls from a staff station. In addition the duty station provides audible and visual annunciation of calls placed from any other station in the system. Normal and emergency calls are distinguished by a distinct difference in signal rate. Duty stations should be located in clean and soiled utility rooms, medication rooms and other areas staff members are likely to be when not at the nurses station.

(6) *Master Station Annunciator.* The master station annunciator can be used to call or receive calls from patient stations, staff stations, duty stations, or other master stations. Toilet emergency station calls are also annunciated at the master station.

When a call is placed on the system the room number and bed number are flashed or steadily illuminated depending on the priority level of the call. Answering a call is accomplished by depressing the station button on the master station annunciator corresponding to the calling station. Two-way voice communication can then take place via the speaker microphone utilizing the talk-listen bar or via a handset. If calls are not answered immediately the tone signal is repeated unless the nurse is in the process of answering other calls.

If the patient stations are equipped with a call selector switch, switches should also be provided in the master station to indicate by bed which stations have the call selector switches placed in the "Patient Priority" and "Personal Attention" positions.

Zone monitoring and paging of several stations simultaneously can be accomplished from the master station. When the system is installed patient stations should be grouped separately from staff and duty stations on the annunciator key bank so staff areas can be paged separately from patient areas. Master stations in other areas can be connected together to provide intercom capabilities between them.

(7) *Nurse Assist Button.* These wall mounted pushbutton stations should be located in ICU (intensive care units), CCU (coronary care units), surgeries, recovery rooms and other hospital areas in which the staff may need to request additional assistance in a hurry. Depending on local codes and the facility's requirements, it is recommended that this level of call be annunciated differently than a standard patient or toilet emergency station call. The installation of a separate power supply and annunciators to achieve this differentiation may be required. Nurse assist calls shall be annunciated at the unit's nurses station and optionally at adjacent nurses stations from which additional help can be obtained.

(8) *Code Blue Button.* See 8.5 for design criteria. These stations may be part of the nurse call system to initiate the highest level of call within the hospital to signal the resuscitation team that a patient is in cardiac or respiratory arrest.

(9) *Dome Lights.* Dome lights are located in the corridor above the patient room door or above the patient's bed in recovery and holding areas. These lights indicate which room, or bed, initiated the call and the level of call. Dome lights can be multi-sectioned (maximum of four) with different colors to indicate different types of calls from each room. For example, a four-section, four-color dome light can indicate the following calls from each room:

Call Type	Priority Level	Dome Light Indication
Code Blue	1	Flashing Red
Nurse Assist	2	Flashing White, Steady Green
Toilet Emergency	3	Flashing White
Patient—Priority	3	Flashing White
Patient—Personal Attention	4	Steady White
Patient—Normal Call	4	Steady White
Nurse Service		Flashing Green
Aide Service		Flashing Amber

These recommended colors vary depending on the scheme previously established in the facility. The same dome light color scheme should be utilized throughout the facility.

(10) *Zone Dome Lights.* Similar in appearance to dome lights these devices should be located at corridor intersections to indicate the areas or zone that the call is coming from.

(11) *Nurse Call System Options.* There are several optional features that are available on most nurse call systems. The options that are included will depend on how the hospital intends to operate and staff the nursing unit. Some of the optional features are described briefly as follows:

(12) *Nurse Service.* This feature allows the nurse at the nurses station to answer a patient's call and if the nature of the call cannot be satisfied from the nurses station, i.e., the patient requests a glass of water, then a nurse service reminder can be initiated at the master station annunciator. Depressing the

nurse service button will flash the green section of the corridor dome light and flash the green section of any associated zone dome lights. If service is not provided by the circulating nurse or other staff member, and the nurse service call not reset at the patient bed station within an adjustable time period (3 to 10 minutes) another patient call is automatically initiated. This feature allows the staff member answering calls to remain at the nurses station while the patient's needs are being satisfied by others.

(13) *Staff Locator.* This feature utilizes buttons in each patient room which are activated whenever the staff member enters the room. A switch on the master station annunciator will illuminate the room numbers in which nurses or aides are located. The nurse at the nurses station can then locate the closest staff member that can respond to a nurse call from an adjacent room and direct him/her to it. This feature provides for more efficient use of staff members; however, it may not always be desirable because it requires staff members to check in and out of each room, and patients trying to rest may be disturbed by calls from the nurses station directing staff members to respond to calls from another room.

(14) *Nurse Follower.* During night and off-peak hours the nurse at the nurses station may transfer calls to another location in which he or she intends to be. This feature allows the staff more mobility because they do not have to be at the nurses station to answer nurse calls; however, transfer of all nurse calls to a patient's room may be disturbing to the patient in that room.

(15) *Call Transfer.* In some units there may be a requirement for nurse calls to be transmitted to different nurses stations at different times. For example, there may be swing rooms that can be a part of two adjacent nursing units depending upon the number of beds required in each unit. Calls from these rooms have to be transferred from one nurses station to another on an individual room basis. Another example is when an entire group of rooms have to be transferred between two nurses stations.

Call transfer may be accomplished several different ways depending upon the sophistication of the nurse call system. A hardwired basic system requires transfer switches in each swing room or a bank of transfer relays activated by a switch at the nurses station. A microprocessor-controlled system can be programmed from the master station to assign patient rooms to a particular nurses station on an individual room basis.

8.4.5 Centralized Nurse Call System. Some hospitals or nursing homes may want to have all patient calls for the entire facility answered at a central location, either on a full-time or nighttime basis. The staff locator feature is desirable in a centralized nurse call system so the person answering calls can locate the staff members closest to the room initiating the call and direct them to the correct room. Staff members can also be directed to the calling room via a pocket paging system. See 8.7.

8.4.6 Central Processor Controlled System. The more sophisticated nurse call systems can provide information storage and retrieval capabilities which can be used for drug, dietary and other patient data. Printers can also be included with these systems to provide a hard copy printout of patient data and traffic patterns on each nursing unit which can be used to determine staffing requirements. A pocket paging system can also be integrated with the nurse call system. For example, when a patient initiates a call the nurse assigned to care for that particular patient receives a beep on his or her pocket pager plus the room and bed number of the patient calling.

8.4.7 Psychiatric Nurse Call System. The nurse call system for psychiatric patient facilities serves a different role than those installed in a general care nursing area. In a psychiatric unit the nurse call system usually serves primarily as an alarm system for staff to request additional assistance in a hurry as well as providing for standard patient calls.

(1) *Room Entrance Station.* In a basic psychiatric nurse call system, room entrance stations are located in the corridor outside each patient room. These stations contain one or more keyed switches that can be used to activate or deactivate the patient station and nurse assist station within the room. When these switches are in the off or deactivate position the patient cannot initiate nuisance calls on the system. Room entrance stations can also be used to signal the nurse at the nurses station that a staff member is about to enter the patient's room. The nurse at the nurses station can then monitor the conversation within the room and send assistance if required.

(2) *Nurse Assist.* There are systems available that were originally developed for installation in prisons that may satisfy the nurse assist requirements. These systems utilize an ultrasonic receiver in each room and the staff members carry an initiation device with them at all times. If a staff member requires help, he can initiate an alarm by actuating the initiation device. The signal is picked up by the receiver and the call is annunciated at the nurses station to indicate the room location. This type of system has some advantages over a standard psychiatric nurse call system in that staff members always carry the initiation device with them and they cannot be blocked away from the nurse assist button.

8.4.8 Medical and Dental Offices and Clinics. Variations of a visual nurse call system can be utilized in clinics and offices to provide a variety of signals. Some examples include the following:

(1) *Exam Room Status System.* Multisection colored dome lights are located above the corridor door into each exam room with corresponding switches in each room. One illuminated color may signal that the patient is ready to see the doctor. Another color may indicate the room is vacant and needs to be prepared for the next patient and/or another color may be used to signal the room has been prepared and is available for the next patient. A central annunciator may be located at the reception desk to indicate the status of each exam room.

(2) *Doctor and Dentist Offices.* Different colored lights may be used to provide rapid, discrete interoffice communication between the doctor and his or her staff. Messages will vary between offices, but some typical messages are: doctor's next patient has arrived, doctor is wanted on the telephone, doctor would like to see his assistant or laboratory technician, hygienist wants doctor to check patient.

8.4.9 Design Considerations. After the engineer has talked with the facility staff and has determined what type of nurse call system best meets the hospital's needs, he begins to lay out the final system.

(1) *Patient Bed Stations.* These stations can be mounted in the wall behind the patient bed, in a patient headwall unit, in the patient's bedside cabinet, or in some cases in the handrail of the patient's bed. The station should be located to allow the call cord to be draped to the patient bed. Locating the patient station in the bedside cabinet or bed handrail may not be the best location because this would inhibit later changing of the furniture, and the multi-pin receptacles required for portable beds and bedside cabinets with nurse call stations can be a maintenance problem.

(2) *Toilet Emergency Stations.* These stations should be positioned in such a manner so they can be activated by a patient seated on the toilet and/or by a patient who may have fallen forward on the floor. In combination toilet/shower rooms one station may be sufficient provided it meets the location requirements described above and the cord is long enough to drape into the shower to a maximum of 6 in above the floor.

(3) *Staff and Duty Stations.* Sometimes rooms such as staff lounges and utility rooms serve more than one nursing unit. If so, two or more duty or staff stations should be installed and connected to the nurse call system in each unit. Be sure each station's nursing unit is identified.

(4) *Master Station Annunciator.* These stations can either be wall mounted or desk mounted. It is recommended that visual system master stations be wall mounted to provide as much desk space as possible. Audio-visual system master stations should be desk mounted to allow the nurses answering calls some flexibility in their location. Be sure that the room numbers on the master station match the final room numbers assigned to each room by the facility.

(5) *Psychiatric Patient Stations* installed in ambulatory patient rooms must be tamperproof for the patients' safety. Call cords should not be located in patient bedrooms and tamperproof pushbuttons should be specified for toilet emergency stations in lieu of pull cords.

(6) *Central Equipment and Power Supplies.* Nurse call systems shall be connected to the critical branch of the emergency distribution system in hospitals or to other emergency power systems in other health care facilities. Be sure to coordinate the ventilation, wall space and wall depth required for these cabinets.

8.5 Code Blue Systems

8.5.1 Introduction. Code blue alarms are the highest level of emergency call in a hospital. When a cardiac arrest or other emergency occurs, the system is used to alert the person who is responsible for the delivery of the crash cart to the point of need and notify the resuscitation team as to the room or area that initiated the alarm. Different hospitals may call this alarm level something other than code blue, such as code 199, code 99, Doctor Heart, crash unit, etc.

8.5.2 Design Criteria. A code blue alarm system is required by hospital regulations. Typically, code blue buttons (or other initiation devices) are located in intensive care and coronary care patient rooms, emergency rooms, recovery rooms, labor and birthing rooms, surgery suites, and other areas required by the hospital. Annunciators should be located at the central control center so the telephone operator can announce the code blue alarm either via the public address system or by radio paging, or both. Annunciators may be desirable at adjacent nurses stations, anesthesia office, and the nurse supervisor's office. In some hospitals the staff members may want the code blue alarms from the patient's room to go to the local nurses station. If the alarm is a true code call and not a false alarm initiated by a visitor, the nurse at the nurses station can forward the alarm via the telephone or separate code blue button.

8.5.3 System Types and Selection

(1) *Nurse Call System.* A separate hardwired visual nurse call system with code blue buttons and annunciators can be installed to serve the code blue system requirements. Code blue alarms can also be incorporated into some microprocessor-controlled nurse call systems; however, there is some advantage to keeping the systems separate so one can be serviced without affecting the other.

(2) *Telephone System.* A code blue call system can be set up as a separate direct line to the central operator via the hospital telephone system. The major advantage of this type of installation is that a code blue alarm can be initiated from any telephone within the hospital. If the particular phone system is equipped with direct access paging, the code blue alarm can be directly annunciated via the public address system, thus bypassing the telephone operator. Code blue pages must have priority over all other paging calls.

(3) *Radio Paging.* Code blue alarms can be transmitted to the resuscitation team members via the radio paging system, provided the system has the capability of group paging calls together so the proper people are notified with just one call from the telephone operator.

8.5.4 Design Considerations. A code blue alarm system should always be designed with system reliability in mind. The power supply for this system must be connected to emergency power.

8.6 Paging and Voice Paging Systems

8.6.1 Introduction. The objective of the paging system is to aid in locating persons who do not have a fixed location within the facility. It generally augments the telephone system, in that it notifies persons who are not at a fixed telephone number to contact another person inside or outside the facility. In order to be effective, it should reach all the locations in the facility where these people are likely to be.

8.6.2 Design Criteria. Paging systems increase the efficiency of communications in most health care facilities. There are three types of systems:

(1) *Flashing Annunciator Paging.* This system provides a silent, visual, coded message by repeatedly lighting numbers on annunciators located throughout a facility. It is not recommended because of the excessive number of annunciators required before the coverage provided is compatible with other types of paging.

(2) *Radio Paging System.* This system transmits messages over a radio frequency channel and is preferred where cost is not an obstacle. Coded signals can be used for messages, or one-way or two-way voice transmission can be provided.

Installation costs are low, no corridor wall space is required, and there is no disturbance to other personnel. Radio paging is effective in many areas where visual or voice paging is not practical, for example, it often covers restrooms, utility and nearby outdoor areas with radio signal. However, equipment is costly and maintenance costs can be high since pocket-carried receivers are subject to damage. Radio paging can be tied into the telephone system so that staff telephones allow paging by other than the telephone operator. This system can also be tied into a doctor registering system. Refer to 8.7 for Design Criteria.

(3) *Voice Paging System.* This system uses loudspeakers to transmit voice or audible coded messages. It is recommended for all facilities. Even if a radio paging system is installed a voice paging system should be provided as a backup.

A large number of low power speakers are used to keep the sound well distributed but at a low volume. They may be used for voice signals, background music, sound masking noise, security tones, or any combination of these. The voice paging system may be connected to the building telephone, intercom or visual annunciator systems as part of an overall building communication system. Voice paging systems are required for issuing instructions during emergency conditions, code blue and instant contact of personnel. It is important that these systems are not abused causing a noisy atmosphere for staff and patients. The facility should develop a policy limiting when and why personnel are paged. Paging should not be permitted on speakers in surgery, delivery or recovery rooms. The rest of this section discusses voice paging systems.

8.6.3 Voice Paging System Design Criteria

(1) *General.* Audio components (amplifiers, equalizers, mixers, etc) are almost all solid-state, analog devices. A few audio control devices and several time delay units utilize digital logic; however, all components can be treated as building blocks for audio systems in a similar manner. Performance is not measured by broad band or hi-fi principles, but rather in terms of correct distribution and syllabic articulation of voice. It is not essential that the system reproduce the entire audible spectrum for best results, and quite often it is necessary to make compromises with performance in order to justify economics.

(2) *Priority.* Voice paging systems often feature several types of control for audio sources (microphone, tape deck, tone generator, etc). Operators generally have manual control of most sources while links from other communication systems are automatic.

In both small and large voice paging systems, the relative signal priority determines the control requirements. A background music and paging system with one paging microphone location may mute the background music when the microphone is activitated. When several paging sources or a paging source and an emergency signal source are used, a priority system should be set up to accommodate each level of importance.

The sound volume at a listener may be changed to suit varying work conditions, changing personnel, background noise, etc. Also, it may be changed with each change of source signal. In a background music and paging system, the listener may want local control of the music volume and full volume paging signals. The various volume levels should be consistent with each signal's priority.

(3) *Zoning.* In large installations, and in small installations where specific activities vary from area to area, zoning of the public address system is recommended. Each zone may require volume and local paging controls. Priority controls for both source selection and volume are designed to include zone paging and local sources. In some installations, local pages are given priority and, in others, general pages have priority, so each installation must be looked at individually.

(4) *Talk-back.* Single-zoned systems may include talk-back. Either by push-button control or by automatic means, talk-back allows the listener to respond to the operator via the public address system. Talk-back complicates the electronics of a public address system when it is employed in multi-zoned systems with several signal sources. Also, alternate means of listener response (telephone, intercom, etc) usually provide more efficient systems in large installations.

(5) *Complexity.* The simplest voice paging system may consist of one microphone, a mixer/power amplifier and several speakers in the area served. As systems become larger, alternate music sources, frequency shaping, compression and priority logic may be added to the system. In the largest of systems, the audio equipment may be located in several locations with audio and priority lines running between equipment racks.

(6) *Distribution.* In music and paging systems, there are several ways to distribute audio signals. The simplest involves one set of audio lines run to each speaker zone with background music and paging levels set at the amplifier.

When local control of music volume is desired, the audio lines may be run to a local volume control equipped with a bypass relay (priority relay). The relay coil is connected to a priority control pair to bypass the volume control for paging announcements.

(7) *Muting.* When two sources, one with priority, are available to a voice paging system, two common methods are used to accomplish the signal level changes required. First, the priority signal may be set to a higher volume than the other signal. This method is limited to circumstances where the nonpriority signal is low level so the priority signal is not too loud. Second, the initiation of the priority signal may mute the nonpriority signal either by relay contacts or solid-state devices. The same circuit may drive the priority relay at local volume controls. This is the standard method used in most public address systems.

(8) *Volume.* The required volume determines electronic component ratings and dimensions. The system should be louder than the ambient noise. Sound with a signal-to-noise ratio of 25 dB (decibels) and an appropriate frequency response and low distortion usually provides clearly audible signals. Room acoustics should be considered in every case. Small rooms with low ceilings consisting of acoustic tile are not a problem. Rooms with acoustically hard surfaces (plaster walls and ceiling, and tile floor, for example) have a high reverberation time that will contribute to poor intelligibility; however, special installations are seldom required for hospital systems.

(9) *Frequency Response.* Many paging systems, especially those using a telephone system as the audio source, do not require frequency shaping electronics

because the electronics and speaker system will present the full range of telephone or microphone frequencies to the listener. Where particular rooms present acoustical problems or where music or a natural sounding voice page is important, an equalizer may be used. See 8.17.3(7).

(10) *Compression.* Audio signal volume varies from one source to another. Paging announcers may produce a difference in voice levels greater than 20 dB depending on their voices and how they use the microphone. In some cases, variations in signal levels of 20 dB are unmanageable and, in many cases, variations of that magnitude are annoying to some listeners. Compressors may be employed to help reduce large sound level variations. They are usually located at the microphone inputs and at telephone/intercom paging interface inputs because the volume of these sources varies the greatest. Pre-recorded music sources, radio receivers, tone generators and noise generators usually produce a consistent signal level or are equipped with their own compressors (automatic gain control, etc). Where paging signals originate from trained operators, compression is not required.

(11) *Source.* A voice paging system signal is never better than its source. Pre-recorded messages, music sources and radio receivers are satisfactory sources; however, the quality of microphone sources should be considered. The quality of the microphone itself is usually satisfactory, but the location should be considered. Using the microphone very close to the mouth (several inches) helps reduce problems of room noise and reverberance. Telephone handsets and headsets with direct access to the paging system provide both efficient operator access to telephone and paging systems, and very close microphone use for noisy environments.

8.6.4 Design Considerations

(1) *Interfacing.* Telephone, intercom, and tone generating systems may be connected to the voice paging system. The priority and zoning of each system should be determined. A telephone or intercom system may utilize several lines to provide both general and zone paging.

(2) *Coverage.* Basically two types of speaker layouts are used for voice paging systems. Each room or open space may utilize either a central or a distributed speaker system. Central speaker systems are usually applicable to large spaces with high ceilings and are often used in sound reinforcement systems. See 8.17.

A distributed speaker system (typically recessed ceiling speakers) should provide even coverage of direct sound at the proper frequencies and at sufficient volume to be heard above the ambient noise. High volume distributed systems are required in noisy areas and in situations where the speaker spacing is too great (poor design). Most applications involve low level, closely spaced recessed ceiling speakers.

The best recessed ceiling speakers have a high frequency distribution angle of about 90° which requires about a two-to-one spacing-to-height ratio where the height is measured from ear height to ceiling. With ceilings at 9 ft, spacings of 9 ft center-to-center for sitting listeners and 7 ft for standing (or walking) listeners are recommended.

(3) *Equipment.* Voice paging equipment can be as small as a small file cabinet or as large as a small room. Its location is flexible but the equipment requires access and a cooled or ventilated space. Speaker wiring requires one pair of conductors for a single-zoned page only system, two pairs for a single-zoned music/page priority system, and many pairs for a multi-zoned multiple-page priority system with local volume controls. Priority logic pairs will often be 22 AWG (American Wire Gauge) and audio signal pairs will be anywhere from 20 AWG to 14 AWG depending on the speaker load and system voltage.

(4) *Installation.* Nearly all sound system components on the market today exhibit low noise, low distortion, flat frequency response and high continuous power ratings; however, the performance of sound systems is rarely limited by individual component ratings.

Solid-state audio components are manufactured for specific input and output levels, so cascading components (for example, a mixer, an equalizer and a power amplifier) require that the output level of one unit match the input level of the next unit. The mismatch of these levels will degrade the overall system signal-to-noise ratio or reduce its maximum output. Adjustment of all controls by experienced technicians, using calibrated test equipment, will result in proper component matching.

Audio signals are generally found at three levels: microphone level, line levels (for lines between various pieces of equipment) and high level (the output of the power amplifiers used to distribute audio frequency energy to the speakers). The microphone and line level signals are susceptible to pickup of hum, noise and crosstalk from higher level lines and power cables. Microphone level lines should never be run in the same raceway with other audio lines or power cables and each type of audio line should be bundled separately in each equipment rack.

When an audio system includes an equalizer, the frequency response of the system must be properly measured and corrected to match the desired response curve. Improper system response may cause a loss of speech intelligibility or make the system sound unnatural.

Proper use of a voice paging system is as important as its initial installation. Operating personnel should be instructed in the system's use by people familiar with the equipment. Often this instruction is specified as part of the system installation.

(5) *Reliability.* Backup inputs (a second microphone or a microphone as backup to a telephone system) and backup electronics (amplifiers, etc) may be included in a system where reliability is a must. See 8.1 for power connection requirements.

8.7 Radio Paging Systems

8.7.1 Introduction. Radio Paging Systems transmit messages over a radio frequency channel. This section discusses on-site and off-campus radio paging systems.

8.7.2 Design Criteria. Refer to 8.6 for a discussion of the criteria for radio paging systems. The following functional factors should be considered to define radio paging system performance: number of active radio pager users, average system call rate, desired grade of service, average input waiting time, and maximum message storage time. The following equipment factors should be considered when designing radio paging systems:

(1) *System Input or Encoder*. On-site and off-campus paging systems are often interfaced with one or more of the telephone, intercom, staff register, nurse call and code blue systems. Telephone interconnected systems provide almost unlimited access to the paging system. With voice messages, it is probable that voice message storage equipment may be required to increase system voice traffic capacity. Display message systems may also use message storage. This and high speed message transmission can provide high system pager capacity. It is recommended that the engineer read reference [16] that deals with this difference. Interconnection with staff in/out register systems, intercom systems and nurse call systems is unique to each supplier and should be reviewed in detail with their representatives.

An encoder or paging terminal may be any kind of device, manual or automatic, from which a radio paging message may be originated. The following is a typical list of such devices:

(a) *Manual desktop (or flush mounted) keyboard console*. (Frequently located at the telephone operator position, although parallel units may be located at several sites throughout the facility.)

(b) *Telephones*. May be dial or touchpad type and either dedicated or part of the facility's telephone system.

(c) *Intercom stations*.

(d) *Automatic alarm stations*. (Any contact opening or closing device may be utilized to initiate an emergency or routine radio page message. This might include such functions as elevator stoppage, security door openings, boiler temperature limit switches, chiller failure, oxygen low pressure, etc.)

(2) *System Type*. On-site pagers, in the SERS (Special Emergency Radio Service), like the systems that control them, come in many different types. Pagers may be classified by type of modulation (AM or FM); frequency band (VHF lowband, VHF highband, UHF and 900 MHz); type of encoding (two-tone or five-tone analog and digital); and type of message capability (tone, voice, LED's, LCD's, digital display and alphanumeric display).

Generally speaking, there has been a gradual shift from inductive loop paging to AM and then to FM paging technology. Inductive loop paging is a low-frequency radio technique, and its employment has largely been discontinued in favor of AM and FM radio equipment for reasons of better coverage both within and throughout a hospital complex of buildings. The recent development of display pocket pager technology has added to the tone-only and tone-and-voice types of paging systems. The availability of this new technology and additional frequencies in the 900 MHz band increase the variety of systems available for on-site and off-campus radio paging system implementation.

(3) *Frequency Selection*. For on-site systems, the frequency selected is largely a matter of determining which available frequency is the least crowded, although in an on-site mode, carefully designed systems on the same frequency can operate

without any interference with each other, even when only a very few miles apart. In SERS, the VHF lowband and UHF bands are the least crowded. Transmitters for on-site radio paging systems are either AM or FM and set to the FCC assigned frequency of the system. The FCC has set aside eleven one-way paging frequencies in the SERS for which all hospitals are eligible. Business frequencies may also be used; these include four VHF high-band frequencies and nine UHF frequencies for paging only. The paging-only frequencies in the business service are coordinated by NABER, the National Association of Business and Education Radio users. The FCC has also authorized paging frequencies in the 900 MHz range for which all hospitals are eligible. Frequencies in the 900 MHz range are also coordinated by NABER.

The VHF lowband frequencies and UHF frequencies are generally much less congested than the VHF highband frequencies and, therefore, represent a better potential for fewer problems in sharing the frequency. The FCC does not coordinate the SERS frequency assignments and will authorize whatever is requested. It is suggested that you borrow frequency monitoring equipment from a potential supplier to monitor the frequency band selected. Or, if hospitals in the area have formed a frequency coordinating committee, the best frequency can be determined by contact with such organizations. Note also that the 157.450 MHz frequency is limited to 30 W maximum. On-site radio paging systems, however, particularly for tone-only or display messages, require much less power than voice or wide area paging, and 30 W may be entirely adequate. It is imporant to note that transmitters may only be set up, serviced and adjusted by persons holding a first or second class FCC commercial license.

(4) *Type of Encoding.* Again, the gradual shift from two-tone and five-tone to digital encoding has paralleled the growth of radio and electronic technology. Most equipment installed today is either two-tone or five-tone, but new paging systems are more and more likely to use digital encoding. Digital encoding is extremely fast, that is, approximately one and one half seconds for the transmission of a battery saver preamble and alerting signal, and approximately one third of a second for transmission of the alerting signal versus as much as five seconds for two-tone systems. In a low traffic, small paging system, the latter would be no problem. But with today's larger systems, high traffic loading dictates that transmission time be as short as possible. Digital encoding also permits multi-digital and alphanumeric display paging messages, and these too can be transmitted in a total of two seconds or less. Voice messages generally require at least five to ten seconds, depending upon the operator. Traffic capabilities in display message systems can be up to ten or more times that of voice systems. Digital encoding, because of high speed multiple transmissions and built-in code checking techniques, reduces "falsing" (pager receives a message designated for someone else or pager receives a false alert tone where no message was transmitted) to an absolute minimum.

(5) *Message Type.* Radio paging messages may consist of tone(s), light emitting diode (LED) or liquid crystal display (LCD) signals, voice, vibrations, digital display (one or more) and alphanumeric display (up to eight or even eighty

characters — and combinations of all of these). Which one or ones you select will depend upon how the paging system will be used, the number of pagers (and the need always increases), the expected message traffic and your budget. A few guidelines on each type may be helpful. Tone-only pagers should not be ignored. Staff members who will receive a minimum number of messages can effectively use a tone-only pager. For example, one tone would mean "call your office," and another tone might mean "return to your work station." A change in the tone may signify the level or urgency. More sophisticated tone-only pagers may have multiple address, that is one address number for individual calls and one for a group call and display signals to visually indicate which address number has been called. Many different message types may be transmitted in this way. Voice pagers provide unique message content. Although most paging messages contain number information such as "call extension 386," some emergency messages may be difficult to transmit without voice. Display pagers, particularly those with eight or more digits or alphanumeric characters, can provide surprising amounts of information, and all display pagers on the market today (at least six brands now available) have message memory. If a seven-digit telephone number is transmitted, it will be stored in the pager's memory for recall. This provides high message accuracy and confidence during busy times, and eliminates the need to call the operator for verification. Display message systems may need message storage equipment, and messages may be printed on a logging printer together with the time of transmission and the pager address. Vibration alert or "wiggler" pagers are becoming more widely used because of the silent alert, and because they are a natural adjunct to the inherently silent nature of the display paging. Night shift personnel carry such pagers to avoid noise on patient floors.

(6) *Pager Batteries and Chargers.* There are two types of batteries: disposable batteries and rechargeable batteries with various types of chargers.

The decision between the two types is a function of battery life inherent in the design of the pager selected, the average number of calls per pager per day, average call duration and the type of message, that is, tone, voice, display, etc. The longer the expected life, the more practical it is to use disposable batteries. A pager with a battery life of 1500 hours would strongly suggest the use of disposables. Factors that reduce battery life are: average message duration of ten to twenty seconds, voice messages, more than eight to ten calls per day, vibration alert and whether or not a pager is left "on" during hours when it is not used. "Battery saver" circuits are effective in some pagers, but this benefit decreases as more pagers are added to the system. The choice between disposable batteries and rechargeable batteries should be based on the type of usage and the economics over a significant period of time, for example, a week, month or year. Convenience and cost must be balanced by the user. The alternative is to charge batteries in a rack or in individual chargers. This requires someone with the time and expertise to switch the batteries. In some installations, secure storage of pagers in a rack is combined with the charging function. A keypad or magnetic card reader provides access to the secured pager storage rack. This function is sometimes linked to a staff in/out register system.

8.7.3 Design Considerations

(1) *Encoder Location.* Locations of telephones, intercom stations or automatic alarm station type encoders may be almost anywhere in a facility. However, FCC regulations require that there be one so-called "control point" in every radio paging system from which the entire system is monitored and controlled. This particular encoder or paging terminal is most commonly located at or immediately adjacent to the telephone operator's position. This location is generally the focal point for radio paging and other types of message functions and is the recommended site for the control point.

The control point encoder generally consists of the following: a keyboard to enter the address of the pocket pager to be paged (may be a telephone dial or standard twelve-button keypad or other button configuration); an emergency switch to interrupt a message placed from another parallel encoder (required by FCC regulations); an emergency message button or capability; a microphone with hand or foot switch (if voice messages are to be provided); a small loudspeaker with volume control (part of a frequency monitoring system to allow cooperation in the use of the FCC assigned transmitting frequency); and an "in-use" or "busy" signaling lamp (illuminates when other encoders or input devices are using the system). Depending upon the particular brand of encoder selected, a variety of other special control buttons, lamps and displays may also be provided. Parallel encoders (that are not a "control point"), if provided, will omit the emergency interrupt switch.

(2) *Base Station Configuration and Location.* The base station may include a computer or central processor unit; voice or display message storage capability; an automatic paging terminal; pager address translation circuitry and other special circuits depending upon the system supplier. The central unit of a radio paging system contains the control circuitry of the system. All manual or automatic encoders (sometimes both types) normally terminate at the central unit. Also connecting to the central unit may be inputs from a telephone system or intercom system and an output to the system transmitter.

The location of a central unit is largely a matter of choice, but it is usually preferable to select an air conditioned space which may be keylock secured. Systems with tape recorder(s) voice storage capability may require especially clean or dust-free space.

Central units are commonly housed in a 19 in (½ m) rack mount or other similar configuration. Computer bus technology with a mother board and plug-in PCB's (printed circuit boards) are currently state-of-the-art. PCB's are provided for control of sequencing and prioritization of connected encoders, automatic alarm devices, intercom stations and telephones if the system is interconnected. The mother board also accepts PCB's for connection of speech enabling circuitry, display message control, automatic system supervision or diagnostic circuitry and interface of staff registration and message management systems. Power requirements are normally nominal, usually requiring only a 117 V ac, 60 Hz, 20 A circuit. If voice message storage or automatic paging terminal equipment is included, power requirements may need to be increased. The engineer should check carefully with the supplier to ascertain exact requirements. It is strongly suggested that the selected system include a battery backup capability or be connected to the facility's emergency power system. Radio paging systems with either multiple dispatch points or with interconnection with the hospital's telephone system will include a monitoring circuit with output to the control point encoder. This allows the telephone operator to meet the FCC requirement of monitoring all dispatch points' transmissions and to be able to interrupt such transmissions for priority page messages or to prevent illegal transmissions.

(3) *Transmitter Location and Configuration.* Transmitters are generally located as close to the antenna as possible to reduce signal losses. However, consideration is also given to location for easy service access, security, and, generally, air conditioning. Regarding the latter, it is important to consult with the supplier's technical staff or to review technical literature, or both, to determine the requirements. On-site systems utilizing slotted, radiating coaxial cable for the antenna system may require transmitter location centrally to provide equal cable runs to all parts of the building.

A wide range of transmitter configurations are available based on particular supplier requirements, range of coverage, type of antenna and method of signal coverage within the building(s) and hospital complex. Transmitters are frequently mounted in a 19 in (½ m) standard rack with a secured door. Transmitters generally contain the following modules: a power supply (connected to the building emergency power system); the transmitter itself, an automatic carrier-operated relay circuit (inhibits transmission when carrier signal is detected from another transmitter on the same frequency and assures compliance with the FCC requirement to cooperate in the use of the assigned frequency); and an automatic station identifier (eliminates the need for the telephone operator to transmit the station call letters periodically as required by the FCC). An ASI (automatic station identifier) may transmit either a voice message or Morse code, the latter being more common in new systems. The ASI makes the identification at prescribed intervals, but it will not interrupt a transmission to make such an "announcement." While primary power requirements vary depending upon transmitter power, generally one 20 A, 117 V ac, 60 Hz circuit is adequate.

Improved "coverage" of an on-site system is obtained by some suppliers by the use of master and slave transmitters. This technique accomplishes several things: lower total radiated power (reduces interference with other possible users on the same frequency and reduces the possibility of interference with sensitive or unshielded bio-medical electronic equipment); more even signal coverage within the building(s); improved coverage of a multiple building complex; and better coverage of below grade floors.

(4) *Antenna Systems Selection.* The conditions governing the installation of an on-site paging system antenna are quite different from those applying to a mobile radio system. The main objective is not to cover as large an area as possible but to ensure full and uniform coverage within the defined paging area.

Ideally, signals are dispersed uniformly in all directions and decrease linearly at increasing distance from the antenna. In practice, however, antenna radiation is not uniform, primarily due to attenuation caused by screening or reflection.

To a certain degree, radio waves are attenuated by all sorts of materials, but antenna radiation is affected most by metallic objects between the antenna and the receiver, such as in steel reinforced concrete buildings. It is obviously undesirable to place the antenna on the roof of such a structure, in all instances, as the radio waves might have to pass through several screening floors before reaching the receiver. Also, the signal strength is generally at its lowest directly below the location of most antennas.

When radio waves reach a surface, part of them will pass or be absorbed, while others will be reflected. When the reflected radiation mixes with the direct radiation, interference will occur which may amplify the signal at some places but weaken and perhaps extinguish it at other places. A special risk of such dead zones is present at elevator or stairwells or between thick pillars. Dead zones may be eliminated through change of antenna location or type, but may then arise at other places instead.

The on-site paging receivers are generally designed for best reception of vertically polarized radiation. The choice of transmitter antenna is influenced by many different factors, such as the size and shape of the area which is to be covered, the construction of the building where the paging is to be performed, etc. For these reasons, there are several different types of antennas in use. The Tuned Antennas include:

    (a) Ground Plane
    (b) Dipole
    (c) Aperiodic Antennas
    (d) Twin-lead with folded dipole
    (e) Radiating coaxial cable

The first two are used as regular directional antennas while the remaining ones are used as extra antennas. The latter ones are used to improve the reception at places which are out of reach of the radiation of the regular antenna.

It should always be observed that the antenna height should be reduced as much as possible and only cover the required area, thereby reducing the risk of interference with other installations.

The following general remarks may be of assistance in choosing antenna type and location.

The quarter wavelength ground plane antennas are used where wide and mainly circular coverage is desired. Due to the construction, a free area with a radius of about 3 m around the antenna is required for the ground plane elements at the place of installation.

If possible, the antenna should be located above nearby steel or concrete structures and above other antennas which lie within a radius of ½ wavelength. If the antenna is to be installed on a roof, for example, and there are no obstacles nearby, it is, as a rule, sufficient to mount it on a steel pipe at least 15 ft high in order to avoid lobe-lift, that otherwise will decrease the field strength at ground level. Ground plane antennas, because of their radiation pattern, are frequently best located close to the edge of the roof.

Antenna(s) must always be mounted a minimum of 15 ft (4 m) above the ground or roof. The horizontal distance between ground plane antennas and building sides must be at least 50 ft (15 m), this with a view to prevent both reflection and permanent-wave patterns.

In a large building made of reinforced concrete, for example, it may happen that the signal from the regular antenna is so strongly attenuated in one or more parts of the building that reception there becomes unsatisfactory. To improve reception in a single place, a slave transmitter (or multiple slave transmitters) connected to an internally located aperiodic antenna may be installed in the place in question.

Lightning protection for all antennas should be provided; however, the potential for lightning damage is one that is often misunderstood. If a radio antenna suffers a direct hit from lightning, no built-in protection will save it and possibly its transmission line and base station from substantial damage. The 100 000 A and great surge currents encountered in a direct lightning hit will destroy an antenna used in normal radio installations.

Antenna design features that offer lightning protection actually minimize damage from the nearby lightning strikes as well as damage and static that can be caused by various other electrostatic charges in the air. Spark gaps and grounded elements within the antennas themselves are used to provide this important feature.

(5) *Requirements and Licensing Procedure.* In order to operate a radio paging system, the owner/user of the system must obtain a license for the system and be assigned call letters to identify the "station."

An important part of planning a radio paging system involves conforming to the FCC requirements regarding radio system control and obtaining the station license. The following material discusses both the FCC requirements and licensing.

Since paging systems utilize "Radio" transmission, these systems will be governed by FCC Rules and Regulations [10]. Therefore, an Operator's License is necessary to test, adjust and maintain a system. A "Radio Station Authorization" is a license issued by the FCC that authorizes the operation of radio paging systems.

A copy of the appropriate part of the FCC Rules and Regulations [10] should be available at each control point. Part 90 is contained in Volume V of the FCC Rules and Regulations [10]. A copy of the applicable FCC Rules and Regulations [10] should be kept on site during radio equipment operation.

The FCC defines a control point as an operating position under the control and supervision of the licensee where the person immediately responsible for the operation of the transmitter is stationed and where monitoring facilities are located. Authority must be obtained from the FCC for each control point. Every system must have at least one control point.

A dispatch point is any point from which messages may be transmitted under supervision from a control point. Dispatch points may be installed without authorization.

Each control point must have the following facilities:

(a) A visual indication of a "transmitter-on" condition — either a light or a meter.

(b) Facilities to permit the operator to turn the transmitter on and off.

(c) Equipment to permit the operator at the control point to monitor all transmission by dispatch points under his supervision.

(d) Facilities to permit the operator at the control point to take transmitter control away from dispatch points (priority, or supervisory control).

Any operator must be able to monitor the channel to see if it is clear before transmitting.

These regulations determine, to a great extent, what equipment the facility must have in any given system. For example, a special requirement in the FCC license to monitor the channel prior to transmitting means that the system must have either a receiver/monitor or a method of indicating detection of the carrier transmission by others on the same frequency, or both.

No "on-the-air" testing may be started until the station license is granted and Form 456 has been completed and forwarded to the FCC Regional Office.

A station log must be maintained in accordance with the part of the FCC Rules under which the station is licensed. Initial frequency and power measurements must be made and entered in the station log and signed by a technician or engineer holding a first- or second-class radio-telephone operator's license.

Paging systems with voice capabilities must be identified with station call letters every 15 minutes in standard services and every 30 minutes in the Public Safety and Special Emergency Radio Services (FCC 90.425(a)) [10]. However, if there are no transmissions over a 30-minute period, the station may be identified at the end of the next transmission. Stations are not required to go on the air solely for identification. Morse code station identification is now acceptable by the FCC.

When making a change to the system, that is, adding a second control point, the customer may be required to change his license. Any time the user has two (or more) operating points, neither of which has priority, he must obtain authorization from the FCC and specify the number of control points in his license.

8.8 Physician and Staff Register Systems

8.8.1 Introduction. Physician and staff register systems are information systems used to locate staff, deliver messages, provide legal records, and provide personal services to physicians. Messages received before the physician or staff has arrived are transmitted by a recall feature that indicates message(s) are waiting upon "in" activation. Since these systems are now used by both physicians and the in-house staff, they will be referred to generically as staff register systems.

8.8.2 Design Criteria

(1) *General.* Staff register systems are not required by the Joint Commission for the Accreditation of Hospitals (JCAH) but are widely used, partly because of their ability to increase the efficiency of JCAH required functions related to code blue, fire and security systems. Some type of staff register system is needed by virtually all health care facilities. In small health care facilities, the handwritten entry/exit log is useful for purposes of location, message delivery, legal records, and other personal services for physicians and staff. These represent the four basic requirements for all staff register systems, regardless of configuration.

The number of functions to be accomplished by a register system is a function of several factors:

(2) *Size.* The larger the health care facility, the more difficult it becomes to use a handwritten or lighted annunciator type register. The number of entry/exit transactions, roster changes and entry/exit locations make such systems physically unworkable.

With increasing size, message traffic becomes a real problem for the telephone operator. Some facilities try to solve this problem by refusing to handle messages for non-staff physicians when the messages are related to private practice matters. But in the long run, this distinction proves difficult to make and often competes for physician's services. If facility "A" provides good message service, and facility "B" does not, facility "B" may be at a disadvantage.

Facility size also creates problems in locating staff members for both emergency and routine messages. The bigger the facility, the more likely it is that people are going to be away from the "assigned" work station. For example, few facilities can afford to equip every staff member, plus the roster of outside physicians, with pocket pagers. Overhead loudspeaker paging can become almost continuous background noise pollution for both patients and staff. The display of staff location information on video monitors throughout the hospital in key locations can greatly reduce these problems. Register systems are generally agreed to reduce overhead paging by at least eighty percent. The balance of the paging represents information of an emergency or general nature not suitable for register system use. Monitors can also display, via special symbols, the location of a particular member, their pocket pager number, and whether or not there is a message waiting and how urgent it is.

(3) *Number of Hospitals in Proximity.* In larger metropolitan areas, where physicians often see patients in several hospitals, the location problem for routine, urgent and emergency messages becomes critical. Where did Doctor Davis go when he left City General? Did he go to Einstein or St. Anthony's? State-of-the-art register systems can store and display this information quickly and easily. The physician leaving a facility is given several destination choices as part of the registering OUT procedure. This information is stored in the systems' memory and can be retrieved by a telephone operator in seconds.

(4) *Specialization.* If 80 doctors are in the hospital and a specialist is needed in the emergency room, the question becomes, "Is there one in the house?" If not, who is on call, and where are they? With a well-designed register system, these questions can be answered quickly, and the proper person located.

(5) *In-House Staff Location.* In an emergency, it is often the in-house staff that must solve a problem. Locating and assembling the best team can be greatly facilitated by a register system just by knowing who is in the hospital, and who is on call. This is particularly important in teaching hospitals. Some hospitals have display monitors that list outside physicians and in-house staff members separately to simplify this process.

(6) *Incentive to Use.* Because the technology now allows innovative solutions to long-standing problems, needs not previously recognized or addressable can

now be satisfied. However, the overriding need is simplicity. Computer-controlled systems, unfortunately, can complicate even simple functions. Nevertheless, the system is only as good as the people who use it. Many times the advanced features on these systems go to waste because the physicians do not bother to utilize the system. If entry/exit stations in particular (this can also apply to the telephone operator or other control points) are difficult to operate, they won't be used. At entry/exit stations, directions and function labels must be simple, clear, concise and familiar. Displays must be very readable. The entry/exit procedure must be quick and easy to remember. The engineer should insure that the physicians are directly involved in the purchase of the system. The physicians should guarantee their cooperation in utilizing any new system before it is purchased.

8.8.3 System Types and Selection

(1) *General.* In its simplest form, the lighted annunciator type of system, with a toggle switch by each name, has been with us for at least 40 years. Annunciator systems continue to be sold and used effectively by small hospitals, nursing homes and clinics.

The development of microprocessors, personal computers, and mainframe computers has allowed for the expansion of the registering IN and OUT concept to extremely sophisticated systems for literally thousands of physicians and staff members with special functions for message management, voice synthesis, internal and external destination information, location of staff by title or specialty, radio paging, telephone interconnection, multiple video monitor display of staff registration information, displays of code blue or disaster alerts, staff profiles (listing telephone number(s), pocket pager number, date/time last in hospital), system diagnostics, message printers, logging printers, etc.

(2) *Lighted Annunciator Panels.* This is recommended for small facilities. A basic system will consist of a minimum of two panels, one usually in front of the telephone operator position and the other at the doctor's entrance point. Both panels have a switch opposite each backlighted name slot. A staff member or doctor indicates their presence by turning on the switch opposite their name. This, in turn, lights the appropriate name in each panel. Many of these systems have a light flashing circuit activated at the telephone operator position that advises the entering or exiting person of a message waiting. Often, a private telephone or two-station intercom system is provided to obtain messages from the operator.

The installation requires a minimum of a pair of wires for each name to be annunciated. Therefore, a panel for 50 persons requires a minimum of 100 wires and 200 terminations. In a small facility, with stable size and a very slow building program, this works well.

The disadvantage of lighted annunciator panels appears when more names must be added and/or the system must be expanded to add or relocate entry/exit stations. For example, adding one doctor's name (assuming space is available on the panel) requires moving every name in the alphabet beyond the initial letter in the name to be added. If changes occur regularly, and they tend to, this can be a time-consuming process, multiplied by the number of panels in the system. Adding stations requires more wire, conduit space and multiple terminations. Moving a station is the biggest problem because of the cabling, all of which may have to be replaced or extended via a large junction box with terminal strips. Some of these cables in bigger systems get to be several inches in diameter.

Lighted annunciator panels work well, are simple to use and are generally reliable. However, they don't offer the users much incentive to register IN and OUT, and it is expensive to display the data in more than a limited number of locations in rather close proximity.

(3) *Telephone Operated Entry/Exit Station Systems.* The word telephone indicates that some of the systems within this category use private or dedicated telephone (or intercom) type keypads, or their equivalent, to accomplish the register activity.

Keypad or coded button operated register systems deal with the cabling problem detailed above with lighted annunciator panel systems. Further, the stations become much smaller, since the annunciator panel with names is eliminated at the entry/exit station. Note, however, that this deprives the user of knowledge about a colleague's absence or presence. Some systems do allow users to make IN/OUT status inquiries, but this is a time-consuming operation.

Note also that these systems still require a large annunciator display panel at the operator position to keep track of the IN/OUT data.

In use, the staff member enters an assigned two or three digit registration number on the keypad. The entered digits are displayed via LED's in a display window for verification. Then an IN and OUT button (sometimes within the keypad and sometimes separate) is pushed to complete the registration. If a message is waiting, a "message" light will illuminate, and the user can then call the operator with the provided handset. A "message cancel" button is sometimes provided.

Because of wiring simplicity, usually two twisted pairs per station, multiple entry/exit stations can be installed at various entrances and other key locations. However, some systems that are of this type still use as many as 33 pairs of #22 AWG wire for each station. Few of these systems are available today.

(4) *Electronic Systems with Video Monitors.* During the 1970's, a number of companies designed and sold what might be called pre-computer based systems using some magnetic core memories and PROM's (Programmable Read Only Memory). In addition to register functions, these systems have a variety of optical features such as links to radio pocket paging systems, bed status systems and dial and DTMF (Dual-Tone Multi-Frequency) interfaces to telephone PBX's (Private Branch Exchange). Most of these systems have video display monitors, and some have loop tape voice response capability verifying IN or OUT status plus simple messages such as "call records," "call office" and "call home." Dedicated entry/exit stations are operated by keypads and/or punched cards.

Video display monitors show staff registered IN, pocket pager numbers and various abbreviations indicating location in the hospital, message waiting, etc.

These systems are generally complex and expensive when fully configured, but provide significantly greater capability. Being able to use any telephone to access the system is most helpful in determining whether or not a particular staff member is in the hospital and where he or she is located. Video monitors are located at many points, providing a continuous display of registration information.

These electronic systems have now been superseded in the marketplace by computer based systems for reasons of cost, software flexibility and the requirement for more extensive message and other related capabilities in the systems.

(5) *Microprocessor Voice Synthesizer Systems.* A number of voice synthesizer systems are on the market, all of which are quite similar in their functions. A staff member registers into the system from either a dial or DTMF type telephone. First, a two or three digit system access number is dialed; access is indicated by a connection tone. Then, the assigned staff member's two- or three-digit number is dialed into the system. The voice synthesizer in the system responds by repeating the digits dialed and then saying the words "IN" or "OUT," depending upon the current status of the staff member.

The staff member then dials, for example, the number four to register IN or seven to register OUT.

Messages stored in the system are tagged with the extension number of internal departments trying to reach the registering staff member. Depending upon various option selections, these "extension calling" messages may be entered either from the operator position or from any telephone within the hospital. Special number codes are utilized to accomplish these functions.

Additional cost options on such systems increase voice synthesizer message capacity to include a number of "canned" messages, such as "call lab," "call office" and "call records." Video display monitors may be added wherever desired in the hospital and will display staff members' names, pocket pager numbers, location in the hospital, alternate covering physician number, specialty codes and message insertion and retrieval from outside telephones.

An option is available from some suppliers for dedicated telephone "terminals" that do not require the initial dialing of two or three access digits to use the system.

Components of these systems consist of:

(a) A telephone operator 12-button keypad with video monitor.

(b) Video display monitors throughout the hospital.

(c) A microprocessor controller.

(d) Entry/exit stations that might consist of dedicated telephones, telco network telephones and/or hospital telephones.

(e) FCC (Federal Communications Commission) approved telephone interconnect device.

(f) System cabling (generally two twisted pairs).

(g) Message printer option.

The voice synthesizer systems represent an improvement over earlier systems, but some hospitals may find that the realism, intelligibility and general quality or presence of the synthesized voice messages leaves something to be desired. What sounds intelligible in a quiet room during a test demonstration may be very difficult to understand in a noisy corridor when a doctor is in a hurry. These systems do not use the synthesizers (which cost in excess of $100,000) used by telephone companies to handle number changes.

Canned message limitations and the small number of other message management functions may also be discouraging to possible buyers. There are real quality differences in these systems, and the engineer is counseled to make careful comparisons before specifying. These systems will generally be somewhat less expensive than microcomputer-based systems, but the added cost of the latter may seem like a bargain when their additional capability is examined.

(6) *Microcomputer Systems.* The microcomputer-controlled registry systems are now available from five or six different suppliers. With the possible exception of voice synthesis, these systems provide virtually all of the functional capability of prior systems plus some new and useful functions relating to management of the message processing function of the telephone operator position, and related record keeping and staff services. Microcomputer prices are dropping steadily. Coupled with increasing knowledge and sensitivity in the development and utilization of the required software, cost effective, "user friendly" solutions to hospital communications problems are promised.

The primary differences between the microcomputer systems and other systems center around the functional flexibility and adaptability of the system as controlled by the stored program data processor. Functions, instructions, user terminology, nomenclature and vocabulary, display formats, message content and many other variables can be customized for each installation. The better systems allow most of this flexibility to be in the hands of the hospital user. Capable and responsible suppliers provide extensive in-service training in system operation, set-up, modification and testing.

A second major difference exists in the use of printers to provide users with printed messages. There are systems with other types of entry/exit stations using alphanumeric display panels, different configurations and disk drives, keyboards and quantities of standard features, all of which may be modified by both the vendor and the end-user.

A printer for messages received at registration and a logging printer with its system data activity printing capability for legal records free the telephone operator from the enormous chore of logging all page and message information.

The particular system specified allows for display of up to three special alert messages on all video monitors, such as disaster alerts and code blue information.

Messages for staff members may be personal ("YOUR GARAGE CALLED, AND YOUR CAR IS READY"), departmental ("DR. MURRAY IS SICK TODAY"), or general ("GRAND ROUNDS AT 12:30 P.M. TODAY").

The amount of information available to the PBX operator position is relative to each staff member in the roster.

(7) *Combination Systems.* Microcomputers allow staff register systems to be combined with such functions as bed status, dietary programs, automatic paging terminals, patient and staff directories, etc. Although this combination will work, the overall complexity of the resulting system may produce an unusually complex system. Therefore, it is recommended that the staff register system be a standalone system.

8.8.4 Design Considerations

(1) *Entry/Exit Stations.* Entry/Exit stations should be located at all physician entrances, and should include message recall features. The intent is to provide entry/exit station users with a practical, useful and compelling incentive to use

the station. Well-designed systems provide personal, general, departmental and emergency messages. Hospitals with such systems report 95% utilization. Without such an incentive, often less than half of desired staff use is obtained.

(2) *Central Control Equipment.* Control cabinets and power supplies should be located with other communication control equipment. Name indicators with recall activation or operators' consoles are located by the telephone operator.

(3) *Cable Plant.* Well-designed systems use off-the-shelf video and RF (Radio Frequency) monitors or both to simplify service. The same may be said for the microcomputer selected. It should be a well-known national brand with a trackable service history.

Installation of these systems normally requires no more than two twisted pairs of #22 AWG for connection of entry/exit stations to the computer, and coaxial cable for the monitors.

Well-designed units contain a battery backup to retain computer memory of the current day's activity during momentary power losses.

Computers are notoriously susceptible to spike or surge damage to chips and other circuitry. It is recommended that a good quality surge protector unit be purchased to protect the microcomputer portion of the system.

(4) *Software Considerations.* Good programming is required to provide simple user friendly displays and instructions. For a staff registration system, this is apparent from one's comfort in operating the system. If any portion of the program seems awkward, it will be hard to use, inflexible, and staff members may not use it. Quality software programs for staff register systems are available. Such programs come from several years or more of intensive work with customers. Pick a supplier with a visible track record. There are no bargains in good quality microcomputer systems.

The selected system supplier should offer a thorough questionnaire covering all aspects of the operation so that the software program, user vocabulary and screen format on displays will fit individual needs. Startup of the system requires input of all the roster data plus the pre-established message content and other user variables. The system supplier should be required to teach the operating personnel not only how to run the system, but how to change all the variables.

8.9 Dictation Systems

8.9.1 Introduction. Dictation systems are recording systems used for storing voice signals (dictation) for transcription. They are used in the production of patients' medical records and for administrative functions.

8.9.2 Design Criteria

(1) *General.* Health care facilities are required by federal and state laws to maintain a medical record for every individual who is evaluated or treated in a facility. Studies by communication consultants indicate individuals speak six times faster than they write and that memory retention is a function of time since the event. Dictation systems improve the efficiency, productivity and accuracy of producing medical records from medical staff notes. Dictation systems are required when the medical staff chooses dictation over writing of medical records.

Systems should be selected based on performance, which is measured by turn-around time of important dictation, ease with which the system is used (personnel productivity) and dependability as well as overall output. System selection criteria should include the following:

(2) *System Capacity.* An effective dictation system eliminates bottlenecks. The system capacity should be determined by a survey of the dictating load, with consideration being given to the number of persons dictating, amount of dictation, and dictating habits. All systems should allow dictation positions and recording machines to be economically added as system usage expands. While the same amount of dictating may be done, more recording machines will be necessary where dictation cannot be scheduled or occurs during limited peak periods.

(3) *Recording Machine.* Cassette and loop recorders are both employed in dictation systems. Cassette recorders utilize cassette stack loaders to provide a high, unattended recording capacity and allow particular tapes to be saved or moved. Portable cassette recorders with matching cassettes add flexibility. Loop recorders require no tape handling and utilize two tape heads (record and playback) to allow simultaneous dictation and transcription. Different recorders may be used in the same system to get the advantages of each type.

Cassette recorders are best applied where the dictation rate (the number of users) is low but where a large storage capacity (that is, a weekend's dictation) is required. Loop recorders with multiple heads are best applied where the dictation rate is high, but where large backlogs are low because the dictation is rapidly transcribed. The minimum number of recording machines must equal the maximum number of simultaneous dictation sources. Recording machines should have a voice-operated relay so that a machine is activated only when the person dictating speaks. This eliminates pauses on the recording medium. In addition, lights and audible signals should be provided to indicate that a recording machine needs reloading, a recording machine is in use, and intercommunication with the person dictating is requested. Security features should permit only the person dictating to play back during a recording period, and only authorized personnel to play back after termination of dictation.

(4) *Record Keeping.* Many dictation systems include computer-based operating equipment which keeps records for the system. The information may include location of priority dictation; length of dictation recorded on each recorder with system totals; production history of each transcriptionist; doctors' code, patients' code and length of each dictation. Particular record information varies from system to system and should be tailored to each installation. In high volume installations, the record keeping ability of a computer control unit is necessary.

(5) *Supervision.* The supervisor helps both dictation authors and transcriptionists. Supervisor controls should include all recorder controls and an on-line/off-line switch, record keeping controls and intercom or telephone controls (for speaking with the author or transcriptionists). The supervisor's console often includes a CRT, printer, keyboard, and central processor.

(6) *Transcription.* Transcription controls include recorder transport functions and controls for tone, speed and intercom (for speaking with the supervisor).

Transcriptionists' terminals may be equipped with a word processor in any size system.

(7) *Dictation Station Comfort.* A good dictation station makes it easy for an author to record, review and edit his notes. Each dictation station or telephone handset should have controls or codes for rewinding, fast forwarding, quick reviewing, full playback, editing and signaling the operator. Automatic start/stop controls make the system more efficient by eliminating pauses in the dictation; however, manual start/stop controls may be used. Comfort can affect the efficiency of dictation systems. User friendly terminals include features like signal muting during fast forward and reverse, automatic gain control, and clear indication of system functions.

8.9.3 System Types and Selection

(1) *Portable.* A small dictation system may consist of portable tape machines and tape players equipped as transcription terminals. Recorded tapes are carried from the dictation author to transcriptionist.

(2) *Central System — Independent.* A central dictation system allows dictation at any time at various points convenient for the medical staff who will be dictating. Data as it is being dictated is transmitted to a central location for storage until material can be recorded. An independent system requires a separate wiring system and dictating sets. These sets are similar to a desk telephone, with pushbuttons for recording, playback, correction, and other items. Depending on the size of the system, a desk set may connect directly to a single recording machine, or have a selector permitting a speaker to connect to any free recording machine. Because of the additional expense of wiring such systems, their use should be limited to small facilities and to those cases where telephone interconnect is not available.

(3) *Central System — Telephone Access.* Used with telephone systems, a central dictation system transmits over the telephone system by use of that system's desk instruments. Central recording is connected to the telephone system through a link. The person dictating can record, get playback or correction, and other items all by dialing preselected numbers. Dictation systems are available from most telephone interconnect companies as a part of their system or other companies' equipment may be directly connected to telephone company systems.

(4) *Combinations.* These systems have a combination recorder and transcriber, or master recorder, when only a limited amount of dictation is recorded. Use where requirements are limited to a small department, for security, or where specialized dictation material indicates handling by one stenographer.

8.9.4 Design Considerations

(1) *Dictation Stations.* The effectiveness of a dictation system will depend on both the flexibility of the system and on the way the staff uses the system. Simple systems, effective training programs and operator assistance help improve performance. Prerecorded instructions, available each time a system is used, will be useful where staff may work at several facilities and need a reminder of operating codes each time they change systems.

Locate stations for convenience so staff wishing to dictate can do so in a location where he or she has access to all the relevant source material. This includes charting areas at nursing stations, operating and delivery suites, control areas, radiology reading rooms, and pathology analysis areas.

(2) *Portable Recorders.* Portable recorders should be compatible with central system transcribers. Use where requirements call for the person dictating to be in the field or at locations not accessible to the central system stations.

(3) *Off-Site Dictating Positions.* Ability to dictate into the central system from locations off of the facility should be provided when many persons will dictate for short periods and connection costs will not be excessive.

(4) *Network.* When the recorders and supervisors' console are in separate rooms, many cables are required to connect them. When the dictation system operates through the telephone system, cable is required from the console and recorders to the telephone switch. All of this wiring requires raceway systems installed per code.

8.10 Patient Physiological Monitoring Systems

8.10.1 Introduction. A patient monitoring system allows several patient parameters to be monitored by the nursing staff at a central station usually located at the nurses' station. The system provides continual monitoring of several patients from one central location, thus contributing to an increased quality of patient care.

The patient monitoring system consists of bedside instrumentation, interconnection hardware, the central station and optional remote monitors. Bedside instrumentation displays patient parameters such as ECG, pulse, blood pressure, respiration and temperature. Interconnection hardware, consisting in part of a central station junction box and multi-conductor interconnecting cable, connects the bedside instrumentation and the central station. The central station displays the same patient parameters on an oscilloscope or recorder as displayed on the bedside instrumentation. The central station also displays parameters on meters or numerical displays. If a patient's vital signs fall below a preset level, an alarm is initiated indicating which patient is in trouble. Remote monitors are optional and display the same patient parameters as displayed on the bedside instrumentation.

8.10.2 Design Criteria

(1) *General.* Patient physiological monitoring systems with transmission to a central location are usually installed in intensive care or coronary care patient rooms, recovery rooms, and other areas required by the hospital. Local bedside patient monitors may be utilized in emergency rooms, operating and delivery suites, and nurseries.

(2) *Telemetry Systems.* For ambulatory patients a telemetry system may be utilized. This type of system includes a portable transmitter carried by the patient with antennas located throughout the department. A receiver at the nurses station processes the signal and displays the patient's heart rate.

If the hospital considers telemetry, the system supplier will generally make on-site field strength measurements to insure adequate signal coverage. Each installation must be treated on an individual basis as each hospital has specific details of construction, placement of walls and location of electrical equipment along with other factors that can affect telemetry signal reception.

(3) *Computerized Systems.* If the hospital is considering a computerized patient monitoring system, adequate signal and power arrangements should be made during the initial stages of planning. It is suggested that the system supplier medical specialist be contacted as recommendations for computer installation vary with specific situations.

Computer system installations normally require special signal junction boxes and larger diameter or additional conduits. In addition, power requirements for computer-based systems are generally higher so provisions for increased capacity to computer patient monitoring areas must be made early in the design phase.

8.10.3 Design Considerations

(1) *Location of Equipment.* Patient monitoring central stations are usually located at the nurses stations of the units where central monitoring systems are installed. These central stations are located on the counter within easy view for continual monitoring.

Bedside modules can be located on small tables, on mobile instrument carts for freedom of movement to any desired location or ideally on wall mount brackets to keep the bedside area as free of equipment as possible.

Remote monitors may be ceiling mounted at any strategic location in the medical staff flow patterns, such as hallways, where monitoring of patient parameters is desired. These allow observation of the entire unit while staff members are away from the central station.

(2) *Space Requirements.* A countertop or other suitable structure to support the equipment at the central station must be provided. A minimum depth of 6 in from the rear of the instruments to the back of the enclosure is required for ventilation and cable access. The structure should consist of a surface above and behind the monitoring equipment for protection. Custom-built enclosures are often available from the system supplier. The engineer should contact the system supplier for dimensions of these monitors in order to ensure the availability of adequate space.

(3) *Installation Requirements.* Interconnection requirements for the patient monitoring system including sizes and types of raceways, cables and terminating junction boxes at the bed location and central station can be obtained from the system supplier. In general, for interconnection of bedside units with those at the central station, a 1¼ in diameter steel conduit with a 25 conductor, #22 gauge wire is recommended for its superior protection and ease of handling additional monitoring capacity in the future, without the necessity of pulling additional cabling. It is recommended that the conduit be run under the floor to eliminate unsightly conduit runs above the console at the central station. Where conduit installation would be unduly expensive or impractical for other reasons, systems can be interconnected using surface mounted raceway.

Installation of the bedside instrumentation and remote monitors requires the provision of a single outlet and power receptacle adjacent to the equipment. Installation of the equipment at the central station requires the provision of power receptacles along the length of the counter sufficient to power the equipment.

Coordination of the installation is of utmost importance as several different specialties are involved in or affected by the installation of the monitoring system.

(4) *Power Requirements.* A power source of 120 V, 60 Hz should be provided for the patient monitoring system. It is recommended that this be tied to the hospital emergency power source as a safety factor for continued monitoring in the event of a power failure. It is recommended that each bed location have a dedicated (supplied via a separate circuit breaker), 15 A (minimum), three-wire grounded outlet. The dedicated outlet allows the system to remain operative if a failure occurs at one bedside.

Some manufacturers require that all outlets serving patient monitoring instruments be connected to the same power phase in order to assure reliable operation of the patient distress alarm circuits. If the same phase is not available for the entire system, special installation techniques must be used to insure proper operation of the instruments. These manufacturers may also require that each patient station and the central station be provided with a separate grounding wire to a common ground bus in the power distribution panel. They may also require that all monitoring equipment be on a separate grounding system isolated from all other hospital equipment. It is suggested that the system supplier be contacted for further information in this area.

To avoid ac and RF interference problems, conduit and cabling should be located as far away as possible from ac power lines, diathermy cables, etc.

8.11 Emergency Medical Service Communications

8.11.1 Introduction. EMS (Emergency Medical Service) is a system of trained personnel, transportation equipment and communications equipment that provides pre-hospital medical care to patients at a remote accident scene and during transport to the hospital. Emergency transportation includes ambulances, helicopters, and fixed wing aircraft. The communications equipment can provide continuous voice communications and cardiac telemetering between the patient's site and the hospital emergency room. The communications equipment may also be used to coordinate the hospital's participation in regional emergencies. The design, operation and control of EMS communication systems is usually set by state authorities. Special UHF frequencies are set aside by the FCC Rules and Regulations Section 90.53 [10].

8.11.2 Design Criteria. Whenever a health care facility is equipped for emergency care, the engineer should investigate his responsibilities in installation of the EMS communications equipment. Close coordination with the equipment supplier is required.

8.11.3 Design Considerations

(1) *General.* There are many different systems available to provide EMS communications, and the equipment locations and power requirements can vary widely from what is described here. The engineer should carefully investigate the system requirements for each design and insure the reliability of the power supply to this important system.

(2) *Emergency Room Control Center.* The console contains the radio transmitter and receiver equipment, as well as equipment to display the physiological

monitoring signals and to route the voice communications to telephone lines.

(3) *Raceway for Antenna Conductors.* The EMS antennas will normally be located on the roof of the health care facility and the engineer must provide a 1¼ in raceway from the transmitter and receiver to the antennas. The engineer should verify the maximum length of these cables for the system installed.

8.12 Clocks

8.12.1 Introduction. Clocks are required to provide accurate and reliable time indication for legal records, medical procedures, and efficient and safe operation of health care facilities. Clock systems with automatic hourly and 12 hour time supervision and regulation features provide accurate and reliable synchronized time indication. Individual nonself-regulating (nonsystem) type clocks will usually provide reliable individual time indication.

8.12.2 Design Criteria. Clocks are required by health facility regulations.

(1) *Clock Locations.* Clocks should be provided in lobbies, waiting rooms, cafeterias, staff lounges, offices, central control center and elsewhere where time indication is appropriate. Clocks with a sweep second hand shall be located in nurses stations, recovery rooms, scrub sinks, birthing rooms, emergency treatment rooms, intensive care rooms, coronary care rooms, operating rooms, and nurseries. Elapsed time clocks may be required in emergency, surgery and delivery suites depending on local codes and staff requirements.

(2) *Individual Clocks.* Individual nonself-regulating (nonsystem) type clocks will usually provide reliable individual time indication; however, they have the inherent disadvantage of nonsynchronization and they must be individually handset twice a year for daylight savings time changes as well as following power outages. They are recommended only for public areas, offices and general care patient rooms. There are two types of individually powered clocks. One type plugs into a 120 V, 60 Hz receptacle and the other type is battery operated. Battery operated clock prices are decreasing and this, coupled with mobility, accuracy and long battery life make them acceptable. The disadvantages are the cost of replacing the batteries and that they may not be designed for heavy duty cleaning.

(3) *Elapsed Time Indicating Clocks.* Recently, digital direct read displays have become popular, but often these are too small for across-the-room reading. If the readout is large enough (1 in [2.5 cm] acceptable, 2 in [5 cm] recommended), digital direct read displays are preferred over analog dial clocks in the operating and delivery rooms. The time clock should have the capability of immediate automatic time correction in the event of power interruption. The elapsed-time clock is controlled from a control panel, with settings for start, stop and reset from zero or resumption. It is desirable to have both upcount and downcount timer capability with audible signal option at end of downcount.

(4) *Clock Systems—General.* The centrally controlled clock system approach provides the advantages of synchronized, accurate time indication throughout the building and allows quick resetting of all clocks for daylight savings time changes or after a power failure.

Clock systems can also be a source of control signals for time-of-day control of building systems, such as HVAC and exterior lighting. The clock system control unit serves the function of a number of individual time clocks in this mode. Where employee shift changes are supervised by attendance recorders, the recorders may be connected to the clock system to provide accurate operation at the recorders. Time stamps may also be connected to the clock system.

(5) *Clock System — Wired.* There are two types of direct wired systems: wired synchronous and minute impulse. Minute impulse systems are obsolete. Wired synchronous systems require three conductors to be run from the master controller to all of the secondary clocks, with the clocks wired in parallel. The three conductors are labeled clock power, correction, and common, and system voltage is either 120 V, 60 Hz or 24 V, 60 Hz.

(6) *Clock System — Carrier Current.* This system requires connection only to a suitable 120 V, 60 Hz electric circuit, usually the nearest unswitched duplex receptacle circuit. Automatic individual self-correction is provided by carrier current transmitted over the building secondary electrical distribution system. The costs of carrier frequency signal generator equipment makes its use economical only for medium to large facilities and remodels. For systems having over 100 clocks, where either a wired synchronous or carrier current system is acceptable, the engineer could show the wired type on the drawings and provide the non-wired type as an alternate. For systems of over 100 clocks, the carrier current type system is recommended.

8.12.3 Design Considerations

(1) *Size and Mounting.* Clocks are available in a wide variety of sizes, face styles, enclosure styles and mounting methods. The clocks are most commonly mounted on the wall in a semi-flush or surface mounted configuration. In either case a flush outlet box is supplied with the clock to support the clock and to accommodate a concealed attachment plug and receptacle to allow quick disconnection of the clock wiring. The plug and receptacle are three-wire grounding type for carrier current systems, but direct wired system clocks require four-wire grounding type plugs and receptacles.

Clock sizes are determined by maximum viewing distances and relations to architectural designs. Minimum recommended sizes are listed in Table 17.

(2) *Clock System Control Unit.* The clock system control unit contains the time base for the clock system. The time base is usually a quartz crystal oscillator, which is either synchronized with the 60 Hz power line, or is a completely independent, temperature compensated oscillator. The signal from the oscillator is used to drive either a master synchronous motor or a microprocessor-based computer. In the mechanical motor type unit, the system control signals are regu-

Table 17
Clock Sizes

Viewing Distance in feet (meters)	Clock Diameter in inches (centimeters)
100 (30)	12 (30)
150 (45)	15 (37.5)

lated by the rotation of the motor. The microprocessor-based units generate control signals using solid-state counting and signal generation circuits.

One of the main functions of the master control unit is correction of secondary clocks that are displaying the incorrect time due to power failure or changing to or from daylight savings time. Synchronous wired and carrier frequency type systems will provide up to 59 min slow and 55 s fast correction at the end of each hour, and will fully correct the clocks within 12 h.

The master time control unit should be provided with a standby feature to insure retention of the master time during power outages. This device may be either a spring motor or internal battery and should be capable of retaining the master time for a minimum of 12 h.

(3) *Cable Plant.* The synchronizing signals originated by the master control unit are conducted to the secondary clocks either by direct (dedicated) wiring or by carrier current signals over the 120 V, 60 Hz building secondary electrical distribution system. If a carrier current system is selected, the engineer should investigate possible interference with medical instruments and monitors caused by the high frequency carrier current signal. Power line filtering may be necessary for some equipment.

8.13 Fire Alarm Systems

8.13.1 Introduction. Fire alarm systems for health care facilities provide early detection, accurate location of the zone of origin, fire department notification, and automatic control of the heating-ventilating-air conditioning (HVAC) systems, elevators and other building systems necessary to make the building safer for its occupants. The engineer must keep in mind that the fire alarm system is designed to initiate a planned response by the staff and the fire brigade without disturbing patients unnecessarily. The fire must be placed under control quickly, because evacuation of seriously ill patients is not always possible.

8.13.2 Design Criteria. Fire alarm systems are required by Life Safety Regulations. The engineer should meet with the local Fire Marshal to determine the legal fire alarm requirements. Although beyond the scope of this standard, compartmentalization, fireproofing, and sprinklering are essential to adequate fire protection in health care facilities. The electrical engineer is not charged with the responsibility for designing architectural, structural, and fire suppression systems, but he must be aware of their importance in the overall fire protection plan.

There are three building codes generally accepted on a country-wide regional basis. They are:

(1) *Uniform Building Code.* Used by most cities west of the Mississippi.

(2) *Basic Building Code.* Used by jurisdictions east of the Mississippi River and north of the Mason-Dixon Line.

(3) *Southern Building Code.* This covers an area south of the Mason-Dixon Line.

The basic standards of the Fire Alarm Industry are NFPA (National Fire Protection Association) and UL (Underwriters' Laboratories). UL standards are equipment testing standards that are used to determine if equipment meets the functional and operational requirements of the appropriate NFPA standards, and that the equipment does not present a safety hazard if properly installed and maintained.

(a) The following NFPA standards provide appropriate guidelines for the application, installation, maintenance, and use of fire protective signaling systems.

1) ANSI/NFPA 72A-1985 — Standard for the Installation, Maintenance, and Use of Local Protective Signaling Systems for Guards Tour, Fire Alarm and Supervisory Services.

2) ANSI/NFPA 72B-1979 — Standard for the Installation, Maintenance, and Use of Auxiliary Protective Signaling Systems for Fire Alarm Service.

3) ANSI/NFPA 72C-1982 — Standard for the Installation, Maintenance, and Use of Remote Station Protective Signaling Systems.

4) ANSI/NFPA 72D-1979 — Standard for the Installation, Maintenance, and Use of Proprietary Protective Signaling Systems.

5) ANSI/NFPA 72E-1984 — Standard for Automatic Fire Detectors.

6) ANSI/NFPA 71-1982 — Standard for Central Station Systems.

7) ANSI/NFPA 90A-1985 — Standard for the Installation of Air Conditioning and Ventilating Systems.

8) ANSI/NFPA 101-1985 — Life Safety Code.

(b) In addition to codes, the following factors should be considered when designing fire alarm systems:

1) A high percentage of patients in acute care hospitals are not ambulatory. Almost all patients will require staff assistance for relocation or evacuation.

2) Most hospital patients are in a weakened condition, and many have some cardio-pulmonary deficiency. Therefore, the effect of smoke inhalation can be devastating in terms of loss of life.

3) Panic or stress resulting from a poor fire management plan can cause shock, heart attack, and stroke — particularly in the critical patient.

4) Heat from the fire or even the absence of environmental systems can jeopardize the sick patient's life. Extremes of temperature are particularly threatening to the critically ill or postoperative patient.

5) Ambulatory patients may be sedated and may not be able to evacuate or relocate themselves.

6) The high incidence of plastics, volatile liquids, and other combustibles present a unique hazard—supporting combustion and often producing toxic gases.

7) At any given time, a significant percentage of patients cannot be relocated or evacuated, because they are undergoing surgery or some other invasive procedure. For example, a 300-bed hospital can have as many as 30 such patients during a typical morning.

8) The presence of data processing, biomedical, radiological, and other electrical and electronic equipment presents a two-fold problem. First, these items, because of their high use of electricity and combustibles, increase the chances of fire. Second, when a fire starts, the loss of critical, sophisticated and expensive equipment can be great.

9) Health care facilities have a high incidence of low property damage fires which take lives.

10) About half of all hospital fires first start in service areas such as kitchens, general storage, maintenance areas, etc. Fires in patient care areas are most likely to occur in patient rooms.

8.13.3 System Types and Selection

(1) *Hard-Wired.* Hard-wired systems use individual circuits for transmission of alarm initiation signals and fire alarm audible and visual signals.

(2) *Multiplex.* When fire alarm systems are combined with emergency communication and other nonfire related systems, the number of conductors needed to interconnect all the system components is greatly increased. This has resulted in sharply escalating installation costs. Multiplex systems offer a means of reducing the installation costs, though some of the savings are offset by increased equipment complexity and cost.

Instead of requiring two conductors for each zone and four conductors for each additional riser in a zone, a multiplex system only requires a single two-wire, four-wire or coaxial cable regardless of the number of zones or risers in a zone. In addition to reducing the number of conductors required, a multiplex system also simplifies the method of wiring. Instead of requiring, for the purpose of supervision, that all the wiring for a single zone be installed in one continuous loop without any parallel branching, a multiplex system can be installed using parallel branching at any convenient location. This is made possible because NFPA Codes only permit the use of active multiplex systems which report continually the status of each device on a zone within prescribed time intervals, eliminating the need for the conventional method of continuous supervision.

Existing national codes only provide requirements for multiplex systems when used for central station or proprietary protective signaling systems. Since the requirements for these systems are more stringent than those for a local system, a system listed for proprietary system application could be used in a large highrise or multi-building health care facility. ANSI/NFPA 72D-1979 [5] no longer makes direct reference to a multiplex system. Instead, the performance characteristics of different styles of initiating device and signaling line circuits are charted in Tables 2-9.1 and 3-9.2, respectively, in reference [5]. The tables classify circuits based on their ability to indicate troubles and to transmit an alarm during specified abnormal conditions. Multiplex systems can be identified in the tables because of their use of a carrier to transmit information. The capacities of the various styles of circuits are determined by the minimum performance characteristics the circuit can meet. In practice, it is necessary to first determine the maximum number of devices, equipment, buildings, etc, to be connected to a circuit and then use the tables to determine the minimum performance requirements the circuit must meet.

Because many initiating devices in a multiplex system share a common transmission path and each device transmits its status sequentially, it is not always possible for a change of status indication to be received immediately at the control panel. Codes permit a delay, not to exceed 90 s, from the time a fire is sensed by an initiating device until it is displayed at the control panel. Since requirements can vary with each application, the acceptability of the system delay time should be determined before a particular system is specified or accepted.

Because multiplex systems offer the advantages of lower installation costs, a greater variety of features and computer compatibility, they are being used extensively in all types of buildings and should be given consideration in systems with more than 15 zones.

(3) *Combination Systems.* Codes now permit fire alarm systems to be combined with other systems not related to fire emergencies. These would include building management systems and combination communications/fire alarm systems. When these systems are used, fire alarm signals shall be clearly recognizable and shall take precedence over any other signal, even though the nonfire alarm signal is initiated first. The nonfire alarm functions of the system shall not degrade the integrity of the first alarm functions. Circuits and components which are common to fire alarm and nonfire alarm functions shall be installed and supervised in accordance with fire alarm system standards. It is most important that combination systems are listed by a nationally recognized testing laboratory for fire alarm use. When combination systems can meet the above requirements, significant cost savings can be realized when the systems are installed. Because of the importance of the fire alarm system for life safety and property protection, combination systems should be installed and serviced by trained fire alarm personnel.

8.13.4 Design Considerations

(1) *General.* Both manual and automatic fire alarm initiation should be used in health care facilities. In order to provide the best coverage, at the most reasonable cost, and with a minimum of nuisance alarms, detection should be well planned and selective.

The complete system should consist of ceiling or spot type smoke detectors, duct type smoke detectors, manual stations, and sprinkler water flow switches. Heat detectors are used selectively in place of smoke detectors where conditions may tend to cause a false alarm from smoke detectors.

(2) *Smoke Detectors.* In terms of sensitivity and number of devices, the smoke detector is the first line of defense in a health care facility. Ceiling detectors are recommended for use in corridors spaced no more than 30 ft apart or more than 15 ft from any wall. Applicable codes govern spacing at doors and dead ends. Corridor detectors serve a twofold purpose. They control the operation of cross corridor smoke doors and provide hospital-wide coverage, detecting smoke from adjacent spaces. Since fire and health codes insure that no area will be far from a corridor, all spaces are near a detector. In addition to corridors, smoke detectors should be used in high fire risk areas where false alarms are not likely, in areas requiring very early detection such as medical records, electrical rooms and computer rooms, and in areas without sprinkler heads. As mentioned before, health care facilities should be sprinklered but sometimes it is considered unwise to sprinkler areas such as intensive care units, electrical rooms or radiology rooms where an accidental discharge may jeopardize patient safety or expensive equipment. In these areas the engineer should consider using a smoke detector operated pre-action sprinkler system.

Suppliers of photoelectric and ionization type smoke detectors have long de-bated the advantages and disadvantages of their detectors for health care facili-ties. Accepted wisdom has been that hot, invisible products of combustion are detected faster by ionization detectors, and cold, visible smoke from a slow, smol-dering fire is detected better by photoelectric detectors. Photoelectric detector suppliers argue that fires likely to occur in hospitals are of the slow, smoldering type. They also contend that photoelectric detectors are best in large buildings where smoke cools when it must travel great distances before detection. It is accepted in the industry that ionization detectors are more likely to false alarm from cooking fumes, ozone produced by electrical arcing, steam, and engine exhaust. ANSI/UL 268-1981 [8] now requires all detectors to pass the same fire tests including the slow, smoldering fire test originally used only to test photo-electric detectors. This has improved the performance of the ionization detectors, but for some models it has made the detector even more sensitive and subject to more false alarms. Suppliers of ionization detectors argue that quick burning fires are more dangerous and do not produce the visible products of combustion needed for photoelectric detector operation, making their detector the logical choice. The specifier should make his or her choice based on the above factors, local and state requirements and the requirements of the particular facility. Detectors selected for use in health care facilities should be listed under ANSI/UL 268-1981 [8] and not one of the earlier standards (UL 167-1974 or UL 168-1976). Residential single or multiple station detectors listed under ANSI/UL 217-1979 should not be used.

Codes often permit smoke detectors in patient rooms, at smoke barrier doors and horizontal exits to be used in lieu of corridor detectors on patient sleeping room floors. When door closers are required, smoke detectors can be provided as a part of a combination holder/closer.

(3) *Door Closers.* The use of closers on patient room doors is a controversial issue. The use of closers almost demands that holders be provided, because nurses cannot function with all patient room doors closed at all times. If closers are required, detector control of closers can be handled in a number of ways.

(a) The smoke detector can be installed as an integral part of the holder/closer. This location permits detection of smoke in both the room and the corri-dor, but its position makes for poor detection in either case.

(b) A smoke detector can be installed in the patient room. If a fire starts in the room, the door closes and a general fire alarm is initiated, but without annunciation (usually at the nurses station or over the door) the location of the fire cannot be quickly determined and the patient can be asphyxiated before the fire is discovered. This represents a sacrifice of the patient to impede smoke spread to the corridor. Individual annunciation of each patient room is an alter-native, but an expensive one.

(c) Holders can be operated from corridor smoke detectors by zone or by individual detectors. Another alternative is to close all patient doors in the build-ing for any general alarm. However, the problem of identifying the patient room which is on fire continues. If all doors are closed, a problem with evacuation and relocation of patients is also created.

Because all of the above methods are unsatisfactory, door closers are not recommended for patient rooms. Patient room detectors offer an additional measure of protection, but at substantial increase in cost. Corridor detectors, fire rated trash cans, non-combustible mattresses and fixtures, and vigilant supervision by the nursing staff may provide adequate protection against the patient room fire.

(4) *Heat Detectors.* Heat detectors should only be used in lieu of smoke detectors in places likely to provide false alarms due to the normal occurrence of combustion products. The designer should keep in mind that sprinkler heads operate only a little slower than heat detectors and, in addition to extinguishment, provide alarm initiation and general location annunciation through flow switches. The only advantage added by the heat detector is that it can provide better annunciation. Heat detectors, flame detectors, and other special detectors are not used extensively in fully sprinklered facilities.

(5) *Sprinkler System Water Flow Switch.* In a fully sprinklered facility, the next line of protection is provided by sprinkler water flow switches. The importance of flow switches comes from the fact that virtually every space in the building has a sprinkler head that is heat actuated. If there is a problem with using the sprinkler system to detect fire and initiate an alarm, it comes from difficulties with providing accurate location annunciation. For several reasons, it is not always possible to make sprinkler zones coincident with smoke detector or building zones and smoke and fire compartments. Often, sprinkler systems are hydraulically calculated by the fire protection contractor and zoning becomes a matter of optimum water flow and lowest cost rather than conforming with building geography. If it is not possible for sprinkler zones and other zones to coincide, the engineer should ensure that:

(a) The sprinkler zone on the annunciator coincides with locations of the heads monitored by the flow switch—not the location of the flow switch itself. Sometimes, the sprinkler flow switch is not located in the same area as the sprinkler heads it monitors.

(b) The limits of the sprinkler zone are properly identified. In all cases, coordination is required among subcontractors to ensure the proper location of annunciation for alarms initiated by the sprinkler system.

(6) *Duct Detectors and Fan Shutdown.* Air conditioning and ventilating systems can potentially transmit smoke, toxic gases, and fire from one building compartment to the other. They may also provide oxygen to sustain combustion. For this reason, duct smoke detectors are generally installed in HVAC ducts to automatically exhaust smoke-laden air or to shut down air handling equipment and to provide an additional measure of detection. Duct detectors are required in supply and return plenums of air handling units 2000 ft^3/min capacity or larger but can be omitted in systems of less than 15 000 ft^3/min capacity under certain conditions. The main purpose of duct detectors is to ensure that smoke-filled air is not recirculated by air handling equipment. It is recommended that these detectors be tied into the fire alarm system to initiate a general alarm. To provide early warning, duct detectors should be used in addition to a complete area smoke detection system and never in place of area detectors. A large amount of

smoke will generally be required to activate a duct detector because the smoke-filled air entering the duct from the fire area is mixed with and diluted by large volumes of clean air entering the duct from other areas. Duct detectors should be installed in the return duct at a point before the return air is exhausted from the building or the introduction of outside air. Duct detectors in the main supply duct are installed downstream from the last filter (to detect smoke from a filter fire) and upstream from humidifiers (to prevent false alarms). Some local or state authorities require additional detectors in the duct system to detect smoke before it is diluted. Additional supply duct detectors provide little or no additional protection and are not recommended. Additional detectors in the return exhaust ducts can provide additional protection when installed in the duct system at dampers or other strategic locations to detect smoke near the source before the air is diluted by air from collateral ducts. Although providing an additional measure of protection, it is questionable whether additional detectors are worth the additional investment — particularly in a fully sprinklered building or buildings with area smoke detectors mounted on 30-foot centers in the corridors. Most codes dealing with duct detectors in the duct system (not at air units) are not specific and only imply intent. Therefore, local interpretations vary widely. It is recommended that all detectors (both duct and area) in a system serve to shut down all fans and close all dampers in the affected system. The simplest and most reliable mechanism for this purpose is a pneumatic electric valve used to close pneumatic smoke dampers. Each duct and area detector zone module in the fire alarm control panel is wired back to a fan control circuit and serves to shut down the fans serving the fire alarm zone when smoke is detected. When the fans shut down, the PE (Pneumatic Electric) valve is deenergized and dampers close. If electric dampers are used, wiring must be provided for each damper. Again, it is recommended that every detector in the system — both area and duct — serve to shut down the fans and close all dampers on the affected HVAC system only.

Facility-wide fan system shutdown is not recommended, but shutting down only fan systems which serve the affected building zone is preferred. HVAC systems not only provide heating and cooling, which are especially important to critical patients, but also humidification and proper air balance, which are crucial to infection control. It must also be remembered that parts of the facility not directly affected by the fire must continue to function normally as patients are relocated and efforts are made to control the fire.

(7) *Smoke Evacuation Systems.* Smoke evacuation systems are becoming increasingly popular in commercial and institutional buildings. These systems use return and exhaust fans to evacuate smoke-filled air with the outside air dampers fully open to provide makeup air. Several things should be considered before designing a smoke evacuation system into a health care facility as follows:

(a) Is a smoke evacuation system required by state and local codes?

(b) Will patients be subjected to sudden, significant changes in temperature from the outside air? As mentioned earlier, the lives of critically ill patients can depend on favorable environmental conditions.

(c) Extremely cold, outside air can freeze coils in the duct system — especially cooling coils.

(d) Smoke evacuation systems tend to complicate the HVAC control system.

(e) Additional generator capacity may be required to serve the fan loads.

It is recommended that warnings about subjecting patients to cold outside air and the potential for freezing the coils be included on the smoke evacuation control panel.

(8) *Manual Pull Station.* The final measure of protection in a fire detection system is provided by manual pull stations. In addition to those placed at exits and in corridors as required by codes, it is recommended that manual stations be provided at all nurses stations. It is quite likely that the nurse will either see fire or smoke in his or her patient care area or the first report of fire will come over the patient nurse call system. Since the nurse's job is to assist with patient evacuation, he or she will not want to walk to an exit in order to initiate an alarm. Breakglass stations (stations with a glass restraining rod) are recommended as a deterrent to false alarms. Recent requirements for the handicapped prohibit mounting manual stations out of the reach of children. Manual stations are an important part of the fire alarm system and should not be left out no matter how sophisticated the automatic system. In addition to exits and nurses stations, pull stations should be installed so that horizontal travel distance to a pull station is never more than 200 ft.

With more reliance being placed on automatic detectors instead of manual stations, the trend in recent years has been away from coded fire alarm systems. Coding of automatic detectors is usually done by zone using transmitters located in the system control panel. Manual stations usually generate a coded signal mechanically utilizing a coding mechanism located within the station. Coded systems require more maintenance than noncoded systems and are more expensive. Instead of relying on coded signals to inform the fire brigade of the fire location, facilities generally use a continuously monitored annunciator. The annunciator station has access to telephone, paging, or other communication systems to inform the fire brigade and others of the fire location. Normally, persons responsible for evacuation of patients and in-house fire suppression can be notified within seconds after an alarm is received. Therefore, a coded alarm is not generally required. Still, some fire alarm engineers and facility personnel feel a coded system can save additional seconds in responding to a fire because a coded alarm system permits the fire brigade to dispatch immediately to the affected area without waiting for a call from the telephone operator or for paged instructions. All things considered, the noncoded system with annunciation is recommended for most health care facilities, particularly if there are more than 10 fire alarm zones.

Audible alarm signals can be chimes, small bells, or electronically generated sounds such as the slow whoop. The slow whoop is not recommended for health care facilities because it can be frightening to patients. Visible alarms are required and shall be installed with all audible alarms.

Since the fire alarm signal is primarily used to initiate a planned response by the staff, it is important for the alarm to be heard in all parts of the building, including mechanical rooms. This might require the use of different types of audible signal devices in different locations (for example, chimes in nurses stations, horns in mechanical rooms). However, this is not always possible because some authorities require the alarm sound to be the same throughout the system. The engineer should also consider that horns in mechanical areas adjacent to patient care areas may alarm patients unnecessarily.

(9) *Alarm Signals.* Presignal, zoned voice alarm, and other systems which do not provide facility-wide general alarm signals are not recommended for health care facilities unless there are some unusual circumstances. These systems may be considered for the campus-type facility where there is no chance of a fire spreading from building to building. Facility-wide alarm signals may also be undesirable in the extremely large facility where the number of occupants makes the building-wide evacuation or relocation of patients, visitors, and staff undesirable or the sheer number of automatic devices makes the incidence of false alarms high. The decision to go with something less than a health facility-wide general alarm is one that must be taken up with inspection authorities and accreditation agencies.

Presignal systems are no longer common but voice alarm systems which automatically direct prerecorded messages to selective parts of the building are becoming increasingly popular — especially in high-rise buildings. Most building codes require voice alarm systems for high-rise business and residential occupancies, but do not require them for high-rise institutional occupancies. The voice alarm is intended to relocate or evacuate occupants of a large building one, two or three floors at a time — thus avoiding a panic situation in crowded stairwells. A voice alarm system also assumes that the building's occupants can respond to voice instructions under their own power, which is not true for health care facilities. Since patients must rely on staff help to relocate or evacuate, voice alarm systems are not always recommended for health care facilities that have an adequately trained staff and a well-maintained paging system. If the paging system is used to broadcast instructions during a fire situation the engineer should verify that paging speakers are located in all areas of the facility.

(10) *Elevator Control.* Standards for elevator installations in multi-story buildings require the elevator controller be interlocked with the fire alarm system to provide elevator recall. Although these standards intend for the elevator to be controlled by elevator lobby smoke detectors, many authorities require elevator recall to be initiated by any general fire alarm. As stated before, health care facility fires are unique in many ways. The fire brigade attempts to control the fire while relocating patients to safe areas of the hospital. Although there may be a fire in one wing of the hospital, operation of the hospital must continue in other areas. Elevators can be very useful in relocating patients and dealing with other emergencies. So, the automatic controlling of elevators from the fire alarm control panel on any general fire alarm is not recommended, but may be required by code.

Requirements for a vertical fire alarm zone, incorporating all of the upper (second floor and above) floor lobby smoke detectors for a particular elevator bank are frequently encountered. With all lobby detectors on a single initiating circuit, elevator recall can be indicated on the fire alarm annunciator. However, the floor of the fire would not be known unless adjacent smoke detectors sense the fire and make the proper annunciation. Therefore, the vertical zone is not recommended unless other detectors connected to the floor zone are installed in the vicinity of the elevator lobby to provide floor annunciation. An alternative to the vertical zone would be to use lobby detectors with auxiliary relay contacts and to place each lobby detector on the same zone with other detectors on that floor. Each lobby detector's auxiliary relay contact would be used for elevator recall. These contacts are connected in parallel and two wires connected to the elevator bank control circuit.

Elevator control systems are designed so that smoke detected on any upper floor will cause the elevator control circuit to go into the recall mode. All elevators in the elevator bank return to the ground floor and cease operation with the doors open. The elevators can only be returned to operation by means of a fireman's key. If an elevator is on an upper floor when the sequence begins, its door closes and will not be permitted to open until the elevator reaches the ground floor. The drawback with this system is that the elevator passengers could be exposed to danger if the first floor elevator lobby were involved in the fire. For this reason, newer systems are available which stop the car on the second floor if a first floor lobby detector senses smoke. The system would stop the car on the third floor if the first and second floor lobby detectors senses smoke, and so forth.

(11) *Emergency Communication Systems.* Emergency communications systems can be useful in high-rise health care facilities. These systems usually consist of a central control station, usually located on the ground floor, portable telephones, and strategically located telephone jacks for firemen's use in stairways, at exit doors, at sprinkler system valves and hose connections. In addition, a corridor and lobby paging system is used for transmitting "live" or prerecorded messages to the building occupants. These systems are generally required by building codes for high-rise residential and business occupancies. Although they are not always adopted for institutional occupancies, state authorities frequently require them. These systems can be a valuable tool for firefighters if the firefighters desire to use them and are properly trained in their operation.

(12) *Annunciation.* Although a requirement for location annunciation in health care facilities is not apparent, it is strongly recommended that a zoned, backlighted or graphic annunciator be installed where it can be monitored 24 hours a day. This location will usually be the telephone operator location, a nurses station, or a security office. This location should have access to a telephone and a paging microphone. Duct detectors for each fan system, each manual station, and each sprinkler water flow switch should be separately zoned and annunciated by a separate light on the annunciator. Smoke detectors should have a light for each building zone as a minimum. Graphic annunciators are preferred if the graphics are prepared with sufficient detail and areas of the facility are properly labeled. Graphic annunciators can be confusing if sufficient detail is not included or if the person doing the monitoring is unfamiliar with the facility layout. Graphic annunciators tend to be more expensive than backlighted annunciators and are difficult

and expensive to modify when expanding the facility or changing the fire alarm system. If zones are properly labeled, backlighted annunciators are adequate for most health care facilities.

(13) *System Integrity.* Applicable codes deal with requirements for protection and supervision, so these aspects will not be dwelled on here. It should suffice to say that all alarm initiating and indicating circuits must be supervised to detect a single ground or open fault in the circuit wiring that would interfere with normal operation. Most fire alarm systems used today utilize Class B circuits that may not be capable of initiating or sounding an alarm when the initiating or indicating circuit is in a "trouble" condition. Class A circuits are designed to deliver alarms even with a single grounded or open conductor and are therefore recommended. This is generally accomplished by using special zone modules in the control panel and looping the circuit conductors back to the control panel instead of terminating it with an end-of-line resistor after the last device.

Health care facilities generally have a large number of area type smoke detectors on ceilings — especially in corridors. Class B initiating circuits go into trouble (from an open circuit) when a smoke detector is removed and may not be able to initiate a fire alarm signal. This is of particular significance if initiating circuits combine several types of devices such as smoke detectors, pull stations, and flow switches. In a large hospital, there is high probability that at any given time a detector will be out for repair or a circuit will be otherwise in trouble alarm. Combining devices can mean that all alarm initiating devices in a particular building zone may be incapable of initiating a fire alarm signal when that zone is in trouble. It is recommended that each type of device within each building zone can be placed on a separate initiating circuit, so a trouble condition on one circuit will not affect the operation of other types of devices in that part of the building. If devices are to be combined, it is recommended that a Class A circuit be installed.

Placing different types of devices within each building zone and each sprinkler system valve status switch on individually supervised circuits with proper location annunciation can increase the speed with which the staff can respond to a trouble condition.

If an annunciator is required to be installed by the authority having jurisdiction, the annunciator must be fully supervised. Supplementary annunciators are not required to be supervised.

(14) *Power Supply.* Fire codes require that all fire alarm systems have a primary power supply and a trouble signal power supply (usually taken from a different phase of the power system from the primary power supply using two single-pole circuit breakers). If systems are used to automatically notify the fire department, a secondary power supply shall be provided and sized to operate under normal load for 60 h. Codes for health care facilities require the fire alarm system to be connected to the life safety branch of the emergency system, which is supplied by the primary and secondary power sources. When this is done, batteries are not generally required. Since there is some controversy concerning the need for batteries with generators, the designer should check with the authority having jurisdiction. If batteries are required, they must have 4 h capacity.

8.14 Security Systems

8.14.1 Introduction. Electrical and electronic devices that provide monitoring and security detection are used primarily to supplement passive physical and staff monitoring provisions. Intrusion devices are used to monitor the security of property within the facility in areas where high risk of theft is probable.

8.14.2 Design Criteria. Security systems are not required by codes but are justified for personal safety of staff, patients, and public from violent or criminal acts and to reduce property loss. The following relates to application of devices to solve security problems:

(1) *Metal Detectors.* These are intended to prevent inadvertent or premeditated loss of valuable hardware, instrumentation, movable equipment, etc, which may be intermixed in soiled linen or refuse being removed from a facility. Metal detection, X-ray, or other detection systems which are not labor-intensive may be considered at all loading (discharge) platforms which would screen all carts or material handling equipment carrying material from the facility.

(2) *Intrusion Detectors.* Intrusion detector equipment should be considered for pharmacy dispensing areas, drug vaults, narcotic cabinets, radiology, silver recovery, bulk storage rooms, gas storage rooms, cashiers, emergency exits and medical records.

Movable protection devices can be any number and kind of security sensors which are removed from their circuit during times the protected area is occupied. This is done so that they do not constantly signal the presence of authorized personnel working in the area. Examples are switches on doors, relay contacts of motion detectors, capacitance detectors, or photoelectric beams, pressure mats, etc.

(3) *Closed Circuit Television.* Television systems are used for monitoring personnel to help control access to facilities. Security guards monitoring television systems may have an opportunity to locate or identify intruders and prevent violent or destructive activities. Television cameras are located in high traffic areas like main lobbies where door switches are useless. They are commonly used in waiting areas, cashiers counters, at loading docks and in parking areas. Television security electronics usually provide remote control of cameras and switching control of video signals. Refer to Section 8.16 for design criteria.

8.14.3 Security Sensors. A security sensor is any detection device ranging from a simple door switch to a sophisticated solid-state motion detector. Examples of security sensors are as follows:

(1) *Mechanical Switches.* Switches, generally with spring-loaded levers or plungers, that operate when a door, window, or cabinet cover is removed or opened.

(2) *Magnetic Switches.* These are used to supervise the position of movable openings such as doors and windows. A magnet on the movable portion operates a switch on the fixed or frame portion. Reliable operation can be expected.

(3) *Balanced Magnetic Switches.* These utilize a bias magnet inside the switch housing along with the standard magnet on the movable portion. They will respond to an excessive magnetic field imposed on them as well as a reduced field. They are most difficult to compromise with an external magnet.

(4) *Foil (Tape) and Screens.* Foil is a thin strip of low ductility tin-lead material adhered to a glass surface to detect breakage. Cracking or breakage of the glass interrupts the circuit current flowing through the foil. Screens are grids built with wooden dowels containing a groove in which a fine hard-drawn copper wire is embedded. The grids are used as an electrical barrier over openings. If a dowel is broken, the wire breaks, interrupting the circuit current in the same manner as foil.

(5) *Pressure Mats.* When stepped upon, these devices close an electrical contact. They make an excellent intrusion detection device since they can be concealed under carpeting or scatter rugs. They are stable and reliable devices and when used properly, have an extremely low false-alarm rate. They have SPST switching action, providing only a cross (short) on the protection circuit.

(6) *Photoelectric Beams.* Beams of light (usually infrared) which, when interrupted, cause an alarm, since a relay in the photocell receiver will deenergize.

(7) *Laser Beam Devices.* These operate somewhat like photoelectric beams, except that the light sources are solid-state devices (such as light-emitting diodes [LED's] or gallium arsenide laser sources).

(8) *Audio Detection.* Sensitive microphones are installed in the area to be protected to detect sounds of intrusion. Sounds that are picked up are amplified and operate an alarm relay if they are loud enough and are repetitive beyond a preset count. Audio detection operates best in quiet areas such as vaults.

(9) *Ultrasonic.* This system fills an area with high-pitched sound waves (above human hearing) and detects the disturbance of the sound pattern when motion occurs in the area.

(10) *Infrared Body Heat Detection.* This motion detection system is basically optical since the detector "sees" a moving human source of infrared energy (98 °F) against a background at room temperature (usually around 72 °F).

8.14.4 Design Considerations. Intrusion detectors should have:

(1) An internal, automatic charging dc standby power supply with primary ac power operation.

(2) A remote, key-operated activation/deactivation switch installed outside protected areas adjacent to the room entrance door frame.

(3) An integral capability for the attachment of wiring for remote alarm and intrusion indicator equipment (visual or audio) to provide annunciation at a security office or central control center.

Where security systems affect personnel safety or protect valuable items or information, the engineer may specify a supervised security system. The electronics of these systems indicate trouble when shorts or open wires develop. The sensitivity to supervisory current changes may be increased to make these systems difficult to compromise.

8.15 Facility Monitoring

8.15.1 Introduction. Health care facilities contain complex systems critical to patient care that need to be monitored. This section discusses the code required and optional monitoring systems.

8.15.2 Medical Gas Alarms

(1) *Introduction.* Medical gas alarms are a required part of a hospital's system for distribution of nonflammable medical gases. The requirement is established by ANSI/NFPA 56F-1983 [2], which states: "A master alarm system shall be provided to monitor the operation and condition of the source of supply, the reserve (if any), and the pressure in the main line of the medical gas system."

The gases covered by this standard include, but are not limited to, oxygen, nitrous oxide, medical compressed air, carbon dioxide, helium, nitrogen, and mixtures of such gases. The alarm system is required to detect two classes of system problems: abnormal line pressures (high or low) and low gas supply.

(2) *Design Considerations.* Alarm equipment such as alarm panels and actuating switches are normally supplied as part of the medical gas distribution system (piping, manifolds, gas columns, etc). The engineer should closely coordinate his work with the supplier of the gas distribution equipment. The engineer's responsibilities normally include the following areas:

(a) Alarm system ac power

(b) Alarm panel locations

(c) Interconnecting alarm signal wiring

ANSI/NFPA 56F-1983 [2] requires the ac power source for the gas alarm system to be the life safety branch of the hospital electrical system.

All medical gas alarm systems are required to include two master alarm signal panels, which will display alarms related to the source of gas supply for the entire system. ANSI/NFPA 56F-1983 [2] requires one master panel to be located "...in the office or principal working area of the individual responsible for the maintenance of the medical gas system..." such as the maintenance supervisor or hospital engineer. The second panel shall be located "to assure continuous surveillance, at the telephone switchboard, the security office, or at another suitable location." The intent of these requirements is to insure "continuous, responsible surveillance" of the medical gas system, since the life of the hospital's patients may well depend on continuous delivery of the medical gases.

In larger hospitals, where medical gases may be distributed to widely separated areas of use, an area alarm panel will be required. ANSI/NFPA 56F-1983 [2] specifically lists areas where medical gas may be supplied, and where an area alarm system must therefore be installed:

(a) Anesthetizing locations

(b) Vital life support areas

(c) Critical care areas

(d) Intensive care areas

(e) Post-anesthesia recovery

(f) Coronary care units

(g) Operating and delivery rooms

The area alarm panel shall be installed "...at the nurses station or other suitable location near the point of use which will provide responsible surveillance."

The engineer must make provisions for the signal wiring between the alarm panels and the actuating (pressure sensing) switches. The switch locations will be determined by the supplier of the gas distribution equipment. The engineer's responsibility will normally be limited to providing support and protection for the signal wiring in the form of raceways and cable trays.

ANSI/NFPA 56F-1983 [2] contains these additional provisions which should be noted by the engineer:

(a) Air compressors and vacuum pumps shall not be installed in rooms or enclosures used for the storage of gas cylinders.

(b) Electrical equipment and fixtures located in cylinder storage areas shall be located at least 5 ft above the floor, to avoid damage from the cylinders.

8.15.3 Refrigeration Alarms

(1) *Introduction.* Hospitals will frequently contain one or more of the following items of refrigeration equipment: blood bank refrigeration, donor organ refrigeration, pharmacy refrigeration, laboratory refrigeration, kitchen refrigeration, kitchen freezer, and morgue refrigeration.

Effective operation of a hospital will depend on continuous and proper operation of these refrigerators, and the installation of refrigerator alarms is an important step toward insuring proper operation. The alarms can provide an indication of loss of power, as well as internal temperatures that are too high or too low.

(2) *Design Considerations.* Alarm equipment locations and power requirements should be obtained from the refrigeration equipment supplier. Separate alarm systems will normally be furnished with each type of refrigeration equipment. The master monitor station and its associated temperature sensor are normally located at the refrigeration enclosure while remote monitors are normally located where continuous surveillance is available, such as at the hospital control center. The engineer should provide raceway for the multiconductor cable between the master and remote monitor stations. Power for the alarm system should be obtained from a critical branch circuit, and in the case of blood bank and organ bank refrigerators, this is required by code.

8.15.4 Emergency Generator Monitoring.

An emergency generator monitoring system is required by ANSI/NFPA 99-1984 [6]. The annunciator shall be located at the central control center. See 5.4.5 for design criteria.

8.15.5 Energy Monitoring and Control Systems

(1) *Introduction.* EMCS (energy monitoring and control systems) are being used as the key to a successful energy conservation program. Such systems, in addition to saving energy, may: protect and limit damage to equipment; allow malfunctions to be corrected with minimal service interruption; operate equipment only when necessary, thus extending equipment life; cut down on the number of operating personnel required; improve maintenance management; and perform other related functions such as fire alarm annunciation, security, life safety, and other real time event-initiated functions.

Various levels of control are available as follows:

(a) Basic local controls. These are equipment control systems supplied/ recommended by the equipment system supplier. These systems turn equipment on or off depending on sensor (temperature, humidity, pressure) activated messages. A larger, more sophisticated EMCS should incorporate local controls into its system.

(b) Single building system. A microcomputer is used to control the independent local controls of several pieces of equipment in one building. In the event of a failure of the microcomputer, the local controls shall control the equipment.

(c) Distributed processing control systems. These systems employ a minicomputer that controls numerous limited area systems or the single building system or both. Mass storage of information is used to keep records and support a sophisticated software system. In the event of minicomputer failure, the basic local controls will control the equipment.

(2) *Design Considerations.* Refer to ANSI/IEEE Std 241-1983 [1] for design of ECMS.

8.16 Television Systems

8.16.1 Introduction. In its most general form, a health care television system is utilized to transmit visual and, when desired, audio data over cable circuits, rather than via antennas. In addition to the cable plant and receivers, a health care television system will usually include a master antenna or a connection to a local cable franchise to obtain commercial entertainment programming or both. Portable video cameras and video tape recorders are occasionally used as program sources. This describes a fairly simple MATV (Master Antenna TV) system, that would be installed in a nursing home or small hospital.

Television systems in larger clinics and hospitals become more complex with the addition of specialized CCTV (Closed Circuit TV) systems. Such systems may include a central control and equipment room, production studio, fixed video cameras, or a satellite earth station.

Health care applications of television systems may be categorized as follows:

(1) Entertainment and Education Programming. This system distributes entertainment programming from a number of sources to patient rooms and visitor areas. A secondary function is the distribution of educational programming to patients and staff.

(2) Interdepartmental Communication. There are a number of specialized CCTV systems in this category that provide two-way, audio-visual communication between physicians and support departments, such as pathology and radiology.

(3) Patient Monitoring. This category also includes several specialized CCTV systems. Such systems provide visual contact with patients in intensive care units, emergency treatment rooms, and in certain areas of radiation therapy units.

(4) Security Monitoring. A CCTV system, with fixed video cameras and a central monitoring point with continuous surveillance augments security systems.

8.16.2 Design Criteria

(1) *General.* Television systems are not required by codes. Rapid changes are taking place in the whole field of television that are affecting its use in health care facilities. A vast number of new program services are becoming available, not only to the general public, but also to special groups through the new technical facilities such as satellite earth stations, microwave interconnections, and improved videotape distribution. Viewing is shifting to new program sources and to Pay-TV.

(2) *Entertainment and Education Programming.* Television systems consisting of a TV signal distribution system are recommended in virtually all health care

facilities for distribution. The usual programs from local broadcast systems are available.

(3) *Controlled Viewing.* Some form of directed programming, sometimes referred to as addressable terminals, is essential to the needs of Health Care Facilities. The concept of individually addressable television receiving sets clearly matches the need to limit the viewing. The question is cost and the maturity of the design. It is recommended that the health care facility use the channel blanking feature of the TV receivers that provide manual means to control the reception of up to 36 channels with a system of 54 to 300 MHz bandwidth. The active channels on television receivers can be selected at the lower front panel. This method can provide a simple and inexpensive method of manual selection of the channels allowed for reception at any receiver. The disadvantage is that a member of the facility's staff must go to each patient room to make the manual selection, which can be time consuming in a 300-patient-room facility.

(4) *Computerized Directed Programming.* This system provides a central control panel where one can direct programming to each television set in the health care facility. In addition, the system can keep track of time used and provide a printout for billing information. Patients can be billed for full length movies and patient education programs. It is recommended that computerized directed programming be purchased when it is cost effective. This means that it will pay for itself within three years from manpower savings, and new revenue from movies and patient education. This will happen when the designs have matured and the system costs have decreased. However, the engineer should consider specification of TV sets for near-term use, which incorporate compatability with computerized directed programming.

(5) *TV Sets and Recorders*

(a) Color Television Systems. Use color television systems only for broadcast systems, for hospital surgery, or where color need has been justified.

(b) Television Projection Systems. Television projection systems are used for large group viewing for staff education. The type of lighting should be adjustable. These systems will accept signals from MATV antennas or from a connected closed-circuit system.

(c) Recording Equipment. Use video tapes where instant playbacks are desired, for further studies, or permanent records. Use broadcast type cameras or high quality two-to-one ratio interlaced cameras to send signals to video tape recorders.

(6) *Medical Staff Education.* The health care facilities size and teaching requirements will determine the criteria for Educational TV. Pictures of surgical procedures have long been an important educational tool among surgeons. It has been traditional to cut and edit these films to make them fit into a suitable time frame or subject category for showing at professional meetings. In recent years live television has been a feature of national or regional meetings, by which means a large audience, usually situated in a hotel lecture room or other meeting hall, can watch a surgical procedure being carried out at a remote hospital. Modern television techniques such as split-screen, instant replay, slow motion, and added animation, enhance the educational value of these showings. With the advent of

lower-priced equipment, surgical television is beginning to take a more prominent place as an intramural or institutional educational instrument. With standard equipment, operative procedures can be transmitted live or shown as taped films in the hospital auditorium, classroom, and at department meetings. Cineradiography done during surgical procedures can be shown in continuity with the operative film. Tapes of such procedures, combining views of the operation, the pathologic section, intraoperative X-rays, and noncommitant commentary of the surgeon, and his or her team and consultants comprise a record unsurpassed by any other medium. Appropriately edited, this type of audio-video record may form the basis of a teaching library, especially valuable in instances of rare or unusual cases, and possibly in medicolegal situations.

(7) *Pathology Consultation.* A two-way audio-video system between the frozen-section laboratory and the operating room can enable the surgeon to communicate directly with the pathologist and permit examination of a microscopic slide in consultation with the pathologist by video without leaving the operating table. It also provides the pathologist with a view of the pathologic lesion *in situ* without entry into the operating room. A television camera may be mounted in or on the surgical light for this purpose. With a camera situated over the cutting table, the surgeon can direct the pathologist or technician as to precisely how to section a specimen, if necessary, without leaving the operating room. In general, a two-way audio-video system between operating room and the frozen-section laboratory should eliminate the need to bring the pathologist into the operating room; it should permit the surgeon, by simply viewing the video screens in the operating room, to supervise the sectioning of a specimen and to peer into the microscope without leaving the operating room.

(a) *Radiology Consultation.* As an aid to diagnosis, an audio-video hook-up between the operating room and the X-ray department permits X-rays to be viewed on the television screen in the operating room. This method holds several distinct advantages over the present practice of locating the films, carrying them into the operating room, sorting out the most appropriate films to mount on the view box, and risking such annoyances as not getting a good view from the operating table, mounting the wrong films, possibly contaminating clean objects by inadvertent contact, and misplacing films in transit between the operating room and X-ray department. Where fluoroscopy X-ray equipment containing a video camera is employed in surgical procedures, the X-ray image may be displayed on a monitor in the Radiology Department for interpretation.

(b) *Staff Bulletin Board.* The hospital should first evaluate the doctor's register system as these systems overlap. The videotext concept should be considered, by which literally hundreds of pages of printed or graphic information could be called up individually at many receivers.

(8) *Patient Monitoring*

(a) *Intensive Care Unit.* Hospital regulations require that each ICU patient be visible from a nursing station; however, it is possible to meet this regulation and still not have a clinically useful view of the patient. Although one can argue that there is very little useful information derived from a televised view of the patient, as compared to information provided by the physiological monitors, the fact is that many nurses feel more comfortable with closed-circuit television. The video picture of the patient is a reminder that the patient is a human being, and it can be particularly useful in large units. When provided, the general room illumination should be adjustable with a dimmer control switch to enable the lighting level to be reduced at night for patient comfort.

(b) *Radiation Therapy*. Some radiation therapy procedures require the use of heavy shielding between the patient and the equipment operator. At the same time, it is important to position the patient precisely with respect to the radiation beam, and insure that the patient does not move during the exposure. This problem is often resolved with a monochrome CCTV system, installed to give the equipment operator a clear view of the patient and the beam reference marks. It is desirable to furnish the video camera with a zoom lens, and the camera resolution should be adequate to allow precise determination of the patient's position. The camera and monitor locations should be coordinated with the hospital. The installation of the video cable between the camera and the monitor shall be designed to preserve the shielding performance of the radiation shielding.

(9) *Satellite Receiving Station*. A satellite station is recommended when revenue is generated from satellite receiver programming. For example, movies could be shown to patients for a fee.

(10) *Security*. The criteria for security surveillance by camera is determined by the size of the facility. See Section 8.14.

8.16.3 Design Considerations

(1) *Cable Plant*. Basic CATV (Community Antenna TV) design concepts are recommended for the television distribution system as distinguished from the somewhat simpler concepts sometimes used in small MATV (Master Antenna TV) systems. The added costs of the CATV methods are insignificantly small because materials cost 20% more but labor costs are less for a 10% net additional cost. The advantages are that the system can be extended or otherwise added upon without redesign and a minimum disruption of the plant or its operation. Leakage of signals (in or about) is minimized and interaction between receiving sets is minimal.

The signal distribution system should consist of a cable network with .412 in trunk/feeder cable providing the main signal path. At appropriate intervals, the cable will have directional taps spliced in to provide a tap-off point for the drop cables, which are the final link to the television receiver. A distribution amplifier may be necessary to distribute the signals at the proper level. Each directional tap will require two .412 in connectors. The number of outlets of each tap will be determined by the location in the building. Also, the attenuation of the tap is determined by the signal level at the tap location.

The type of amplifier will be determined by the signal level that can be delivered to the central control and equipment room.

(2) *Master Antenna*. The engineer should make a list of signals to be received, and design accordingly. The type of antenna required is determined by the frequencies covered and their signal strength. Several antennas may be needed to cover all required frequencies.

(a) *Location and Orientation.* The exact location and orientation of antennas are determined by a signal strength survey.

(b) *Lightning Protection.* Follow requirements for lightning protection given in ANSI/NFPA 70-1984 (Article 810) [3]. Where lightning protection must be installed, use arresters and ground them effectively.

(3) *Amplifiers.* Use preamplifiers and amplifiers as follows:

(a) *Preamplifiers.* Use preamplifiers when incoming signals are too weak to be accepted by the amplifier.

(b) *Amplifiers.* Use amplifiers for signal amplification as required to overcome distribution system losses and provide suitable output. A broadband amplifier may be suitable if it can cover all incoming channels and maintain adequate signal level inputs to the distribution system; otherwise single channel amplifiers for each input may be necessary.

(4) *CCTV Camera Selection.* A modern camera is a small, compact unit with a minimum number of circuits and comprises a self-contained, one-package system providing the following features as appropriate:

(a) *Interlace.* Interlace describes the condition where the lines in the second of two successive fields in a picture tube are spaced between the lines in the first field. Use this action where fine details are read. Use interlace wherever a system supplies standard TV receivers (antenna systems).

(b) *Random Interlace.* Use a random interlace camera (self-contained unit) where lines in successive fields may or may not be spaced between each other. Use the camera in all applications where detailed observation is not required, or where videotape recorders will not be used.

(c) *Picture Details.* Picture details (resolution) are expressed in "lines." Commercial television in the United States uses a 525-line system which is one whose distinguishable details are based on 525 horizontal scans of each picture. This is the minimum amount of resolution to be provided. Provide more resolution only where required for acceptable viewing, such as the necessity of 800 lines for surgical observation.

(5) *Camera Mounting.* Use indoor and outdoor mountings as follows:

(a) *Indoor.* Use an air-cooled housing where temperatures exceed those of camera specifications. In studios, the heat from the stage lighting makes air conditioning necessary. Use explosion-proof housings for viewing hazardous areas. Use pan and tilt mounts (manual or remote) when cameras view more than one area. Use standard tripods on cameras for portable use.

(b) *Outdoor.* Always use a weatherproof housing. Never face cameras toward the sun at any time of the day. Avoid picking up reflections from glass or water, if possible.

(6) *Subject Viewing.* Locate a camera so that desired areas, objects, or subject receive the maximum benefits from available lighting.

(a) *Lens Selection.* Choose a lens that fits the scene. A fixed lens limits the field of view to one scene. Lens turrets have the advantage of handling three or four lenses with varying focal lengths (normal view, wide angle, and varying degrees of telephoto). A zoom lens permits varying the focal length without loss of subject viewing during the change.

(b) *Operation.* Cameras which are easily accessible may be controlled manually. The more expensive remote control should be provided where local operation is not feasible. Remote control should be located and coordinated with other operating devices involved in the application being viewed on an adjacent monitor.

(c) *Video Switching.* Provide video switching where more than one camera must be viewed on a monitor.

(7) *Subject Lighting.* Distinguishable details depend on scene contrasts, camera resolution, and monitor resolving powers.

(a) *Required Lighting Levels.* Use the same light levels needed by the human eye for clear visibility. Minimum lighting incident on the scene should be at least 20 fc (20 dekalux).

(b) *Additional Lighting.* Plan lighting so that a minimum number of "hot spots" are seen from camera locations. Illuminate the complete scene for viewing.

(c) *Automatic Iris.* An automatic iris is necessary on the camera to control amount of light focused on the picture tube or vidicon. It automatically compensates the camera gain for illumination increases from 10 to 10 000 fc (10 to 10 000 dekalux).

(8) *Monitor Selection.* Monitors should have the same resolution and type of interlace as cameras. Locate monitors for minimum light reflections on tube faces. Avoid vertical mountings. Use circular polarized face plates where ambient lighting is high. For distances between monitors and viewers, see Table 18. Use multiple monitors for large group viewing.

(9) *Studio.* The studio layout should be arranged for efficiency and storage considerations. The studio should be large enough to show a patient in bed. The design must consider acoustical criteria. Lighting should include track lights and some floor pedestals, which will flexibly provide key, fill and backlighting for various sets. Selective dimming will be needed on certain circuits. Special cooling will be required.

(10) *Chapel.* If the camera in the chapel is to be used several times a week it should be permanently mounted with a remotely controlled zoom lens on the camera. If the camera is used in the chapel only once per week it should be easily detachable from its wall mounting so that it can be used the rest of the week in other places.

(11) *Operating Room.* In recent years, the camera on a floor-standing boom and the hand-held camera have been replaced by more appropriate installations.

Table 18
Recommended Minimum Monitor Sizes

Number of Viewers	Distance in feet (meters)	Monitor Size in inches (centimeters)
1	10 (3)	8 (20)
2	15 (4.5)	14 (35)
3	20 (6)	17 (43)
4	30 (9)	21 (53)
5	35 (10.5)	24–27 (60–70)

The television camera over the operating table may be mounted on an extension arm attached to the stem of the surgical light and outfitted with sterilizable detachable handles. Some manufacturers of surgical lights provide a model with a television camera mounted in the center pod of the light.

Another approach for surgical suites of any size is a portable unit, consisting of a console containing videotape recorder and viewing screen on which is mounted an adjustable boom to hold the television camera. The camera should be remotely controllable for pan, tilt and zoom.

(12) *Satellite Receiving Station.* The satellite receiving station can be located either at ground level or on the building roof with a clear view of the satellite arc. Cable trays or ducts are required from central control to the roof and to a convenient outside location at ground level. If roof mounting is selected, structural reinforcement will probably be necessary because it weighs about one ton.

8.17 Sound Reinforcement Systems

8.17.1 Introduction. Sound reinforcement systems are electronic systems, providing sound pickup, processing, amplification and reproduction, intended to reinforce an acoustic sound source within the room or space where the source is located. Many sound reinforcement systems also reproduce recorded material during slide or movie productions.

8.17.2 Design Criteria. A system is required to improve signal intelligibility where distances, obstructions or acoustical conditions limit the intelligibility of an acoustical source (that is, talker, performer, etc). The sound system shall maintain adequate direct sound to reverberant field ratio (for clarity) and improve the signal to noise ratio (volume). A good sound system should provide a natural sound that appears to originate at the acoustic source.

Sound reinforcement systems are required in auditoriums, meeting rooms, lecture rooms and chapels. In special cases, a large space may be used for several purposes and a sound system may be required, for instance, in a cafeteria or large lobby.

8.17.3 Design Considerations. Sound reinforcement systems consist of one or more microphones, a mixer, processing electronics, amplifier(s) and one or more speakers. The proper operation of a sound system depends primarily on the location and application of the microphones and speakers within the reinforced space.

(1) *Room Acoustics.* Many small auditoriums and lecture rooms designed with optimal acoustics do not require sound systems except for projector sound, etc. Many highly reverberant rooms and rooms with echos have such poor acoustics that a typical sound system will not improve intelligibility. However, most gathering spaces benefit from a reinforcement system that aids the quiet talkers and helps lecturers with noisy audiences. The usefulness of any sound reinforcement system depends, to a great extent, on the space where the system is installed.

Room finishes vary in the amount of sound energy they absorb. Hard surfaces such as concrete, plaster and tile reflect the majority of sound energy that reaches them. Soft surfaces such as carpet, acoustic tile, batt insulation behind cloth, etc, absorb a large portion of the sound energy that reaches them. Sound energy in rooms with mostly hard surfaces will dissipate more slowly than sound energy in rooms with soft surfaces. Thus, rooms with low sound absorption have longer reverberation times.

The optimum reverberation time of a room varies with its size and its use. Optimum reverberation time is close to one second in lecture rooms and meeting rooms. Auditorium reverberation times may vary from one and three-tenths to one and nine-tenths seconds, depending on the primary use. Some auditoriums are equipped with movable curtains or absorptive panels so the reverberation time may be varied for different uses. The specific room conditions are a function of the architectural design.

The design (or existing conditions) of a project may result in a reverberation time longer or shorter than optimum for the project's intended use. Sometimes corrections to the room acoustics are appropriate but often the sound system must be designed to accommodate imperfect conditions.

(2) *Speaker Location.* When an amplified sound reaches a listener within 30 or 40 ms of the original sound, the sounds appear to blend and reinforce each other. Sound waves in air travel at about 1120 ft/s. Therefore, the best location for a central speaker cluster is above the acoustic source (lecturer, etc) such that the sound path to a listener from an acoustic source and from the speaker cluster differ by less than 30 ft. This condition should be met for every listening location in the room.

The best reinforced sound is reproduced at one location. When a listener receives sound from two sources, interference patterns result, reducing its clarity. A typical auditorium stage with a speaker on either side is an example of a poor sound system.

Sound energy should always be directed at an audience. When misdirected, it serves to increase the reverberant field or aggravate an echo in the space, thus reducing the overall intelligibility of the signal.

(3) *Centralized, Distributed and Precedence Systems.* A centralized system reproduces sound at one location; a distributed system reproduces sound at several locations; and a precedence system utilizes a central system and a distributed system in combination. Properly employed, a precedence system seems like a central system to the listener. This is accomplished by delaying the signal to the distributed speakers via a time delay unit and separate amplifiers.

Centralized systems are used in spaces where sound may be directed to the audience from one location. Distributed systems are used in locations with low ceilings or where the stage location may change. Precedence systems are used where the stage (or front) is permanent, but a central speaker cannot reach the whole audience, either because of low ceilings or obstructions. Centralized and distributed systems are used more often than are precedence systems.

(4) *Volume.* Sound reinforcement systems shall maintain sufficient volume to provide a satisfactory signal to noise ratio at each listener location. The amplifier power and speaker ratings may be chosen to provide nearly any volume level desired, but the overall system gain will be limited by the system feedback point. The maximum system gain will be determined by the number of open micro-

phones, their relative location to the speaker cluster, the distance from the talker to the microphone, the distance from the loudspeaker to the farthest listener and the room acoustics.

Usually, the sound reinforcement system will be designed to handle much louder signals than the maximum system gain allows. This permits the presentation of movie soundtracks and other prerecorded information at higher levels than used for sound reinforcement.

(5) *Mixers.* The types of control used in an auditorium system usually depend on its size and complexity, as well as its use. The simplest installation, such as a lecture room with one microphone, uses a preset mixer. It may be adjusted slightly for each lecturer but generally remains the same throughout any given lecture. When several microphones are used, such as at a panel discussion in an auditorium, the relative levels of each microphone may be preset but the system gain is low when all microphones remain open. In situations like this, an automatic microphone mixer may be employed.

(6) *Control Location.* Automatic mixers or mixers that are set once for each event may be located remote from the space. The automatic and preset mixers, however, must be adjusted differently for each event so the equipment rack should be readily accessible from the reinforced space. Controls for projector and auxiliary inputs should be provided at the mixer location.

(7) *Audio Signal Processing.* Several electronic processing techniques are used to improve the sound quality of a reinforcement system in difficult situations. The simpler a sound system is the better it sounds; however, one or more of the following items are often employed:

(a) *Frequency Shaping.* An equalizer may be utilized to correct for microphone, speaker and room frequency responses. A frequency response curve often specified for reinforcement systems is within 3 dB of a flat response from 125 Hz to 1000 or 2000 Hz with a 6 dB per octave rolloff below 125 Hz and a 3 dB per octave rolloff above 1000 or 2000 Hz. The high frequency knee at 2000 Hz is usually used for voice reinforcing systems and the knee at 1000 Hz is used for systems where music will be reproduced by the system. This curve is subject to variations for specific jobs and especially for unusual room acoustics, but will often provide both a natural and highly intelligible sound signal. A "natural" system will not be obvious to the listener.

(b) *Automatic Microphone Mixing.* The maximum acoustic gain of a reinforcement system is limited by the number of open microphones. Installations using several microphones often require an automatic mixer. An automatic mixer opens a microphone line when a sound source excites the microphone. Many automatic mixers reduce the overall system gain when several microphone lines are open. Thus, automatic mixers help maximize gain and prevent feedback.

(c) *Compression.* Dynamic compression is used when sound levels at a given microphone vary greatly during an event and the variation is not desired. Determining the settings required to provide maximum system gain and proper action of the compressor is often difficult. Also, the dynamic range of the sound signal is important to the impact of the material conveyed; therefore compression should only be used where it provides a specific advantage for the users.

(8) *Equipment.* There are many speaker types available for smaller rooms and distributed sound systems. Each type is suited to a specific application and may perform poorly in other applications. In larger rooms, where long throws are required, a large cone driver in a horn or utility enclosure is used for low frequencies and a driver and horn (or several horns) are used for high frequencies. The physical dimensions of horns are determined by frequency and distribution characteristics that are chosen to accommodate the shape and acoustic properties of the space served. Sufficient mounting space must be allowed for the central speaker or speaker cluster. In extreme cases, long throw horns may be over 4 ft long and a cluster may contain several horns.

Cardioid (directional) microphones and omnidirectional microphones are both used in reinforcement systems. Cardioid microphones are preferred by many performers and production groups for the control they provide. Omnidirectional microphones have a smoother off-axis frequency response and are easier to equalize in permanent installations. They are preferred for most lecture and auditorium reinforcement systems. Dynamic (non-powered) microphones are preferred since they simplify system installation.

Wiring for a reinforcement system involves separate cables to each microphone input, cables to projector and auxiliary inputs, cabling to and from a control console when required, and wiring to the speaker cluster. Power is required at the control console, equipment rack and projector locations. Wires for the inputs to the sound system are small, but several pairs of #12 or #10 AWG wire may be used to drive the speaker cluster.

(9) *Installation.* The installation practices are crucial to good sound reinforcement system performance. All of the concerns listed in Section 8.6.4 (4) Installation (Voice Paging Systems) are applicable to sound reinforcement systems. In addition, the following items are potential problems:

(a) *Microphone Balancing.* Where several open microphones are used for an event, the microphones levels must be balanced specifically for each talker. Microphone balancing usually changes for different events. This is the responsibility of the system users.

(b) *Speaker Distribution.* The distribution of a low frequency speaker (a cone driver in an enclosure) is typically 120° or more and its pointing is not critical; however, a high frequency driver-horn combination is manufactured with a specific distribution pattern and must be properly directed towards the listener if it is to serve its purpose. Typical distribution patterns include 90° by 40°, 60° by 40°, and 40° by 20°. Every listener in a space should be included within the distribution pattern of one horn, and the patterns should overlap about 20% horizontially and 10% vertically to provide even, high frequency coverage.

(c) *Speaker Weight.* A speaker cluster for a large auditorium may be very heavy. A check with the structural consultant is recommended. Secure but adjustable mounting should provide for each high frequency horn and low frequency driver.

8.18 Data Processing Systems

8.18.1 Introduction. For purposes of planning, it is prudent to assume that sooner or later computer terminals will be installed in a number of areas of the health care facilities. Today, computers are already being used for accounting, inventory, and patient management work. A growing number of hospitals have a computer-assisted laboratory data system which transmits laboratory data to appropriate nursing stations as it automatically enters charges for the procedures or tests. In a limited number of hospitals, computers are being used in the the care of patients, in situations such as anesthesia, intensive care, and special care of other types. A number of feedback programs are now in use in the treatment of patients in need of blood and liquids, as well as for patients with a variety of metabolic and endocrine disorders. Computerized diagnoses of electrocardiographs, electroencephalographs, and other graphic or numeric readouts are in widespread use. The use of computers in medicine appears to be growing; their use in support services such as surgical scheduling, materials handling, administration, and order of supplies is well established.

8.18.2 Design Considerations. Cable plant capabilities for present and future data processing facilities shall be provided to all central control stations, nursing stations, laboratories, administrative areas and departments.

8.19 Telewriter and Facsimile Systems

8.19.1 Introduction. Telewriter equipment allows transmission of handwriting to remote stations, where it appears exactly as written. Facsimile equipment offers a more powerful system for transmission of any fixed graphic material, including printed material and pictures.

8.19.2 Design Criteria. Within hospitals, telewriter terminals are used to transmit three basic types of data: requests for information, reports, and authorizations. The terminals are commonly placed at the following locations:

(1) *Nurses Stations*
(2) *Pharmacy*
(3) *Dietary Office*
(4) *Medical Records*
(5) *Laboratories*
(6) *Admitting Office*
(7) *Business, Administration Offices*
(8) *Maintenance*

A second category of use for telewriter equipment is communications for the deaf. A telewriter terminal may be connected to a telephone so as to answer an incoming call and provide two-way written communications with any caller equipped with similar equipment.

Facsimile equipment is used both for interdepartmental communications and for communications between hospitals. The most common interdepartmental application is the daily transmission of patient drug requirements from the nurses stations to the pharmacy. Facsimile communication makes the best use of staff time in this situation, since the equipment operates unattended and is much quicker than batch orders conveyed by messenger. When the facsimile equipment is selected for this application, the hospital should also consider placing terminals in the dietary office and laboratory areas.

Where a hospital is a member of a hospital association, facsimile communication may be used to transmit inventory and administrative data between hospitals.

8.19.3 Design Considerations. The selection and location of equipment will normally be accomplished by the architect or system supplier. The engineer should obtain the list of terminal locations with a notation as to whether the terminal is a sender, receiver, or both. At each location, a power receptacle should be provided. Dedicated telephone type cabling is required between each terminal.

8.20 Pneumatic Tube Systems

8.20.1 Introduction. The system consists of an interconnecting tubular network through which small-size containers travel. The container movement is powered by compressed air. These containers, or carriers, as they are referred to, can be dispatched and received at different stations in the system automatically or semi-automatically. The system can thus transport material between points which are horizontally or vertically remote. The carriers are designed to transport items such as paperwork, pharmaceuticals and medical supplies, small tools, IV bottles or bags, production parts, sealed food items, etc. The main advantage of the pneumatic tube system is that it provides fully automated small piece distribution for least cost when compared to other systems. It is the lowest-cost fully automated material handling device available to a large facility that can travel vertically or horizontally and provide the fastest delivery time.

8.20.2 Design Criteria. The system configuration including piping layout and equipment locations is usually designed by the system supplier or architect. The electrical engineer must verify equipment locations and provide power connections. Control wiring between stations is usually in the system supplier contract.

8.20.3 Design Considerations. The engineer should verify the requirements of the system to be installed. The following are general guidelines for power requirements.

(1) *Station.* Stations require a 115 V ac power source from a dedicated circuit breaker.

(2) *Diverters.* Diverters require a 115 V ac power source from a dedicated circuit breaker.

(3) *Blowers.* Blowers require a 3-phase, 208 V ac or 480 V ac circuit for 2 to 15 hp to the motor starter and connection from the starter to the motor. A manual disconnect is recommended within sight of the blower. The starter requires a 115 V ac coil which is connected to the blower control panel.

(4) *Computer Control Terminal.* The computer control terminal requires a 115 V ac power source from a dedicated circuit breaker.

8.21 Disaster Alarm Systems

8.21.1 Introduction. A disaster alarm system alerts the central control center as to the status of disasters, either natural or man-made. Signals must be coordinated with local civil defense and disaster area authorities and design must follow their system.

8.21.2 Design Criteria. Disaster alarm systems such as civil defense alerts and weather alerts are required in health care facilities by civil authorities. The engineer should check local requirements.

8.21.3 Design Considerations

(1) *Actuating Devices.* Actuation can be local or remote. Data can be furnished directly or via telephone, radio, or microwave channels. The number of channels and their coding should meet the requirements of civil defense and local disaster area authorities. Signals are originated by remote control from the offices of civil authorities, or by local pushbuttons. Each coded channel requires a signal cancelling button with a pilot light.

(2) *Annunciator.* The annunciator shall be located at the central control center. Annunciator panels should have a circuit supervisory feature to indicate alarm, operational faults, trouble buzzers, silencing switches, and pilot lights. Test buttons are necessary to verify readiness of equipment and for use in training drills.

8.22 References

[1] ANSI/IEEE 241-1983, IEEE Recommended Practice for Electric Power Systems in Commercial Buildings.

[2] ANSI/NFPA 56F-1983, Nonflammable Medical Gas Systems.

[3] ANSI/NFPA 70-1984, National Electrical Code.

[4] ANSI/NFPA 72A-1985, Standard for the Installation, Maintenance and Use of Local Protective Signaling Systems.

[5] ANSI/NFPA 72D-1979, Proprietary Protective Signaling Systems.

[6] ANSI/NFPA 99-1984, Standard for Health Care Facilities.

[7] ANSI/NFPA 101-1985, Code for Safety to Life from Fire in Buildings and Structures.

[8] ANSI/UL 268-1981, Safety Standard for Smoke Detectors for Fire Protective Signaling Systems.

[9] ANSI/UL 1069-1982, Safety Standard for Hospital Signaling and Nurse-Call Equipment.

[10] CFR (Code of Federal Regulations), Title 47: Telecommunications, published by Office of the Federal Register (FCC Rules and Regulations are contained within this document).[29]

[11] KAUFMAN, J. Planning Communications for Modern Hospitals: A Professional Approach. *Construction Products & Technology*, November 1969.

[12] KREAGER, P. *Practical Aspects of Data Communications.* New York: McGraw-Hill, 1983.

---

[29] This document is available from the Superintendent of Documents, US Government Printing Office, Washington, DC 20402.

[13 LAUFMAN, H. *Hospital Special Care Facilities: Planning for User Needs*. New York: Academic Press, 1981.

[14] NASH, Jr, H.O. Fire Alarm Systems for Health Care Facilities. Conference Record, Industrial Applications Society, IEEE-IAS 1982 Annual Meeting.

[15] SMITH, J.R. *Hospital Paging Systems in the Special Emergency Radio Service*. A technical and regulatory review before the American Society for Hospital Engineering of the American Hospital Association. Update on Hospital Paging Regulations Meeting, April 23, 1980, Dallas, Texas, April 25, 1980, Chicago, Illinois.

[16] SMITH, J.R. Paging System Capacity, Instructions for Estimating Channel Capacity and Delay. *Communications Magazine*, June 1980.

9. Medical Equipment and Instrumentation

9.1 Introduction. In a modern hospital the selection and purchasing of equipment and the care and maintenance of that equipment is an important everyday task facing hospital administration and maintenance staff. The act of selection and purchasing necessary medical equipment is no small matter. The process should follow a set pattern such as the following:

9.1.1 Need. Department head or staff member in charge of project or task should request purchase of a new piece of equipment after investigation into its use in hospital. Will it enhance the state of the art? Will it produce the specified results? Will it reduce costs? Will it save time? Should it be purchased or leased? How long will it be before it is outmoded? Will it help patient care or in diagnostic procedures?

9.1.2 Cost

(1) Does equipment need to have more than one supplier or manufacturer?

(2) Has equipment cost been checked from all suppliers?

(3) Can cost be capitalized and over what time period?

(4) Are funds available at this time?

9.1.3 Space Requirements

(1) Does institution have available space for new piece of equipment?

(2) If new space is required or area needs remodeling, will cost of this work be prohibitive?

(3) Are utilities available at location?

9.1.4 Utilities

(1) Along with space requirements above, the next most important factor to consider is: Are the utilities needed to operate equipment?

(2) Equipment may require hot or cold water or both; air, gas, steam, and, of course, electrical service.

(3) Electrical service and availability should be checked for:

    (a) Voltage (special voltages).

    (b) Capacity (amperes).

    (c) Hertz (frequency).

    (d) Protection.

    (e) Control.

9.2 Equipment Selection

9.2.1 Pre-Purchase Evaluation Form. Many hospitals use a pre-evaluation form before purchase to assure equipment will meet all of the institution's requirements.

9.2.2 Example of Pre-Purchase Evaluation Form

(1) *New Equipment Pre-Purchase Evaluation Form.* This form is to be completed by the manufacturer and returned to the Director of Purchasing with manuals and attachments as indicated below. This form must be completed by an employee of the manufacturer with sufficient technical information or knowledge to provide answers to the items below. If the manufacturer is uncertain about specific portions, it is suggested he send available material promptly so further communication, if needed, will not be delayed. Refer questions to the Director of Purchasing and/or to _____.

Information detailing specific hospital requirements is outlined in the specification requirements. Additional copies of this form are available on request from the Director of Purchasing.

1. **To:** _____   **Date** _____

   Item: _____   **Project #** _____

2. **Listings:**

   Is unit listing with UL? ☐ Yes ☐ No

   If yes, please specify UL listing #

   _____

   Is equipment listed with other certifying agencies? Please give specific standards/listing # _____

   _____

3. **Line-Operated Equipment, Including Battery Chargers:**

   Line voltage limits for stable operation:

   From _____ To_____ V ac

   Phase: _____

   _____

   Frequency limits:

   From _____ To_____ Hz

   Normal Operating Current: _____ A

   Surge Current: _____ A

   How will safety and/or operation be affected if the voltage goes outside the range of 100–130 V? _____

   _____

4. **Battery-Operated Equipment:**

   Type of Batteries or Packs: _____

   Number per Unit: _____

   Recharge Time: _____
   (where applicable)

   Discharge Time: _____
   (under specified load)

   Can unit be line-operated when batteries are fully discharged?
   ☐ Yes ☐ No

   Will batteries charge while unit is line-operated?   ☐ Yes ☐ No

5. Power Cord:

Required minimum is an 18 gauge, three-conductor industrial or hospital grade cord at least 10 ft long with a Hubbell lock or hospital grade U ground type plug.

Does your power cord meet these requirements?   ☐ Yes ☐ No

If not, specify differences and indicate cost of modification in Section 13.

---

6. Power Switch and Overcurrent Interrupters:

Type of Power: _____   _____ Single Pole

_____   _____ Double Pole

Switch (i.e., toggle, slide, etc): _____   _____ Three Pole ☐ SN

_____

Type of Overcurrent Protection: ____

Is power switch clearly labeled?
☐ Yes ☐ No

_____

Ampacity: _____

Is power switch in line of sight from operator position?   ☐ Yes ☐ No

Enclosure: ☐ Surface ☐ Recessed Class_____

Shall protect all line (hot conductors) to all parts of unit. Shall be easily accessible. If fuse, the size shall be marked beside the holder and a clearly marked spare provided. If overcurrent protection does not conform to these specifications, see Section 13.

7. Mechanical Design for Physical Protection:

Unprotected openings on exposed horizontal surfaces not allowed.

Other openings shall be guarded against spillage.

Small appliances used in patient's bed shall be immersible in conductive fluid without macroshock hazard.

If design does not conform to these specifications, see Section 13.

8. Environmental and Interface Characteristics:

Temperature Limits

For Operation:

From _____ To_____ °F

For Storage:

From _____ To_____ °F

Humidity Limits

For Operation:

From _____ To_____ % RH

For Storage:

From _____ To_____ % RH

Maximum allowable storage time: _____

Sensitive to RF interference?	☐ Yes ☐ No
Known to generate RF interference?	☐ Yes ☐ No
Sensitive to power line transient?	☐ Yes ☐ No
Known to generate power line transient?	☐ Yes ☐ No
Known to require other utilities?	☐ Yes ☐ No
Are exposed metal surfaces ungrounded?	☐ Yes ☐ No

If answer is "yes" to any of these questions, give details on separate page.

Specific sterilizing procedures to be used? _____

Type of labeling for O_2 and flammable location: _____

Quantity of radiation emission: _____

Type of shielding: _____

9. **Provide the Following Manuals and Technical Information:**

   Operator's Manual   Block Diagrams
   Wiring Diagrams   Preventive Maintenance Program
   Schematic Circuit Diagram   Operational Tests
   Parts List   Performance Specifications
   Statement of Known   User Performance Test
     Potential Hazards   Service Manual

   One set to be provided with this form. One additional set upon delivery.

10. **Warranty/Guaranty:**

    Warranty will start after delivery and initial installation (if applicable).

    If modifications are made to conform to our specifications will warranty be violated? ☐ Yes ☐ No

    Length of warranty: _____

11. **Service and Training Information:**

    Estimated response time for service calls from time of notice: _____ hours.

    Is local service available? ☐ Yes ☐ No

    Give location and working hours of nearest service facility: _____
    _____

    A replacement unit is available in _____ hours.

    Are training programs available for   Are training programs available for
    service personnel? ☐ Yes ☐ No   users? Yes ☐ No

Give location, schedule, cost and instructor's qualifications for both types of training programs on a separate sheet.

12. Leakage/Risk Currents:

Acceptable Limits

Measurement Site	Device for Patients with Intracardiac Leads	General Patient Devices	Nonpatient Devices	Typical Device Values Indicate Worst Leakage Current
Patient leads or attachments to ground	10 μA	50 μA	Not applicable	
With 120 V applied to patient leads	20 μA	Not applicable	Not applicable	
Worst case to ground	100 μA	500 μA	500 μA	

13. Modifications/Comments:

Please list description and cost quotations for any modifications, accessories, or other items necessary to fulfill the requirements stated. Cost of upgrading unit will weigh heavily on our decision to purchase.

1. _____

2. _____

3. _____

4. _____

14. This form is to be completed and signed by the manufacturer's product manager or his equivalent.

Completed By:

Name _____   Title _____

Address _____   Date _____

_____

Signature _____   Telephone _____

9.3 Equipment and Area Served

9.3.1 Patient Care

(1) *Patient Connected Measurement, Monitoring and Data Acquisition Equipment.* Management of patients has been significantly aided by measurement, monitoring and data acquisition systems. These devices are located in Coronary Care and Progressive Care Units, Operating Rooms, Intensive Care Units and General Care areas. Coronary Care is a self-descriptive term for areas devoted to patients with heart problems. As recovery takes place, limited movement becomes beneficial and they "progress" to a Progressive Care Unit. Here, monitoring takes place with individually carried telemetry units. Intensive Care Units are for patients requiring very special attention, such as recovery from surgery. These areas frequently employ extensive measuring and data acquisition equipment.

Proper care requires information about heart and lung performance, the medication provided and any notes made by the nursing staff. There are a myriad of other observations and actions to be taken with all types of patients. This section covers that class of equipment generally known as patient monitoring equipment and is the type of equipment usually found in Coronary Care, Progressive Care, Operating Room and Intensive Care Units.

Figures 71, 72, 73, 74, and 75 illustrate patient monitoring systems. This equipment collects and displays information on heart and lung performance. Heart rates, systolic, diastolic and mean pressures, cardiac outputs, respiratory waveforms and rates and temperatures are measured and displayed. Because of the large amount of information gathered, computer systems are also sometimes employed to help in the assimilation of the large magnitude of information. Alarms may be provided at the bedside instruments for parameters deviating below or above certain set points. Additionally, computers can be programmed to analyze cardiac arrhythmias, the term given to significant random abnormalities of the heart waveform. Trends of events can be stored and recalled for later observation. Figures 76 and 77 illustrate instruments in Operating and Intensive Care areas. The parameters are typically the same as for the Coronary Care Units but it is more likely that measurements will be made from transducers or electrodes placed inside the heart chambers. Because of patient status, more capability is provided in such instrumentation and it typically contains additional controls, features, precision and accuracy. Extensive use of computer systems is made during catheterization procedures. Catheterization is the process of collecting data from inside the heart chambers for the purpose of determining the details of heart performance and whether surgery can be effective in correcting deficiencies with blood flow or other heart abnormalities. Figure 78 shows such a system.

As heart patients regain their strength, many are allowed considerable freedom in their daily activities but still require close monitoring. Such patients are found in Progressive Care Units. These units employ telemetry systems for monitoring heart rates and waveforms as the patients are allowed to walk within a prescribed area. Figure 79 shows this type of equipment.

(2) *How Does the Equipment Work?* In the general sense, all of the equipment can be described by the aid of the block diagram in Fig 80. A transducer, either

on the surface or inside the body, picks up the signal of interest. These signals range from a few μV to several mV, depending upon the parameter of interest. Bandwidths range from dc to approximately 100 Hz. The output of the transducer is converted to an electrical signal that undergoes certain processing depending upon the end purpose of the data. Typically, filtering will be employed for the purpose of removing as much noise and patient induced artifact as possible. There will be processing for indicating deviations from either high or low alarm settings, waveform presentation and A to D conversion for the computer data management systems.

Patients are relatively large volume, complicated electrical sources. The instruments connected to these patients should be able to provide acceptable information in the presence of large amounts of electrical noise and deliberately induced signals that have been applied for other reasons. Examples of large noise sources are electrosurgery, defibrillation and pacemakers. The spectrum covers amplitudes from a few microamperes to several amperes, frequencies from a few cycles per second to many MHz and voltages ranging to a few kV. The patient is a con-

**Fig 71
Patient Monitoring System, Central Station**

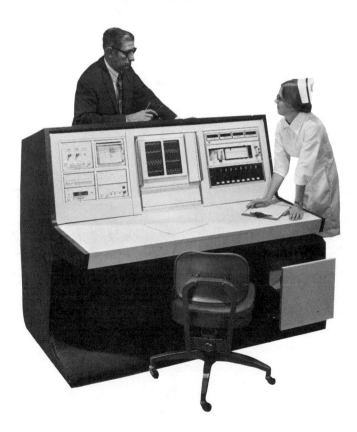

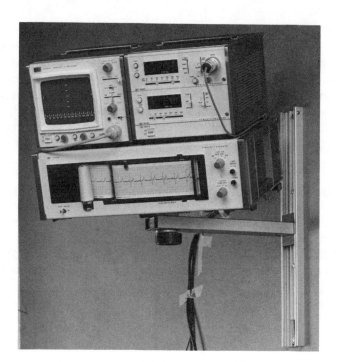

**Fig 72
Patient Monitoring System, Bedside Station**

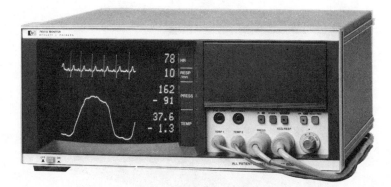

**Fig 73
Patient Monitoring System, Bedside Station**

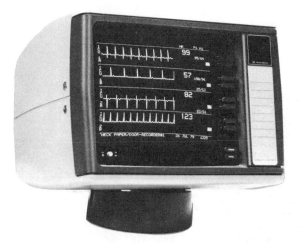

Fig 74
Patient Monitoring System—Table or Console, Mounted

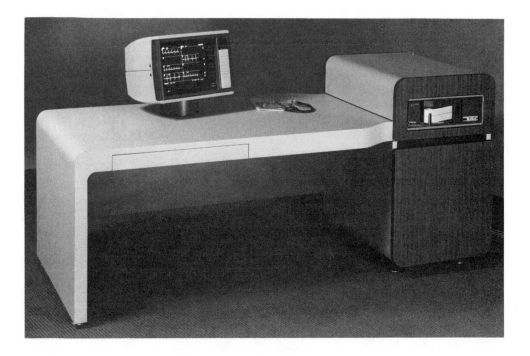

Fig 75
Patient Monitoring System, Central Station

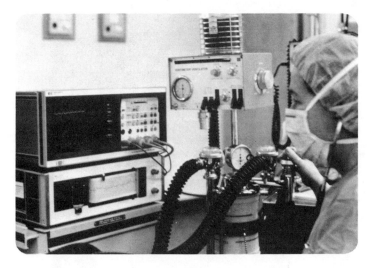

Fig 76
Instruments in Operating and Intensive Care Areas

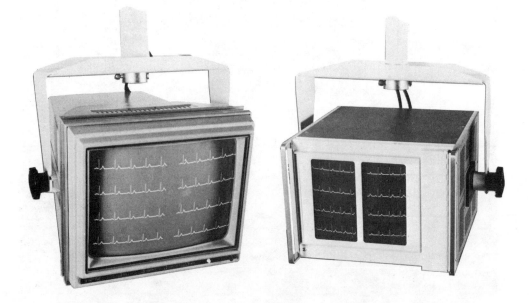

Fig 77
Instruments in Operating and Intensive Care Areas and Catheterization Labs

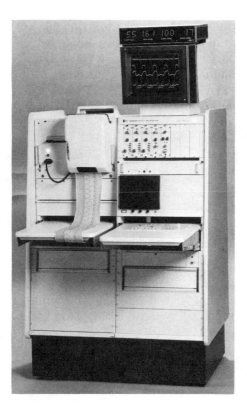

Fig 78
Catheterization Computer System

venient pick-up for 60 Hz and electromagnetic signals. Patient and electrode impedances are complex resistive-capacitative combinations that make the generation of unwanted signals an easy matter.

Defibrillators apply large energies, ranging up to 400 J, for the purpose of converting a fibrillating heart to normal sinus rhythm. A fibrillating heart beats in a random manner such that the net blood flow is close to zero. Normal sinus rhythm is the rhythm of a heart that is pumping adequately. The defibrillation pulse can have durations ranging from about 3 to 30 ms and the voltages reaching electrodes attached to the patient can range as high as a few kV, differential or common mode. Thus, adequate protection should be afforded to the devices connected to the patients. They may be disturbed by the large amount of energy applied but should recover quickly and not be damaged.

Pacemakers apply currents of a typically rectangular shape to the heart for the purpose of compensation for a chronic abnormality. Electrodes are imbedded inside the heart and stimulated by means of pulses ranging from a fraction of a mA to a few mA and with durations ranging from a few tenths of a millisecond to 2 ms. Equipment used in determining and displaying heart rate is asked to

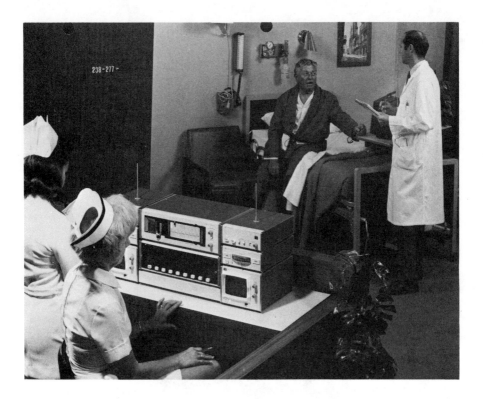

Fig 79
Progressive Care Unit

display these pulses in order to determine if the heart has responded properly to the stimulus but, at the same time, must not count these pulses in case the patient's heart should fail to function. Alarm circuits should be able to discriminate between the absence of a heart beat and the presence of the artificial stimulus. Since the artificial stimulus is orders of magnitude greater than the few mV of electrocardiograph signal, the design task is formidable. Typically, some compromise must be reached and information is provided to the user with respect to the care that must be exercised when pacemakers are involved.

Electrosurgical devices are cutting tools employing large magnitudes of high frequency current. Kilovolts, A and MHz signals are involved. The equipment tied to the patient must not be damaged by such signals and, in the case of surgery, useful data is expected in the presence of these large disturbances.

(3) *Patient Safety.* Some knowledge of electrical safety considerations may be helpful when designing hospital installations. Patient safety is viewed in terms of the small amount of 60 Hz currents that, if allowed to flow through the heart, could induce fibrillation. [6], [10] This is the same condition that can occur when a person comes close to electrocution by touching a high-voltage power line. In

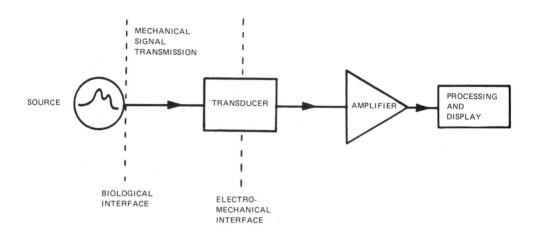

Fig 80
Patient Measurement System

the broad sense, patient safety also includes protection from erroneous data due to electrical noise. The lack of information due to noise conditions or the generation of erroneous data can make diagnosis difficult or impossible under critical conditions and potentially puts the patient into jeopardy. Electromagnetic interference has been reported as causing defibrillators, pacemakers and ventilators to malfunction. [7], [8], [9] It can also add noise that will either obscure data or make it difficult to interpret. High density currents flowing through electrode or transducer sites may also injure the patient by causing serious burns.

(4) *The Microshock Hazard.* Figure 81 illustrates the conditions that could arise due to the flow of 60 Hz leakage currents as a function of poor input isolation of the measuring equipment or poor grounding of the primary circuits. A fault in the ground line will allow leakage current to flow through the path indicated. One such path encompasses electrodes or transducers placed inside the heart. If the input circuits of the instruments involved are adequately isolated, the current that flows can be kept to a very low value under the worst possible case — full line voltage being the direct source, for example. The exact distribution of 60 Hz currents that will cause fibrillation with a high degree of predictability has not been determined. However, the results of various experiments have resulted in an upper limit of 20 μA, 60 Hz being considered as the threshold for fibrillation. Currently, UL 544-1976 [5],[30] CSA C22.2 [4], and ANSI/AAMI SCL 12-78 [1] all require a 20 μA limitation for input circuit isolation for the condition of the direct application of 120 V.

---

[30] The numbers in brackets correspond to the references at the end of this chapter.

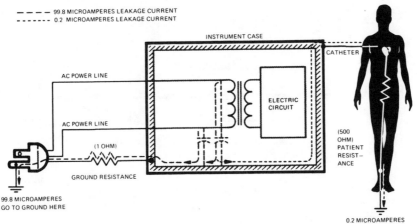

Normal Path of Leakage Current

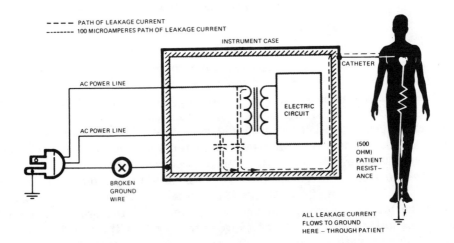

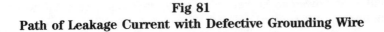

Fig 81
Path of Leakage Current with Defective Grounding Wire

These documents also require that the chassis leakage current in Fig 81 be held to 100 μA, or less. This limitation essentially eliminates a shock being felt by personnel caring for the patient and is a reasonable compromise between safety and the extra cost of providing unnecessarily low chassis leakage currents.

Figure 83 illustrates a commonly used method of isolation.

(5) *60 Hz Noise.* Figure 84 indicates how stray currents coupled to the body generate common mode voltages that must be accommodated by the measuring instruments. Such devices must be able to effectively attenuate these signals by

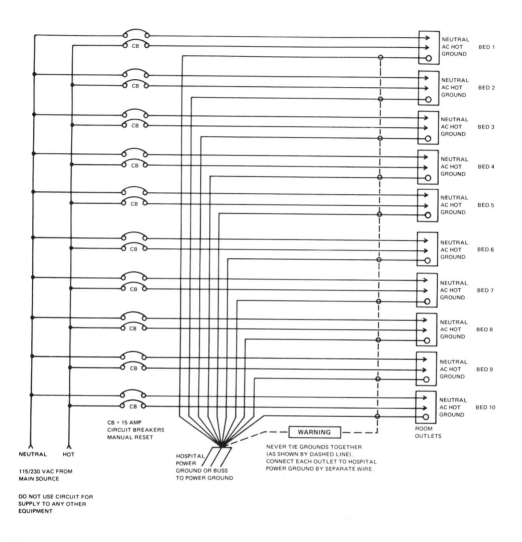

Fig 82
Grounding for Patient Monitoring Bedside Stations in Intensive Care Units

100 dB, or more. Levels of 10 V may exist on the body and yet must not interface with measurements of signals in the mV region.

Figure 85 illustrates the generation of differential voltages from 60 Hz electromagnetic signals. Since these signals are differential and in the passband of much of the measuring equipment, they need to be eliminated or reduced at their source. The patient environment must be one that will restrict the electromagnetic field to low levels. There will typically be an unavoidable area in the electrode system used for measuring heart rate and any signals picked up by this loop will be amplified as a normal signal.

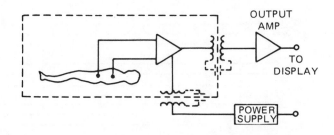

Present practice aims to isolate as much as possible the patient and
instrument front-end from all external electrical sources. Thus input
power and output signals are coupled with high-isolation devices
(high-frequency isolation transformers or opto-couplers).

Isolated Inputs

Fig 83
High Frequency Isolation Transformers

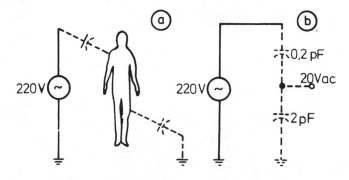

Capacitive coupling to surrounding power sources and
grounds (a) causes the human body to appear electrically
as a 60 Hz noise source (b).

60 Hz Interference

Fig 84
60 Hz Interference Causes

(6) *Burns.* High density currents flowing through electrode sites can generate
burns. The usual source of the energy involved is the electrosurgery equipment.
Figure 86 illustrates the problem and shows that poor contact of the return electrode of the electrosurgical unit may cause the currents to seek an easier path to
ground. This route might be through other electrode sites.

(7) *Electromagnetic Noise.* Electromagnetic interference may be caused by signals coupled to the patient from power lines and high frequency generators such
as radio and TV stations. This noise covers the spectrum from a few Hz to several

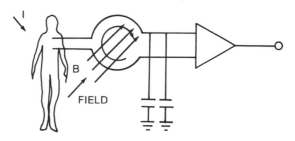

**Fig 85
Generation of Differential Voltages from 60 Hz Electromagnetic Signals**

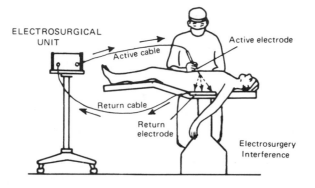

Arrows indicate flow of electrosurgical current in a complete circuit.

**Fig 86
Electrosurgical Current in a Complete Circuit**

GHz. Electrosurgical units, FM, AM and TV transmitters, radar and communication equipment, computer systems and electrosurgical units place noises on the power line that may be sinusoidal, pulse, impulse, as well as other types. The voltages can range from a few μV/m to V/m for noise transmitted through the air. Hundreds of V to low kV for sharp pulses may exist on power lines.

Transmitted interference must be handled by the measuring device involved and requires extensive detail in the design of input filters, shielding and the bypassing of nonlinear elements. Chassis leakage current limitations prevent discriminating against arbitrary amounts of line interference by the use of power line filters. Filter sections tied to ground are generally not usable because they quickly cause the chassis leakage currents to exceed 100 μA. Series inductive elements in conjunction with stray capacities followed by attention to design detail are the methods employed to attenuate the effects of line noise. Hospital power circuits need to be carefully designed in order to avoid patient care area circuits having to accommodate the return currents of noise-producing equipment such as elevators, computers, pumps and the like.

(8) *Environmental Considerations.* Although much of this equipment resides in a fairly benign environment, it may be used in a wide variety of situations. Thus, the equipment will need to operate in the following typical environments:

Temperature — 15–45 °C
Shock — 30 G
Vibration — 15–30 G
Condensation — none
Humidity — 45 °C–90 °RH

Line Voltage — 115 V ±10%, typically. However, many areas of the country are now faced with potential brown-out conditions and much equipment is designed to operate satisfactorily down to 90 V line. Further, many hospitals routinely test their emergency generators. Depending upon how carefully such systems are energized when testing, transients may be placed upon the line that can reach levels of 200 V and more for durations of several ms. The equipment involved is expected to survive such transients without any damage or permanent loss of data.

(9) *Design and Installation Recommendations.* Planning will be a key factor in determining the effectiveness of the unit. Typically, this will include decisions as to size and location of the unit, choice of equipment, financing, selection of the staff, training, maintenance and service. Although it is essential to consider all factors, this section will concentrate on the physical considerations of the unit.

Figure 87 illustrates a possible layout. It shows a nurse's central station, private rooms with individual bedside monitoring and a Progressive Care Unit with telemetry. Each hospital will have its own requirements. Operating Room and Intensive Care areas have not been included. However, similar considerations apply. For an Intensive Care area, nearly all of the equipment will be bedside mounted and may have signals routed to a central station. Operating room equipment may be centrally located, analogous to a central station, or it could be mounted near the anesthesiologist or close to the operating room table. The instruments may be in racks, consoles or individually stacked on bench tops. During the initial planning phases, it will be necessary to work with the hospital and the equipment suppliers in order to fix the locations of the equipment, consider the power needs, evaluate potential noise sources, consider which members of the hospital staff will be using the equipment and what access they must have, including visibility and ease of use of the controls. The cabling must be designed with respect to length, type needed from the point of view of signal transmission, access to ceiling mounts, and any interconnecting hardware. During the planning phase, performance characteristics of different types of equipment can be matched against the desired operation in order to facilitate selection.

Prior to the order being placed, the hospital representative, architect and manufacturer's representative should meet to discuss the locations of the equipment, the power needs and the conduit requirements. It is best to appoint a coordinator so that all involved with the installation will be kept appraised of current requirements and any changes.

During construction or renovation, the hospital and manufacturing representatives should tour the proposed equipment site in order to review equipment locations, mounting hardware, power requirements, conduits and the overall equipment concepts. Prior to installation of the actual electronic equipment, the hospital and manufacturer may wish the cables, wall mounts, shelves, central junction boxes and ceiling mounts supplied in order that they might be more easily mounted before final construction has been completed.

Figure 88 provides an example of the considerations involved and shows the need to consider conduit length and sizes. It is preferable to have installed a conduit that may be a bit larger than needed than find that the one in place is too small to accommodate the wires that have to be pulled.

It will be necessary to make drawings of each and every detail of the installation in order to avoid errors and oversights that can only be remedied by added frustration and extra expense. Large installations can involve two to three hundred separate pieces of equipment and miles of conduit and cable. From a mechanical safety point of view, adequate support should be provided for wall mounted bedside installations and operating room or central station ceiling mounted installations. Typically, the test conditions are four times the load weight for one minute.

A good installation will require a considerable amount of attention to detail.

Fig 87
Floor Plan

Floor Plan

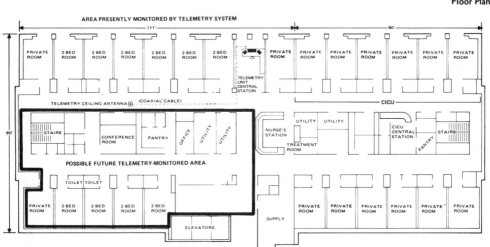

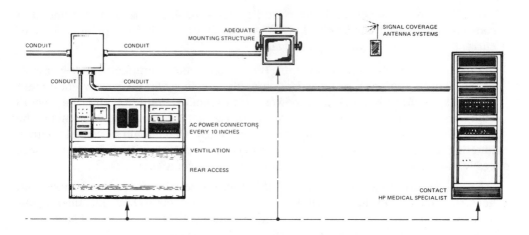

Fig 88
Conduit Lengths and Sizes

Some suggestions follow:

(a) *Bedside.* A typical bedside configuration is shown in Fig 89. For beds where blood pressures will be directly monitored, include transducer mounting poles, etc.

Warning

If wall mounts are used to support the monitors, they shall be capable of supporting four times the specified weight capacity after they have been properly installed. When plaster walls are used, it is recommended that steel or plywood plates (as shown in Fig 90) be employed to distribute the load over a larger section of wall. Expansion bolts are not considered adequate or safe.

(b) *Central Station.* Central station consoles can range from simple tables on which the equipment sits, to a custom-built enclosure. Regardless of the central station console chosen the following minimum features need to be provided:

• AC power connectors every 10 in (25.4 cm), or so, along console's length.

• Cable protecting conduits from central station console to central station junction box.

• A horizontal surface for mounting monitoring equipment. For special consoles, consult the supplier during planning stages.

• A surface above and behind the monitoring equipment, to protect the equipment.

• Access to rear of monitoring equipment at the central station location without the need to move equipment.

• Adequate ventilation (cooling) for the monitoring instruments.

(c) *Remote Areas.* Recent trends in equipping intensive care facilities indicate that remote displays at strategic locations, based upon the medical staff flow

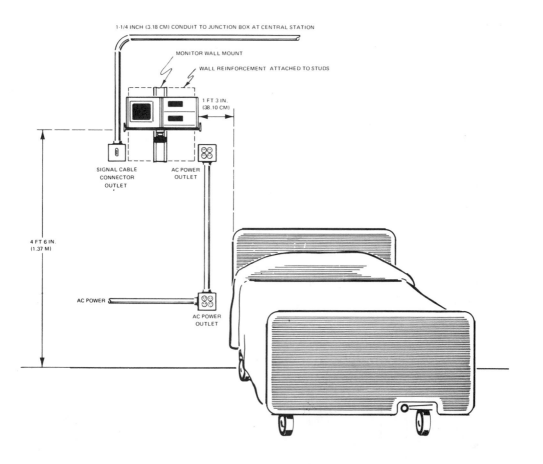

Fig 89
Typical Bedside Configuration

patterns, are desirable. It allows observation of the entire unit while staff members are away from the central station. Whenever displays in these areas are considered, adequate mounting facilities and power and signal distribution, which are the responsibilities of the hospital, must be considered as well. Note that memory oscilloscopes normally require coaxial cables for signal interconnection to the central station.

(d) *Telemetry System.* If the hospital considers telemetry, it may be necessary for the manufacturer to make on-site field strength measurements to insure adequate signal coverage. Because each hospital has specific details of construction, such as placement of walls, location or electrical equipment, etc, that can affect telemetry signal reception, each installation should be treated on an individual basis.

(e) *Computers.* Hospitals that anticipate using a computer in the future should make adequate signal and power arrangements during the initial stages of planning. Recommendations for computer installations vary with specific situations. Consult the equipment supplier as soon as possible in the planning stages of these installations. Figure 91 illustrates one type of computer system.

Note that computer system installations normally require special signal junction boxes and larger than normal diameter or additional conduits. In additon, power requirements for computer-based systems are generally higher and provisions for increased power capacity should be incorporated into the hospital ac supply lines to the proposed computer/patient monitoring areas.

(f) *AC Power.* A separately protected, common power source of 115 V, 60 Hz should be provided for the system, properly tied to the hospital's emergency power system. Each bed should have an individually protected, 15 A, 3-wire grounded outlet. Thus, the system remains operative if a failure occurs at one bedside. Power wiring should never be run in the same conduit or closely parallel to signal wiring from monitoring instruments.

Voltage Requirements — Most patient monitoring equipment operates from single phase 115 V (or 230 V in locations outside of the United States) alternating current, 50 to 60 Hz. Line voltage may vary as much as 10% (for example, 103–127 V or 207–253 V) without affecting operation or accuracy of the instru-

Fig 90
Wall Mounts

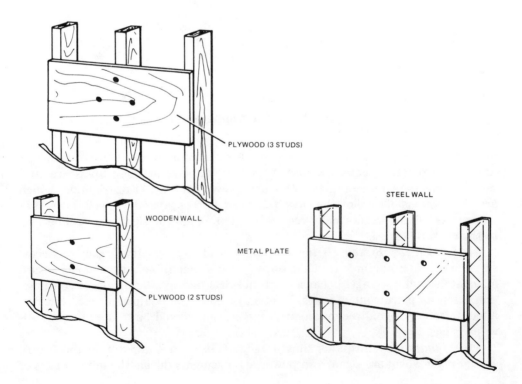

PLYWOOD (3 STUDS)

WOODEN WALL

PLYWOOD (2 STUDS)

STEEL WALL

METAL PLATE

ment. Variations greater than 10% may have to be corrected by a regulating transformer or other means.

Bedside Power—Required power level for each bedside is generally 90 to 200 VA. The following recommendations for bedside stations apply:

- Use only hospital grade acceptable power connectors.
- A minimum of two duplex outlets on each side of patient's bed. The outlets should be breakered in accordance with the ANSI/NFPA 70-1984 [2].
- A minimum of 825 VA for each pair of outlets.
- Provide power outlets within a few feet of the junction boxes and equipment support locations.
- Provide a grounding system in accordance with ANSI/NFPA 99-1984 [3] and the ANSI/NFPA 70-1984 [2].
- Provide an exposed terminal connected directly to the patient common reference bus for testing purposes. These should be within 5 ft (1.52 m) of each bed and each may serve more than one bed.
- Design the system layout to keep power cables to a minimum length as this contributes both to physical and electrical safety.
- Provide for adequate ventilation in areas where the patient monitoring equipment is to be installed.

Fig 91
Computer System

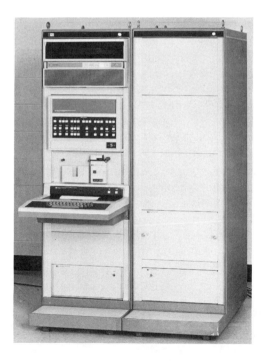

Central Station—Required power level for the central station is about 80 VA for systems of eight or fewer beds. For each eight bed system add 100 VA.

(g) *Conduit and Junction Boxes* (if needed). Elements essential to most ICU installations are the bedside junction boxes, the signal cable conduit or carrier and the central station junction box.

Bedside Junction Boxes—For a new or existing hospital building: NEMA electrical box with plaster ring for standard 1½ in (3.18 cm) conduit. The junction box can be either flush or wall mounted.

One of these junction boxes should be mounted at each bedside station in the ICU area.

Central Station Junction Box—The central station junction boxes provide versatility for an 8-patient ICU area. These boxes will accept conduit and raceway adapters for hidden or surface mounted building cable carriers.

NOTE: Central station junction boxes can be shipped to the building site before the monitoring equipment, if desired by the hospital contractor.

Patient Signal Wiring From Instruments—Hidden 1½ in (3.18 cm) diameter conduit between flush-mounted bedside and central station junction boxes is recommended for maximum cable protection and attractiveness of completed installation.

(h) *Mounts*. Use of a wall mount, ceiling mount, or shelf to mount the bedside modules keeps the area immediately adjacent to the bed free from monitoring equipment, an important consideration when patients require constant attention. The mounting brackets can be installed when the cables are being installed or at the same time as central station, remote and bedside junction boxes are being installed.

Steel or plywood plates should be included in the wall sufficient to distribute equipment support forces over a large section of the wall as required by specific construction. In an arrangement using two wall mounts, the mounting holes between units should be 14 in (35.56 cm) apart, center-to-center. When not mounted directly on the wall surface, it is recommended that the bracket(s) be mounted on a suitable large, ¾-in (1.91 cm) thick plywood sheet prior to wall mounting to make it eaiser to properly space and align brackets. Typically, two half-modules, shelf and bracket weigh approximately 30 lb (13.6 kg), so appropriate fasteners should be used. See Figs 92 and 93.

(10) *AC Power and Grounding*. All equipment should be on a separate grounding system not used by other hospital equipment. Particular attention should be paid to X-ray equipment. X-ray equipment shall not use grounds and power lines for the patient monitoring equipment being described. It is recommended that a grounding system in accordance with ANSI/NFPA 99-1984 [3] be used. Figure 94 illustrates one example of grounding and ac power wiring.

(11) *Central Station*. Central stations may be fairly simple groundings of equipment or they can be quite complex involving twenty to thirty pieces of equipment or more. Thus, careful attention must be paid to the configuration and power and cooling requirements. To protect the hospital personnel and the patient, it is recommended that each instrument cabinet be grounded. This will

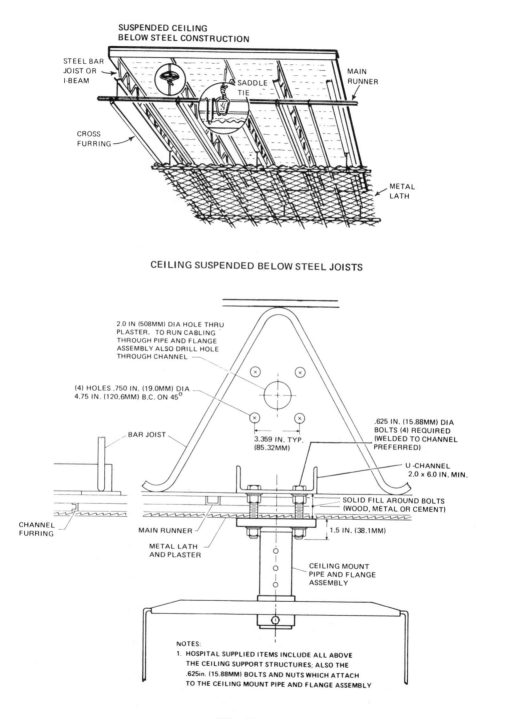

Fig 92
Ceiling Mount Supports for Steel Joist Ceiling Construction

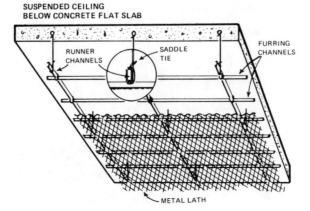

SUSPENDED CEILING
BELOW CONCRETE FLAT SLAB

RUNNER
CHANNELS

SADDLE
TIE

FURRING
CHANNELS

METAL LATH

CEILING SUSPENDED BELOW CONCRETE SLAB

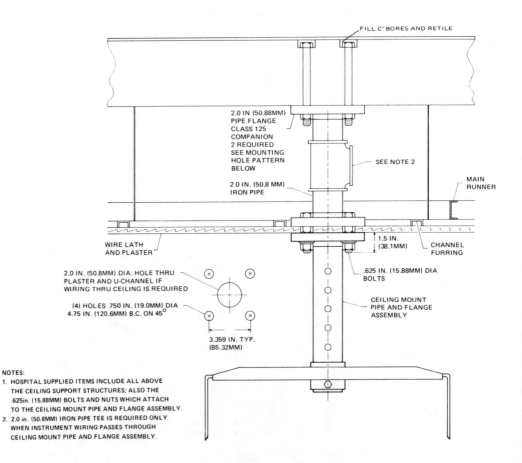

FILL C' BORES AND RETILE

2.0 IN. (50.88MM)
PIPE FLANGE
CLASS 125
COMPANION
2 REQUIRED
SEE MOUNTING
HOLE PATTERN
BELOW

SEE NOTE 2

MAIN
RUNNER

2.0 IN. (50.8 MM)
IRON PIPE

1.5 IN.
(38.1MM)

CHANNEL
FURRING

WIRE LATH
AND PLASTER

.625 IN. (15.88MM) DIA
BOLTS

2.0 IN. (50.8MM) DIA. HOLE THRU
PLASTER AND U-CHANNEL IF
WIRING THRU CEILING IS REQUIRED

(4) HOLES .750 IN. (19.0MM) DIA
4.75 IN. (120.6MM) B.C. ON 45°

CEILING MOUNT
PIPE AND FLANGE
ASSEMBLY

3.359 IN. TYP.
(85.32MM)

NOTES:
1. HOSPITAL SUPPLIED ITEMS INCLUDE ALL ABOVE
   THE CEILING SUPPORT STRUCTURES; ALSO THE
   .625in. (15.88MM) BOLTS AND NUTS WHICH ATTACH
   TO THE CEILING MOUNT PIPE AND FLANGE ASSEMBLY.
2. 2.0 in. (50.8MM) IRON PIPE TEE IS REQUIRED ONLY
   WHEN INSTRUMENT WIRING PASSES THROUGH
   CEILING MOUNT PIPE AND FLANGE ASSEMBLY.

Fig 93
Ceiling Mount Supports for Concrete Slab Ceiling Construction

Heavy Copper Buss Grounding System for Monitoring Equipment Only

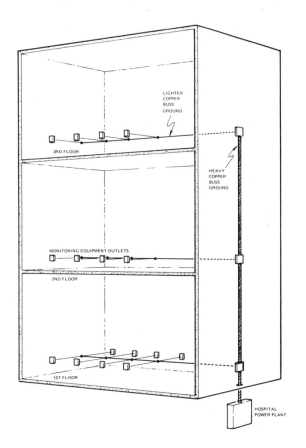

Fig 94
Heavy Copper Buss Grounding System

typically be done through the 3-wire power cord connected to a properly installed electrical system.

(12) *Checks.* It is sometimes helpful to work against a checklist in order to avoid overlooking major items. Following is one set of suggested checklists that might prove helpful:

Prior to Installation

(a) Conference with hospital personnel.

(b) Conference with hospital architect.

(c) Type of patient monitors at bedside and remote areas.

(d) Type of central station monitors/alarms.

(e) Architect aware of number of conduit runs required.

(f) Architect aware of recommended conduit size.

(g) Architect aware that no other wires should be run in same conduit with ICU signal cables.

(h) Architect aware that ac power, diathermy cables, etc, should be run far enough away from ICU to prevent interference.

(i) Architect aware that proper conduit junction boxes are included.

(j) Architect aware that builder must supply and install bedside and remote junction boxes.

(k) Architect aware that manufacturer supplies bedside and remote junction box face plates, if required.

(l) Architect aware that manufacturer will supply central station junction box, if needed, which is to be installed by the builder.

(m) Architect aware that individual 3-wire ac outlets are recommended for each bedside instrument and each central station monitor.

(n) Cables have been identified by bed number and ordered (with noted variations, if any) after cable lengths from point-to-point have been carefully measured. Order 10% longer length to prevent getting a cable too short to do the job.

(o) Confirm day scheduled for cable and patient monitoring equipment installation with person assigned.

(p) That "clerk of the works" has a move-in day assigned for the CCU/ICU equipment.

NOTE: Go over checklist and correspondence again; it will be worth the effort. Oversights will cause delays; delays often run the cost up in an exponential manner.

(13) *Architect Checklist Prior to Installation*

(a) Builder knows number, location and size of conduit runs.

(b) Builder knows location, voltage and number of ac power outlets.

(c) Builder knows location and number of each type of system junction box, if used.

(d) Builder/electrician aware that ICU system conduit and junction boxes, if needed, must be installed.

(e) Builder and electrician aware that only patient monitor signal cables can be run in conduit and that ac power, diathermy cables, etc, should be run far enough away from ICU to prevent interference.

(f) Builder aware of correct conduit junction boxes, if used.

(g) Builder aware that manufacturer will apply bedside junction box face plates, if used.

(h) Builder aware that manufacturer will supply central station junction box, if used.

(i) Electrician aware of recommended electrical requirements and location of each outlet in ICU, that is grounding system requirements, patient safe environment, etc.

(j) Electrician aware of any recommended equipotential test binding post requirements at each patient bedside.

(k) Builder aware of mounting requirements of brackets and shelves if these are to be used.

(14) *Other Important Notes.* Select a site for the equipment as far as possible from the emergency generator power plant, main power service entrance, diathermy machines and units containing large motors. These will commonly produce extremely large amounts of electromagnetic interference and the problem of obtaining high quality data rises exponentially with closer distances to such sources. Keep high current feeder lines away from patient areas.

Although much of the electronic equipment used will be capable of operating over wide temperature extremes, it will be better to design the environment such that temperature variations from day to night can be minimized. This will reduce the probability of condensation forming which may interfere with the operation of some units. Also, any corrosive problems due to moisture buildup will become minimized.

Isolated power centers are not required for electrical patient safety. However, local codes or other hospital considerations may dictate their installation. If such power centers are to be used, or their use is anticipated at a future date, allowance should be made during the initial construction or renovation. Wire lengths need to be considered as well as location. In order to minimize leakage currents, some have recommended that polyethylene insulated wire be used when isolated power centers are involved. This wire has less capacity per foot and leakage currents will be lower. Isolated power centers have received much discussion with regard to costs and any benefits relative to patient safety. Proper equipment maintenance should not be overlooked. Thus, a minimal clearance is needed for cooling and for access to the sides and rear for maintenance.

(15) *Summary.* Equipment used in Coronary Care, Progressing Care, Intensive Care and Operating Room units has proved to be of material benefit in aiding the hospital staff to care for the ill. The installation procedures recommended should be helpful in not compromising the usefulness of this equipment. The following reminders may be helpful:

(a) Generators of electromagnetic and electrostatic noise should not be located near patient areas.

(b) The high current buses that supply the hospitals or large pieces of machinery should not be run through the walls, in ceilings or under the floors of patient care areas and should be as far from these areas as practicable.

(c) Room environment should be designed to avoid temperature extremes.

(d) Wall and ceiling mounts should receive special attention with respect to their load-carrying capacity.

(e) Power and signal wires should be separated as far as possible.

(f) Minimal clearance should be maintained around the equipment from a cooling and serviceability point of view.

(g) Equipotential grounding systems should be used with impedances as low as practicable in order to minimize noise voltages building up and coupling into signal circuits. This refers to both the resistives and inductive property of the ground system.

(h) Provide the necessary amount of time for consideration of all of the details of the planning process. Problems discovered later are often rectified by spending additional sums.

(i) Coordinate such that the builder, manufacturer, architect and hospital administration know at all times what is taking place.

9.3.2 Pediatric and Neonatal

General. The OB/GYN Department in a hospital serves that branch of medicine that deals with the diseases and the normal processes of women, especially in the fields of the reproductive organs and actual child bearing. The Department usually has space provisions for patient rooms, labor room, examination areas, delivery suites and nursery, including neonatal (newborn) section.

During the past decade the delivery suite and its associated labor room and nursery area have been disappearing from local neighborhood hospitals.

Maternity centers have been established in central area hospitals in most major US cities. The neonatal area is a principal element of all these centers.

Basic Equipment in the Neonatal Area

(1) *The Incubator*

(a) Most incubators have two functions: reverse isolation and heat balance. Some are designed only to maintain the infant's temperature (for example, radiant warmers). It is important for nursery personnel to bear in mind that the "isolation" function of the usual incubator is only to protect the infant from airborne infections because his inspired air has been filtered. An infected infant in such an incubator discharges his unfiltered expired air into the nursery; and, other infants are not isolated from him unless they are also in an isolation-type incubator.

Incubators which have been carefully checked and are free from fire and electrical hazards should be available for any infant who needs supplemental heat. There should always be a standby heat incubator or radiant warmer and bassinet for unexpected deliveries or problems. Additional humidity or an oxygen-enriched environment can either be provided by the incubator or, when radiant warmers are used, delivered to the infant by means of a hood over his head.

(b) The incubator contains a small blower, air filtration system, a heating rod device and a water port for humidity control.

(c) Electrical Parameters:

    1) Voltage — 120 V

    2) Frequency — 60 Hz

    3) Amperes — 2 to 5 maximum

(d) Sources of Electrical Problems:

    1) Plug and cord

    2) Corrosion of heating device

(2) *The Patient Monitor.* The typical patient monitor used in the neonatal nursery (or similar unit in ICU or CCU unit) will provide measurements for the following parameters.

(a) The "ECG" or "EKG" electrocardiogram (see Fig 95) is a graphic recording or display of the time-variant voltages produced by the myocardium during the cardiac cycle. The P, QRS and T waves reflect the rhythmic electrical depolarization and repolarization of the myocardium associated with the contractions of the atria and ventricles. The "ECG" is used clinically in diagnosing various diseases

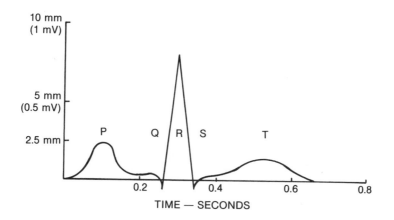

Fig 95
Electrocardiogram in Detail

and conditions associated with the heart. It also serves as a timing reference for other measurements.

(b) Respiration—breaths/minute in the range of 0 to 80.

(c) Blood Pressure—Utilizing a pressure transducer, a carrier amplifier and a display utilizing 2 m showing the systolic and diastolic pressure in mmHg.

(d) Temperature is recorded from the skin, the rectum and the ambient area.

    1) Normal Temperature Ranges:

      a) Oral (mouth) — 98.6 °F (37 °C)

      b) Rectal — Usually one degree higher than the oral reading

      c) Skin Temperature — 70 °F (21 °C)

(e) Electrical Parameters:

    1) Voltage — 120 V

    2) Frequency — 60 Hz

    3) Amperes — mA

(f) Sources of Electrical Problems:

    1) Radio frequency interference.

    2) Patient electrodes (chest, ear and nose clips). There can be twelve (12) electrodes.

    3) Stylus wears out. Driven by servo motor.

    4) Voltage fluctuations from outside sources.

    5) Incorrect grounding.

(g) Design and Installation Recommendations:

    1) Locate receptacles and patient input outlets as close to patient as possible.

    2) Emergency power is essential.

    3) Electrical circuits for bedside (or crib and incubator) patient monitors and central station monitors to be on same phase leg.

4) All receptacles should be hospital grade or equivalent.

9.3.3 Surgery. The surgical suite, whether in a small community hospital or in a major general or teaching hospital, is usually the most complicated in the facility in regard to electrical systems, equipment, patient safety considerations and of course in communications.

The electrical equipment utilized in the surgical suite must be designed for ultimate patient and staff safe use as well as for the surgical procedure it is involved in. The electrical circuiting for the area must be designed for the load served as well as for patient safety. See Chapter 6, Electrical Safety and Grounding, for further details on the correct use of isolated power, equipotential grounding and other special requirements.

9.3.4 Dialysis

(1) *Equipment.* The introduction of maintenance dialysis for the treatment of renal disease with uremia is generally acknowledged as one of the most important advances in medical treatment in the last twenty-five years. This life-saving procedure is used to prolong the life of thousands of patients awaiting kidney transplants or just extending the active life of the kidney patient.

The electrical systems within the dialysis suite must be designed with patient safety as the foremost consideration as well as feeding the equipment utilized. The area is always suspect to moisture from patient waste, the dialysate fluid and other fluids with a salt base. All electrical equipment must be grounded and it is advisable to provide a equipotential grounding system in the suite.

All receptacles should be ground fault interrupter type and all receptacles are to be hospital grade or equivalent.

9.3.5 Radiology

(1) *Introduction*

(a) *X-rays and their production.* The term "radiograph" requires definition. It is a visible photographic record—an X-ray picture—produced by the passage of X-rays through an object or body and recorded on a special film. In medicine it enables the radiologist to study the inner structures of the human body as an aid to diagnosis. How a radiograph is produced—what physical and chemical reactions take place—is the subject of this chapter.

1) *What are X-rays?* The first question that naturally arises is this: What are X-rays—how do they behave? They have two aspects of behavior—as rays and as particles. A *ray* can be defined as a beam of light or radiant energy. (Energy simply means the capacity for performing work.) Light or radiant energy travels as a wave motion and hence one measurable characteristic is its wavelength.

To get the concept of waves and wavelength, think of the disturbance created in a quiet pond when one throws a pebble into it. As the pebble strikes the water, some of its energy produces waves which travel outward in ever-widening circles. Although the water is in motion it does not *travel forward* progressively. This can be seen by the motion of a floating chip of wood or a leaf which rises and falls with the waves but does not progress from its original location. The *energy* of the waves proceeds outward from the center. The *wavelength* of the water waves is the distance from crest to crest or trough to trough. In any system of waves, the distance between two successive corresponding locations in the *moving energy pattern* is the wavelength.

Light, radio waves, X-rays, and so forth, are energy waves of electric and magnetic influence. They are appropriately called electromagnetic waves and travel at tremendous speed — about 186 000 mi/s. All these forms of electromagnetic radiation are grouped according to their wavelengths in what is called the electromagnetic spectrum. It might be interesting to compare some of these wavelengths. For example, the length of 60 Hz alternating current waves is about the distance from coast to coast of the United States. The wavelength of short radio waves is about equal to the height of a man. Medical X-rays — only about 1/10 000 the wavelength of visible light[31] — have a wavelength of about one billionth of an inch. They are ordinarily measured in angstrom units (symbol A) — one of which is equal to 1/100 000 000 cm. The useful range in medical radiography comprises wavelengths approximately 1/10 to 1/2 angstrom unit.

As mentioned earlier, X-rays also act as if they consisted of small, separate bundles of energy — called "quanta" (singular — "quantum") or "photons." Under certain circumstances an action of a beam of X-rays can be better understood if it is considered, not as a succession of waves, but rather as a shower of particles. This does not imply that a beam of radiation changes erratically from particles to waves and back again. Instead, the aspect that is most apparent depends upon the way the radiation is being used or on the method used to detect or record it.

The two "natures" of X-rays are inseparable. For instance, to know the energy in a single *quantum* — that is, in one of the small separate bundles of energy — it is necessary to know the *wavelength* of the radiation. But wavelength is a wave characteristic and must be determined from a consideration of the wavelike nature of radiation.

The experimental facts which prove radiation to be both wavelike and particle-like are well established. All that is necessary for our peace of mind is to admit the dual nature of radiation, not in the sense that it behaves unpredictably, but in the sense that one aspect will predominate under one set of circumstances, the other aspect under another.

Fundamentally, X-rays obey all the laws of light, but among their special properties certain ones are of interest to the X-ray technician:

a) Their extremely short wavelength enables them to *penetrate* materials that absorb or reflect visible light.

b) They cause certain substances to fluoresce, that is, to emit radiation in the longer wavelengths, for example, visible and ultraviolet radiation.

c) They affect photographic film, producing a record that can be made visible by development.

---

[31] The wavelength of visible light at the center of the visible spectrum is about 5.5×10^{-5} cm, while the X-rays used for radiograph — those in the center of the medical X-ray spectrum — have a wavelength of approximately 5.5×10^{-9} cm. Therefore, the wavelength of the X-rays is only about 1/10 000 that of visible light.

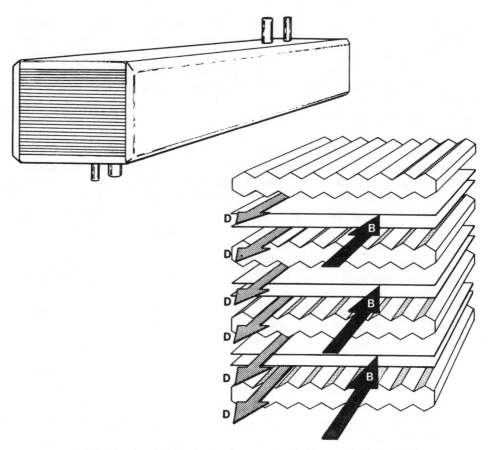

NOTE: Blood and dialysate are always separated by a cellophane sheet.

Fig 96
Schematic Representation of a Flat Plate Dialyzer with
a Magnified Representation of Parallel, Countercurrent Flow of
(B) Blood and (D) Dialysate

d) They cause biologic changes (somatic and genetic), a fact that permits their use in therapy but also necessitates caution in using X-radiation.

These special properties have application in medical and industrial radiography, therapy and research.

2) *The X-ray Tube.* How are X-rays created? When fast-moving electrons (minute particles, each bearing a negative electrical charge) collide with matter in any form, the result is X-radiation. The most efficient means of generating X-rays is an X-ray tube. This is an electronic device that is considerably larger but actually less intricate than the electronic tubes in your radio. In it X-rays are produced by directing a stream of electrons at high velocity against a metal target. In striking the atoms of the target, electrons are stopped. Most of their energy is

transformed into heat, but a small proportion (about 1%) is transformed into X-rays.

The simplest form of X-ray tube is a sealed glass envelope (from which the air has been pumped), containing two important parts—the *anode* and the *cathode*. The anode is usually formed of copper and extends from one end of the tube to the center. A block of tungsten about ½ in square is set in the anode face at the center of the tube. This is called the *target*. Tungsten has been found to be the most efficient target material for two reasons: (a) its high melting point withstands the extreme heat to which it is subjected, and (b) it has a high atomic number, making it a more efficient producer of X-radiation than materials of lower atomic number. The small area of the target that the electrons strike is called the *focal spot*; it is the source of the X-rays. There are two types of anode—the stationary and the rotating. More will be said about them presently.

The cathode contains a tungsten wire (filament) wound in the form of a spiral about ⅛ in in diameter and ½ in long; it is set in a cup-shaped holder (called the *focusing cup*) an inch or so away from the anode. The support for the focusing cup extends outside the tube so that appropriate electrical connections can be made.

The cathode filament is heated to a glow (incandescence) in just the same way as the filament is in an ordinary light bulb. However, the filament is not heated to produce light, but rather to act as a source of electrons which are emitted from the hot wire. The cathode is so designed and located within the tube that the electrons form a stream beamed in the right direction and of the exact size and shape to produce the desired focal spot on the target of the anode.

When a very high potential (thousands of volts) is applied to these two X-ray tube components—the cathode and the anode—the available electrons are attracted to the anode in such a manner that they strike the focal spot with tremendous force. The higher the potential (voltage) the greater the speed of these electrons. This results in X-rays that are of shorter wavelength and greater penetrating power and intensity.

As has been mentioned, the focal spot is the *area of the target* that is bombarded by the electrons from the cathode. The shape and size of the focusing cup of the cathode, the length and diameter of the coil (filament), and the dimensions of the focusing cup in which the coil rests all determine the size and shape of the focal spot.

Heat as well as X-rays are generated by the impact of the electrons. Only a small part (about 1%) of the energy resulting from this impact is emitted from the focal spot in the form of X-rays. Most of the energy is wasted by heating the target. This heat should be conducted away from the focal spot as efficiently as possible. Otherwise, the metal would melt and the tube would be destroyed. Tube manufacturers use a variety of methods for carrying the heat away from the focal spot. The simplest method is to back up the target with a good heat-conducting metal, such as copper, and to extend the copper outside the glass bulb to a fin radiator. In some tubes, water or oil is pumped through internal holes in the copper so as to dissipate the heat more effectively.

The *size of the focal spot* has a very important effect upon the quality of the X-ray image. The smaller the focal spot, the better the detail of the image. But because a large spot can tolerate more heat than a small one, some method of obtaining a practical size of focal spot that would provide good image detail had to be found. These methods are: utilizing the line-focus principle and rotating the anode.

The line-focus principle refers to the fact that the electron stream is focused in a narrow rectangle on the anode target. The target face is made at an angle of about 20° to the cathode. When the rectangular focal spot is viewed from below — in the position of the film — it appears more nearly a small square. Thus, the *effective area* of the focal spot is only a fraction of its actual area.[32] By using the X-rays that emerge at this angle, radiographic definition is improved while the heat capacity of the anode is increased because the electron stream is spread over a greater area. Thus far we have described a *stationary-anode tube.*

To increase further the capacity of the anode to withstand heat, the *rotating-anode tube* was developed. As the name implies, the disk-shaped anode rotates on an axis through the center of the tube during the period of operation. The filament is so arranged as to direct the electron stream against the beveled area of the tungsten disk. Thus, the position of the focal spot (the area of the target the electrons strike) remains fixed in space while the circular anode rotates rapidly during the exposure, continually providing a cooler surface for reception of electron stream. In this way the heat is distributed over the area of a broad ring, and for the same exposure conditions, the focal-spot area can be made one-sixth or less that required in stationary-anode tubes.

Some tubes contain two separate filaments and focusing cups which provide focal spots of different size and capacity.

Manufacturers furnish charts will all types of X-ray tubes to indicate the limits of safe operation — the maximum factors of kilovoltage, milliamperage, and time that can safely be used for a single exposure; some manufacturers also give cooling charts which indicate how rapidly exposures may be repeated. Thus a tube can always be operated within its rated capacity.

3) *Operation of X-ray Tube.* The electrical apparatus that permits the control and operation of the tube consists of a number of basic components: a high-voltage transformer; an autotransformer; a rectifier; a power supply for the filament of the X-ray tube; and a choke coil to adjust the current supply to the filament.

The circuits involving the X-ray tube, rectifier, and high-voltage transformer are arranged so that high *positive* voltage is applied at the anode end of the tube, with the high *negative* voltage applied at the cathode. The electrons from the hot cathode filament are negative charges and thus are attracted with great force to the positive anode. This high voltage is usually expressed in terms of *peak kV* (1 kV = 1000 V).

---

[32] In designating tube size, manufacturers use a dimension that is the effective focus size. That is, a so-called 1.0 mm tube has a *projected focus* 1 by 1 mm.

It is well to understand that kilovoltage has nothing to do with the manner of electrons that compose the stream flowing from cathode to anode. *Kilovoltage controls the speed* of each electron, which in turn has very important effects upon the X-rays produced at the focal spot.

The *number of electrons* is controlled by the temperature (the degree of incandescence) of the cathode filament. This control is accomplished by adjusting the filament current through its own low-voltage electric circuit. The hotter the filament, the more electrons that are emitted and become available to form the electron stream — that is, the X-ray tube current. In the X-ray tube the number of electrons flowing per second is *measured in milliamperes* (1 mA = 1/1000 A). The "quantity" of X-rays produced at a particular kilovoltage depends upon this number. For example, when the number of electrons per second doubles, the current (milliamperage) doubles, and the X-rays produced double. Note: Setting the X-ray machine for a specific milliamperage actually means adjusting the filament temperature to yield the current flow (milliamperage) indicated.

Perhaps it will be easier to understand what takes place inside an X-ray tube if its operation is compared to that of a conveyer system at a sand pit. Suppose that above one end of the conveyer belt there is a hopper full of sand which runs out the bottom through an adjustable opening onto the moving belt. Assume that the grains of sand are the electrons. The number of grains *available* to be carried away each second by the belt depends on the *size of the outlet opening* of the hopper, which can be compared to the degree of incandescence of the cathode filament. The moving belt will carry away all of the sand just as the kilovoltage will move all of the electrons available at the filament that comprise the electron stream.

Now, suppose the belt is speeded up. This is like increasing the kilovoltage. The number of grains of sand (electrons) traveling per second remains unchanged. Only so many get through the opening (the cathode incandescence) regardless of the belt speed (kilovoltage). Those that are available just travel faster. Again, suppose that the hopper hole is opened wider (filament incandescence increased). More grains of sand (electrons) per second fall on the belt. The belt carries a bigger load — more grains per second (greater milliamperage) — but the belt speed (kilovoltage) is the same.

As you consider the effects of milliamperage and kilovoltage discussed on the following pages, it may be helpful to refer again to the "conveyer" diagram and reread the explanation of it. This should help to fix firmly in your mind how these two factors affect the X-ray beam.

(b) *The X-Ray Beam and Image Formation.* Next, let us see what happens when the X-ray beam leaves the focal spot.

Most diagrams of the X-ray tube show X-rays as forming a neat triangular pattern as they are produced at the focal spot. This serves a good purpose in emphasizing the action of X-radiation outside the tube. However, the radiation does not behave in that way. Actually, X-rays are like visible light in that they *radiate from the source in straight lines in all directions* unless they are stopped by an absorber. For that reason the X-ray tube is enclosed in a metal housing that stops most of the X-radiation—only the *useful rays* are permitted to have the tube through a "window" or port. These useful rays are called the *primary beam*. That pencil of radiation at the geometric center of the primary beam is called the *central ray*.

A high voltage must be applied to the X-ray tube in order to produce X-rays. The electrical apparatus is such that the kilovoltage can be changed over a rather wide range—usually 30 kV to 100 or more. When the lower range of kilovoltages is used, the X-rays have a longer wavelength and are easily absorbed. They are termed "soft" X-rays. Radiation produced in the higher kilovoltage range has greater energy and a shorter wavelength. Such X-rays are much more penetrating and are called "hard." It should be understood that the X-ray beam consists of *rays of different wavelengths* and penetrating power.

1) *X-Ray Absorption.* In listing the important properties of X-rays, it was stated that they are able to penetrate matter. That generality must be qualified, because not all the X-rays that enter an object penetrate it. Some are absorbed. Those that do get through form the image—or shadow, as it is frequently called.

The extent to which X-rays are absorbed by a material depends on three factors:

    a) The wavelength of the X-rays.
    b) The composition of the object in the path of the X-ray beam.
    c) The thickness and density of the object.

We have just mentioned that long wavelength X-rays—that is, those produced at lower kilovoltages—are easily absorbed. The shorter wavelength X-rays—those produced in the higher kilovoltage range—penetrate materials more readily.

How does the composition of the object have a bearing on X-ray absorption? This depends on the atomic number of the material. For example, a sheet of aluminum, being of lower atomic number than copper, absorbs a lesser amount of X-rays than does a sheet of copper of the same area and weight. Lead (of still greater atomic number) is a great absorber of X-rays. For this reason it is used in the tube housing and for protective devices—for instance, in the walls of the X-ray room and in the special gloves and aprons used during fluoroscopy.

The relation of X-ray absorption to thickness is simple: obviously a thick piece of any material absorbs more X-radiation than a thin piece of the same material. The density of a material has a similar effect. For instance, an inch of water will absorb more X-rays than an inch of ice.

In considering the medical uses of X-rays, one must understand that the human body is a complex structure made up not only of *different thicknesses but of different materials*. These absorb X-rays in different degrees. That is, bone absorbs more X-rays than flesh does; flesh, more than air (in the lungs, for instance). Furthermore, diseased structures often absorb X-rays differently than normal flesh and bones do. The age of the patient also has a bearing on absorption—for example, in the elderly the bones have less calcium content and hence less X-ray absorption than the bones of younger people.

The relationship among X-ray intensities in different parts of the image is defined as "*subject contrast*." Subject contrast depends upon the nature of the subject, the radiation quality used, and the intensity and distribution of the scattered radiation, but is independent of time, milliamperage, and distance, and of the characteristics or treatment of the film used.

2) Factors Affecting the Image. The image can be affected by three factors: milliamperage, distance, and kilovoltage.

a) Effect of Mllliamperage. You will remember that increasing the milliamperage increases the quantity of X-rays, and decreasing the milliamperage decreases the quantity. It is easy to understand, then, that all the X-ray intensities of this leg pattern, or the "brightness" of the image, will increase as the amount (quantity) of X-radiation from the focal spot increases. Therefore, this *"brightness" can be readily controlled by changing the milliamperage*. However, it should be understood that the various *X-ray intensities will continue to bear the same relation to each other.*

b) Effect of Distance. Again, the X-ray intensities of the pattern can be altered uniformly by an entirely different, *nonelectrical* means—by moving the tube from or toward the object. In other words, *distance of the tube from the object has an effect on the intensity of the image*. You can prove this to yourself with a simple demonstration. With no other illumination in the room, move a single lighted bulb toward this printed page. You will find that the closer the light is to the book, the more brightly the page is illuminated. Exactly the same thing occurs with X-rays — as the distance from the object to the source of radiation is decreased, the X-ray intensity at the object *increases*; as the distance is increased, the radiation intensity at the object *decreases*. This all results from the fact that both X-rays and light travel in diverging straight lines.

A change in distance is very similar to a change in milliamperage in its effect upon the overall intensity of the image. The amount by which the overall image intensity is changed when milliamperage or distance is changed is a matter of simple arithmetic.

c) Effect of Kilovoltage. A change in kilovoltage causes a number of effects. The first to be considered here is the fact that *a change in kilovoltage results in a change in the penetrating power of the X-rays.*

Another fundamental rule of all X-ray technique is that *increasing kilovoltage reduces subject contrast; decreasing kilovoltage increases subject contrast.*

A second effect of increase in kilovoltage is this: *Not only are new, more penetrating X-rays produced, but so are more of the less penetrating rays, which were also produced at the lower kilovoltage*. This occurs with no change in tube current.

The combination of these two effects of increase in kilovoltage is, then, to modify the pattern so that a *pronounced increase in overall intensity* of the pattern would have been noted in addition to the differences in intensity having been "leveled out."

d) Summary. From the discussion thus far, the following conclusions can be drawn: Overall intensity of the image can be controlled by the three factors — milliamperage, distance, and kilovoltage. When millamperage or distance is used as a factor for control of intensity, subject contrast is not affected. However, when kilovoltage is used as a control of intensity, a change of subject contrast always occurs in conjunction with the change in intensity.

3) Heel Effect. For simplicity's sake we have assumed that the intensity of radiation over the entire area covered by the primary beam is constant. This is not quite correct. Actually there is a variation in intensity due to the angle at which the X-rays are emitted from the focal spot. This is called the "heel effect." The following is a description of this effect and the way in which it may be used to advantage.

This so-called "heel effect" is the variation in intensity of the X-ray output with the angle of X-ray emission from the focal spot. The intensity of the beam diminishes fairly rapidly from the central ray toward the anode side and increases slightly toward the cathode side. This phenomenon can be made good use of in obtaining balanced densities in radiographs of heavier parts of the body.

To do so, arrange the patient relative to the tube so that the long axis of the tube is parallel to that of the body part, with the *anode toward the more easily penetrated area*. For example, in radiography of the thoracic vertebrae, the neck should receive the less intense rays from the anode portion of the beam while the heavier chest area should be exposed by the more intense rays from the cathode portion of the beam.

The heel effect is less noticeable in closely coned projections where the X-ray beam is fairly restricted. But where a long area such as the thoracic vertebrae must be included, it is important.

4) Geometry of Image Formation. The purpose of radiography is to obtain as accurate an image as possible. Two factors that contribute to this accuracy are the sharpness and size of the shadow. A demonstration that you can make with light bulbs will make clear how these factors are applied in radiography.

Get a small clear lamp—a 7 W lamp such as is used in a night light will do nicely. Set it up about 3 ft from a wall, turn it on, and place your hand an inch or two from the wall. Notice that the shadow produced by this small light source is nearly the same size as your hand and that the edges are quite sharp. Now move your hand away from the wall—toward the light—and watch how the shadow grows larger, and fuzzier along the edges. Next, substitute a large frosted bulb and notice that the edge of the shadow is a little fuzzy even when your hand is close to the wall. The unsharpness is caused by the larger light source. Again move your hand toward the lamp and see how the shadow enlarges and the unsharpness increases.

So it is with X-rays. The smaller the source of radiation (focal spot) and the nearer the object is to the recording plane (film), the sharper and more accurate the image. Conversely, the larger the source of radiation and the farther the object is from the recording plane, the greater the unsharpness and magnification.

In addition, not only the shadow of the *edge* of the object but all of the shadows of the *structures* within it are involved in radiography, because X-rays penetrate the object whereas light does not. The same laws apply to the shadows of the internal structures as apply to the edges. If one of these structures is farther away from the recording plane than another, the structure farther away will be magnified more, which will result in unequal magnification. This variation from the actual proportions of the object is known as *distortion*. (Distortion and magnification are not necessarily a bad thing. Sometimes this is deliberately done in order to permit diagnosis of an otherwise obscured part.)

All the foregoing may be summed up in five rules for accurate image formation:

a) The X-rays should proceed from as small a focal spot as other considerations will allow.

b) The distance between the tube and the object to be examined should always be as great as is practical. At maximum distances, radiographic definition is improved and the image is more nearly the actual size of the object.

c) The film should be as close as possible to the object being radiographed.

d) Generally speaking, the central ray should be as nearly perpendicular to the film as possible to record adjacent structures in their true spatial relationships.

e) As far as is practical, the plane of interest should be parallel to the film.

5) Scattered Radiation. In discussing X-ray absorption and shadow formation, we have said that when X-rays strike an object, some rays pass through and some are absorbed. In other words, it is implied that all of the rays that come out of the object have come straight from the focal spot (primary beam) and have traveled through the part to form a well-defined, clear-cut image — and that all of the rays that did not penetrate were absorbed and could be forgotten. Unfortunately, this is not the case. Some of the radiation is *scattered in all directions* by the atoms of the object struck, very much as light is dispersed by a fog. The secondary rays thus produced are known an *scattered radiation* or scattered X-rays.

Because of this scattering, the object is a source of photographically effective but unwanted radiation. It is unwanted because it does not contribute to the information of the useful image. On the contrary, it produces an overall exposure superimpsed on the useful image. The effect of this overlying uniform intensity is to *reduce contrast* and hence to decrease the visibility of gradations in the image when viewed on the fluoroscope or recorded on film.

Other sources of scattered radiation are materials beyond the image plane — the table top, for instance. Radiation arising from such sources may be scattered back to the image.

Recurring Scattered Radiation. Obviously it is advisable to minimize scattered radiation. "Back scatter" is readily controlled by placing a sheet of lead immediately behind the film. Another important way to reduce scattered radiation is to confine the primary beam to a size and shape that will just cover the region to be X-rayed. This is done by attaching to the X-ray tube a *cone or aperture diaphragm*.

Cones are metal tubes of various shapes and sizes — some provide circular fields and others, rectangular. Aperture diaphragms consist of sheets of lead with circular, rectangular, or square openings. When these are properly used, the part of the object not X-rayed does not contribute appreciably to scattered radiation. Hence, an overall improvement in image quality is obtained.

It is important to know what area a diaphragm or a cone of given size will encompass at a certain distance. If the cone is too large, it serves no purpose. Some manufacturers specify the projected diameter of their cones at given focus-film distances. For cones that do not carry this information, it can also be determined with test films and the results marked on the cones.

Another way to determine the projected field is to use the following formula:

$$\frac{A \cdot B}{C} = X \qquad\qquad\qquad\text{(Eq 4)}$$

where

A = distance from focal spot to film plane
B = aperture of diaphragm or diameter of cone
C = distance from focal spot to diaphragm or lower rim of cone
X = diameter of projected field at film plane

For example: The focus-film distance A is 36 in; the diameter of the cone B is 4 in; the distance from focal spot to lower edge of cone C is 12 in. What amount of film X would be encompassed by the X-ray beam? Using the formula above, we have:

$$\frac{36 \cdot 4}{12} = 12 \text{ in, diameter of projected field}$$

Remember these two points: The *smallest cone* that will provide adequate coverage should always be used, and care must exercised in centering the tube so that "cut-off" of the image will not occur.

Thick, heavy parts of the body such as the abdomen produce a much higher proportion of scattered radiation than does a thin part such as the hand. Therefore, when radiographing the heavier body parts, an additional means of controlling scattered radiation is necessary. A device called a *grid* is introduced. This apparatus is composed of alternating strips of lead and radiotransparent material, such as wood or aluminum, so arranged that when the focal spot is centered over the grid, the plane of each lead strip is in line with the primary beam. The lead strips absorb a considerable amount of the oblique scattered radiation (that is, the rays not traveling in the direction of the primary beam). The radiotransparent strips allow most of the primary rays to pass through to the film.

The relation of the depth to the width of the radiotransparent strips represents the "grid ratio." To illustrate, if the depth of the transparent strip is eight times its width, the grid ratio is 8 to 1 (8:1); if the depth is six times the width, the ratio is 6 to 1, etc. The greater the ratio, the more efficiently will the grid absorb scattered radiation.

When a *stationary grid* is used, the shadows of the lead strips are superimposed on the useful image. This can be tolerated when a grid with very thin, uniformly spaced strips is used. The very fine lines are not objectionable in the image. To eliminate the grid pattern, however, it is merely necessary to move the grid at right angles to the strips during the exposure; in this way the grid lines are blurred and not distinguishable. A device comprising a grid and the mechanism for moving it is called a *Potter-Bucky diaphragm* or sometimes simply a "Bucky."

The grid absorbs a large part of the secondary radiation and even some of the primary radiation. It is obvious, therefore, that the exposure must be increased to compensate for this loss. The necessary increase in exposure should be determined by trial with the particular equipment. It depends on the grid ratio — the more efficient the grid in absorbing scattered radiation, the greater the exposure increase must be. As a guide for experimenting, a factor of 3 is suggested.

Regardless of the efficiency of the grid in removing scattered radiation, a cone diaphragm must always be used with the Bucky to restrict the primary beam properly. Here again, it is well to realize that with this combination, care should be exercised in aligning the tube so that "image cut-off" will not occur.

In passing, the use of filters must be mentioned. Filters are thin sheets of metal (generally aluminum) inserted at the tube portal to absorb the longer wavelength rays that do not contribute to the image. This is a safety device for protection of the patient.

(c) *X-ray Generating Apparatus.* To complete the story of the production of X-rays, a brief description of the generating apparatus is needed. As has been mentioned, the principal devices, aside from the X-ray tube, are an autotransformer; a high-voltage transformer; a rectifier circuit and valve tubes (when necessary); and a low-voltage transformer for the filament of the X-ray tube.

1) Transformer. A transformer is a device used to transfer alternating current electrical energy from one circuit to another and from one voltage level to another. In the simplest form it consists of two coils of insulated wire wound on an iron core without having any electrical connection between them. The coil connected to the source of power is called the *primary* winding, the other the *secondary* winding. Voltage is *induced* in the secondary when energy is *applied* to the primary. The voltages in the two coils are directly proportional to the number of turns of wire in each — assuming a theoretical 100% efficiency. For example, if the primary has relatively few turns, say 100, and the secondary has many, say 100 000, the voltage in the secondary is 1000 times higher than that in the primary. Since the voltage is increased, this type of transformer is called a step-up transformer. At the same time, the current in the coils is decreased in the same proportion as the voltage is increased. In the example given, the current in the secondary is only 1/1000 of that in the primary. A transformer of this type is used to supply the high voltage to the X-ray tube.

2) Action of Alternating Current. Voltage can be described in the form of a graph which represents the action of an imaginary voltmeter — if such a very fast-acting one could be built — connected to the transformer terminals. When 60 Hz alternating current is used, the needle of the voltmeter would move from zero to a maximum (peak or crest) and back to zero again in 1/120 second. It would immediately start off in the opposite or inverse direction, reach a peak,

and return to zero in another 1/120 second. This action is called a full cycle and requires 1/60 second. Sixty of these cycles are accomplished in 1 second—hence the term "60 Hz ac." For X-ray purposes, the tube voltage is almost always expressed in terms of the *peak* or *crest* value (which is abbreviated *krp*). The X-ray tube receives a series of voltage pulses, one for each useful peak, and therefore produces X-rays in pulses or "bursts."

3) Autotransformer. The usual line voltage supplied for X-ray equipment is 220 V ac. X-ray techniques, however, require a wide variety of kilovoltages. Therefore, the line voltage is adjusted by a special type of transformer—an autotransformer—so that the primary of the high-voltage transformer has a variable and predetermined supply. The result then is that the high voltage to the X-ray tube can be preselected at the autotransformer before the X-ray exposure is actually made. The device is called an autotransformer because the primary and secondary are combined in one winding.

4) Low-Voltage Transformer for Filament. Some means must be furnished not only to light the *filament of the X-ray tube* but to control the degree of incandescence. The requirements for this are a few amperes at 4 to 12 V, that are provided by a step-down or low-voltage transformer. The secondary winding of the step-down transformer is heavily insulated from the primary and the iron core so that the high voltage to the X-ray tube shall not get back into the supply lines of the X-ray machine.

5) Tracing the Generator Circuit. There are a number of auxiliary devices that go to complete the X-ray generating apparatus, such as meters, fuses, and circuit breakers. Tracing the circuit will help to make clear the action of the various parts of the apparatus. Fuses are placed in the incoming line as in all electrical apparatus. The current passes through the switch to the autotransformer. A line voltage compensator at 3A can be adjusted so that the correct input voltage is applied to the autotransformer. A prereading (ac) voltmeter in the autotransformer circuit indicates the voltage applied to the primary of the high-voltage transformer by means of the variable control. A circuit breaker acts when the high-voltage transformer is overloaded. A switch with automatic timer is closed to make the X-ray exposure. The high-voltage X-ray tube current is indicated by the mA.

The low-voltage transformer for the filament of the X-ray tube is supplied from a fixed position on the autotransformer. An ammeter permits the proper setting of the filament voltage control for the transformer. The secondary of the filament transformer is connected directly to the tube filament in the cathode of the X-ray tube.

The terminals of the secondary of the high-voltage transformer are connected in various ways to the X-ray tube, depending on the rectification method.

Modern equipment is so constructed that all parts exposed to high voltage are especially insulated. This includes the high-voltage transformer, the rectifier system, valve-tube and X-ray tube filament transformers, cables, and the X-ray tube.

6) Power Requirements. X-ray machines produce momentary high power factor loads of 20 kVA to 160 kVA. The momentary load usually has a duration of less than 2 s, but 6 or 7 s exposures are not uncommon. In order to perform

properly, X-ray machines must operate with a certain voltage range—sometimes called the absolute line voltage span. Within this range, voltage regulation must not exceed a certain value (usually in the 3%–10% range). A typical 95 kVA (480 V nominal) unit will have a steady-state voltage requirement of from 360 to 507 V. During the X-ray exposure, the voltage must not dip more than 6% and under no circumstances may it dip below 360 V. Some X-ray machines have undervoltage relays which will automatically cut them off if voltage swings outside of the prescribed tolerance. In other instances, the X-ray unit may remain on line, but yield exposures of poor quality.

X-ray manufacturers normally specify minimum feeder sizes for given increments of feeder length. They will also specify minimum transformer sizes and minimum circuit impedence. Because of the high power factor (usually about 95%), X-ray machines do not create great voltage drops across inductive reactances such as transformer and generator windings. However, the resistance of the supply circuit will bear heavily on the total voltage drop. Because of the high power factor, generator loads create heavy real power requirements on standby generators. Because of the high real power requirements for X-ray machines, X-ray exposures can cause slowing of standby generators, reducing the frequency of the supply. Reduced frequency can be a problem for X-ray generators, because some units operate on a resonance principle. Sophisticated X-ray machines, such as C.A.T. scanners and special procedures equipment with microprocessors, can require surge suppressors or other power conditioners. However, the designer should always consult the vendor before applying a power conditioner.

9.3.6 Physical Therapy

(1) *General.* The Physical Therapy Department is usually the prime element of the rehabilitation wing of a hospital. The department provides the patient who has suffered injury to his motor system, or who has had a major or minor stroke affecting use of arms of legs, the re-educating of affected muscles or systems. The department also retrains patients in speech therapy for those who have had brain damage in that communication sense.

(2) *Basic Equipment in the Physical Therapy Department*

  (a) Partial Immersion Baths

    1) Whirlpool Bath:

      a) This bath is given in a metal tub filled with water which is kept in constant agitation. It thus provides both water temperature control plus the mechanical effects of water in motion.

      b) The water is kept in agitation by an ejector, a turbine, or compressed air. The bath provides heat, gentle massage, debridement (the excision of contused and devitalized tissue from the surface of the wound), relief from pain, and muscle relaxation. It also permits active or assistive exercise of the part which is immersed in the tub.

      c) The tub's temperature is maintained constant by a thermostat. Typical temperature settings are 90 to 100 °F for the entire body, 100 to 102 °F for the legs, and 105 °F for the upper extremities. Often, 110 °F to 115 °F are used for therapeutic effects. When the patient has impaired circulation, temperature should not exceed 105 °F. Treatment usually is of twenty minutes' duration.

d) Whirlpool baths are employed in the treatment of chronic traumatic disorders, inflammatory conditions, joint stiffness, pain, adhesions, neuritis, tenosynovitis, sprains, strains and painful stumps following amputations. Adding a small amount of sodium sulfathiazole to the water hastens the healing of infections. The bath may be used preceding, or instead of, massage or other mechanical applications to injured extremities.

2) Contrast Bath

a) Contrast baths involve sudden, alternate immersions of upper or lower extremities in hot and then cold water. They increase circulation because of the contraction and relaxation of the blood vessels as a result of the alternating temperature extremes. One bath container is filled with water at a temperature of 100 to 110 °F, and the other holds water of 50 to 65 °F.

b) The body part being treated is immersed in the baths in a definite, systematic manner. While authorities differ slightly on the actual length of time a limb should be immersed in each tub, there is still fair general agreement. A typical contact sequence might be as follows:

hot for four to ten minutes, cold for one to two minutes;
hot for four minutes, cold for one minute;
hot for four minutes, cold for one minute;
hot for four minutes, cold for one minute;
hot for five minutes

Treatment always begins and ends with immersion in hot water.

c) Contrast baths are therapeutically effective for headaches, arthritis, fractures, peripheral vascular disease, and as a precedent to massage and exercise in cases of sprains and contusions. When treating patients with peripheral vascular disease, care must be taken to avoid great extremes of temperature.

d) In addition to the above there are a variety of other partial immersion or localized baths. These are as follows: The *hot full wet pack*, in which the patient is wrapped from neck to feet in a sheet which has been immersed in water of about 80 to 90 °F and wrung out; *cold, hot or neutral baths for the extremities*, which vary by temperature; *douches and showers*, in which streams of water at controlled pressure and temperature are directed at the surface of the body; *ablutions*, or sponge baths; *leg, foot, arm and hand baths*, which require immersion of the involved body part in small baths of controlled temperature; *half-baths*, in which the patient sits, the water level being at about the level of the navel; *affusions*, where the water is poured on the patient from a basin or a pitcher at approximately 60 to 80 °F of temperature; *sitz baths*, in which the torso, but not the extremities, is immersed in water; *Hauffe baths*, which provide a constantly increasing water temperature; and a number of other kinds. The particular form of a bath employed depends upon the disorder being treated, the body part or parts involved, the patient's physical condition, and the purposes of the hydrotherapy.

(b) Full Immersion Baths

1) Hubbard Tank

a) The Hubbard tank is a full-body therapeutic pool with a water temperature of 98 to 104 °F. The water is usually agitated and aerated, providing both heat and gentle massage. The patient lies on a canvas plinth and is lifted to and from the pool by means of electrically driven overhead cranes. Some tanks have a grating on the floor which permits the able patient to stand. Partial weight-bearing and ambulation can be initiated in the pool which may be prescribed when gait exercises are indicated, but the stress of weight is contraindicted.

b) The Hubbard tank is useful where the patient's disease or disability is manifest in many joints, such as in chronic arthritis or in burn cases when debridement and active exercise are desirable.

c) Exercise in water is indicated for the following conditions: Spastic paralysis, as in paraplegia; marked muscle weakness with the possibility of increasing strength through voluntary motion, such as in partial peripheral nerve lesions (for example, polyneuritis); poliomyelitis; following amputation when muscle strengthening and stretching of contractures in the involved extremity are indicated; chronic arthritis; following joint injuries; for mobilization in the aftercare of plastic and joint operations and tendon transplants; after abdominal fascial transplants; in certain cases of cerebral palsy; extensive skin burns; muscular incoordination; some neurologic disorders; and disorders requiring metabolic stimulation.

d) Water activities are contraindicated for cases of acute joint inflammation or other acute infections, febrile disease, acute neuritis, active pulmonary tuberculosis, and acute stage of poliomyelitis.

e) Other types of full immersion hot baths include: *Full-body hot baths*, with water temperature at 96 to 105 °F, used for brief periods of time in treating chronic, rheumatic joint manifestations, and for the relief of muscle spasm and colic; *chemical baths*, usually involving the introduction of carbon dioxide gas into the water for therapy with patients suffering from chronic heart disease; *oxygen baths*, which pump oxygen into water of about 90 to 95 °F, used for hypertensive and advanced cardiac disease cases; *brine* or *salt baths*, using sodium chloride, primarily for treatment in cases of osteomyelitis, fractures, dislocations, arthritis, myositis, fibrositis, gout and chronic sciatica; *foam baths*; and *sponge baths*.

(c) Electrical Parameters

1) Voltage — Smaller units - 120 V, 1 phase.

— Larger units - 208/220 V, 1 phase or 3 phase.

2) Frequency — 60 Hz.

3) Amperes — Varies.

(d) Sources of Electrical Problems

1) Improper grounding.

2) Corrosion of electrical components.

3) Portable electrical cords.

(e) Design and Installation Recommendations

1) Receptacles (or outlets) should be as close to units as possible. Provide rough-in as per manufacturer's recommendation.

2) All circuits to be ground fault protected.

3) Ground all equipment and adjacent metallic surfaces.

4) For all large tanks and spas, furnish and install outlet in ceiling for patient lift.

9.3.7 Neurophysiological Department

(1) *General.* The Neurophysiological Department in the medium or larger medical center deals primarily in the established knowledge and in new research in the field of brain physiology. The department deals in the areas of brain disorders and in such diverse activities and states of the nervous system as waking, sleeping, dreaming, consciousness, speech, learning and memory. The *Electroencephalogram* is the prime tool utilized by the neuro-physiologist and surgeon. The electrical activity of the brain is used to determine brain death in accident cases, and in certain circumstances can be used as an electrical parameter check in organ transplants.

(2) *Basic Equipment in the Neurophysiological Department*

(a) The Electroencephalogram (EEG) Measurements

1) Electroencephalography is the measurement of the electrical activity of the brain. Since clinical EEG measurements are obtained from electrodes placed on the surface of the scalp, these waveforms represent a very gross type of summation of potentials that originate from an extremely large number of neurons in the vicinity of the electrodes.

2) The electrical patterns obtained from the scalp are the result of the graded potentials on the *dendrites* or *neurons* in the cerebral cortex and other parts of the brain, as they are influenced by the firing of other neurons that impinge on these dendrites.

3) EEG potentials have random-appearing waveforms with peak-to-peak amplitudes ranging from less than 10 μV to over 100 μV. Required bandwidth for adequately handling the EEG signal from below 1 Hz to over 100 Hz.

4) For clinical measurements, surface or subdermal needle electrodes are used. The ground reference electrode is often a metal clip on the earlobe. A suitable electrolyte paste or jelly is used in conjunction with the electrodes to enhance coupling of the ionic potentials to the input of the measuring device. To reduce interference and minimize the effect of electrode movement, the resistance of the path through the scalp between electrodes should be kept as low as possible. Generally this resistance ranges from a few thousand ohms to nearly 100 kilohoms (kΩ), depending on the type of electrodes used.

5) Placement of electrodes on the scalp is commonly dictated by the requirements of the measurement to be made. In clinical practice, a standard pattern called the *10–20 Electrode Placement System* is generally used. This system, devised by a committee of the International Federation of Societies for Electroencephalography, is so named because electrode spacing is based on intervals of 10 to 20% of the distance between specified points on the scale.

6) In addition to the electrodes, the measurement of the electroencephalogram requires a readout or recording device and sufficient amplification to drive the readout device from the mV-level signals obtained from the electrodes. Most clinical electroencephalographs provide the capability of simultaneous recording EEG signals from several regions of the brain. For each signal, a complete channel

of instrumentation is required. Thus electroencephalographs having as many as 16 channels are available.

7) Because of the low-level input signals, the electroencephalograph should have high-quality differential amplifiers with good common-mode rejection. The differential preamplifier is generally followed by a power amplifier to drive the pen mechanism for each channel. In nearly all clinical instruments, the amplifiers are ac coupled with low-frequency cutoff below 1 Hz and a bandwidth extending to somewhere between 50 and 100 Hz. Stable dc amplifiers can be used, but possible variations in the dc electrode potentials are often bothersome. Most modern electroencephalographs include adjustable upper- and lower-frequency limits to allow the operator to select a bandwidth suitable for the conditions of the measurement. In addition, some instruments include a fixed 60-Hz rejection filter to reduce powerline interference.

8) In order to reduce the effect of electrode resistance changes, the input impedance of the EEG amplifier should be as high as possible. For this reason, most modern electroencephalographs have input impedances greater than 10 megaohms (MΩ).

9) Perhaps the most distinguishing feature of an electroencephalograph is the rather elaborate lead selector panel, which, in most cases, permits any two electrodes to be connected to any channel of the instrument. Either a bank of rotary switches or a panel of push buttons is used. The switch panel also permits one of several calibration signals to be applied to any desired channel for calibration of the entire instrument. The calibration signal is usually an offset of a known number of microvolts, which, because of capacitive coupling, results in a step followed by an exponential return to baseline.

10) The readout in a clinical electroencephalograph is a multichannel pen recorder with a pen for each channel. The standard chart speed is 30 mm per second, but most electroencephalographs also provide a speed of 60 mm per second for improved detail of higher-frequency signals. Some have a third speed of 15 mm per second to conserve paper during setup time. An oscilloscope readout for the EEG is also possible, but it does not provide a permanent record. In some cases, particularly in research applications, the oscilloscope is used in conjuction with the pen recorder to edit the signal until a particular feature or characteristic of the waveform is observed. In this way, only the portions of interest are recorded. Many electroencephalographs also have provisions for interfacing with an analog tape recorder to permit recording and playback of the EEG signal.

(b) Electrical Parameters
  1) Voltage — 120 V.
  2) Frequency — 60 Hz.
  3) Amperes — One (1) 20 A circuit.
(c) Sources of Electrical Problems
  1) Radio frequency interference.
  2) Patient lead connections.
  3) Multichannel pen recorder with chart speed of 30 mm/second.
  4) Interconnections to CRT or analog type recorder.

(d) Design and Installation Recommendations

1) Circuit feeding unit should be clear of any other loads.

2) A filtered circuit may be desirable.

3) All fluorescent fixtures in immediate area may be required to be equipped with RFI filters and low leakage ballasts.

4) Room housing unit may require shielding in walls.

9.3.8 Pulmonary Function Laboratory (ICU/Neonatal)

(1) *General.* The practice of rhythmically inflating the lungs by artificial means has been found to be of great value in the treatment of respiratory failure, the causes of which can be caused by many conditions and/or injury. Since it is not practical to do this by hand for any length of time, there are many machines that have been designed for the purpose.

This does not include machines that exert negative pressure externally on the chest, as they are not used much these days. Only intermittent positive pressure machines will be described. The enormous number of such machines available indicates that there are few that suit every possible purpose. There are even fewer that are satisfactory for the special problems presented by infants or the adult with a small chest cavity.

(2) Equipment

(a) Ventilator

1) A ventilator for an intensive care unit must be able to ventilate any patient from birth to adult size, and must be able to work equally well in the presence of normal lungs or highly abnormal ones. Humidification is essential, but apparatus dead space must be kept to a minimum. The dead space in some humidifiers is far too large for use with infants. It must also be remembered that water overload in infants is a real hazard. Accurate control of inspired oxygen concentration is important, because there is evidence to suggest that high oxygen concentrations, combined with pressure on the lungs, may contribute to death from "ventilator lung" (a condition characterized by decreasing compliance of the lungs, increasing opacity on X-ray, associated with small translucent areas, and an "air bronchogram"—microscopy shows hyaline membranes in the alveoli).

2) Since intensive care units tend to be places of stress for both patients and nursing staff, it is helpful if a ventilator is fairly quiet in operation—on the other hand, an alteration in noise may serve as an alarm to warn of machine failure. Ease of sterilization is important, as patients on ventilators are very susceptible to infection.

3) To summarize, some desirable features of ventilator for use in this type of unit are:

a) Ability to deliver accurately a tidal volume of 15 ml to 1000 ml.

b) Ability to deliver this volume against high resistance and/or low compliance.

c) Ability to deliver low flow rates.

d) Rate control from 15/minute to 40/minute.

e) Accurate control of inspired oxygen concentration.

f) A variable inspiratory:expiratory ratio (I:E ratio).

g) Good humidification for all tidal volumes.

h) Ease of sterilization.

i) Quietness of operation.

j) Ability to apply a variable expiratory resistance.

4) The type or types of machine chosen for an individual unit depend on personal preference and also on the conditions treated. Some units may prefer to have all of one type—this certainly ensures that everyone becomes familiar with its operation. It is preferable to have two or three different types, to cope with various problems. A greater variety could become unwieldy.

(b) Monitoring of Ventilation. It is essential to have some method of ensuring adequate ventilation of the patient at all times. For this purpose several devices are used. Most machines incorporate a pressure manometer which reads airway pressure at the mouth, or at the machine; this is connected to the patient by a wide-bore tubing of low resistance. Due to resistance in the airways, the pressure in the alveoli may be very different from that at the mouth. Many machines have a blow-off valve preset at, for example, 70 mmHg, to protect the lungs from excessive pressure.

9.4 References

[1] ANSI/AAMI SCL 12-78, Safe Current Limits for Electromedical Apparatus.

[2] ANSI/NFPA 70-1984, National Electrical Code.

[3] ANSI/NFPA 99-1984, Standard for Health Care Facilities.

[4] CSA Std C22.2, no 125-M84, Electromedical Equipment (Canadian Standards Association).[33]

[5] UL 544-1976, Standard for Medical and Dental Equipment.

[6] BRUNER, J.M.R., MD. Hazards of Electrical Apparatus. *Anesthesiology*, no 2, March-April 1967.

[7] *Health Devices*, vol 5, no 8, June 1976, pp 194-195.

[8] LEEDS, C.J., RN, CCRN; OKHTAR, M., MD; and DAMATO, A.N., MD. Fluoroscope-Generated Electromagnetic Interference in an External Demand Pacemaker. *Circulation*, vol 55, no 3, March 1977.

[9] *Respiratory Care*, vol 21, no 7, July 1976.

[10] STARMER, C.F., WHALEN, R.E., and McINTOSH, H.D. *American Journal of Cardiology*, vol 14, Oct 1964, pp 537-546.

---

[33] In the US, CSA Standards are available from the Sales Department, American National Standards Institute, 1430 Broadway, New York, NY 10018. In Canada they are available at the Canadian Standards Association (Standards Sales), 178 Rexdale Blvd, Rexdale, Ontario, Canada M9W 1R3.

Index

C